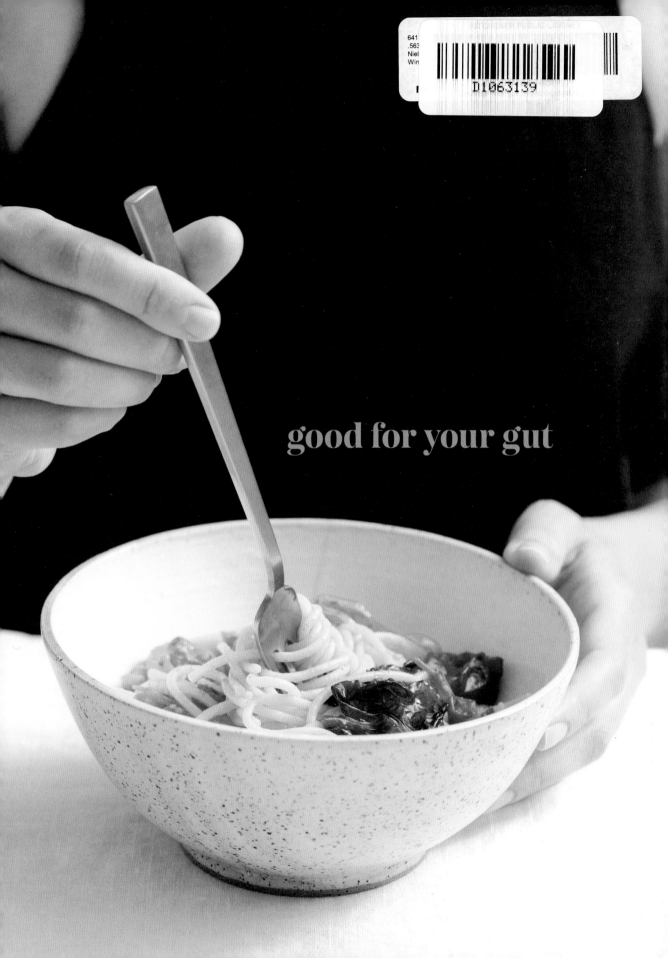

good for your gut

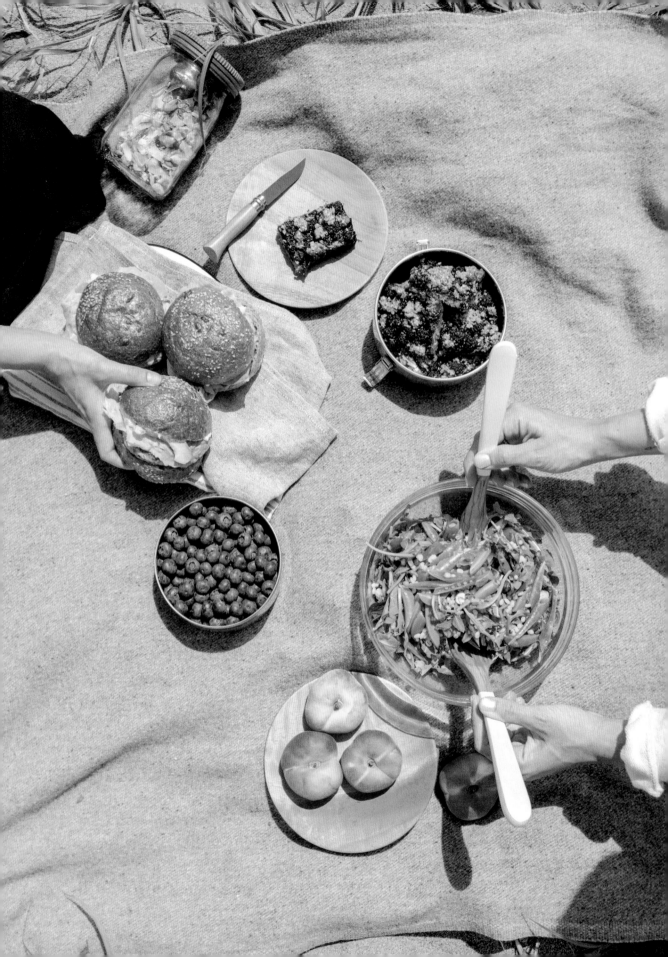

good for your gut

A PLANT-BASED DIGESTIVE HEALTH GUIDE AND NOURISHING RECIPES FOR LIVING WELL

Desiree Nielsen, RD

PENGUIN

an imprint of Penguin Canada,
a division of Penguin Random House Canada Limited
Canada · USA · UK · Ireland · Australia · New Zealand ·
India · South Africa · China

First published 2022

www.penguinrandomhouse.ca

Library and Archives Canada Cataloguing in Publication

Title: Good for your gut : a plant-based digestive health guide
and nourishing recipes for living well / Desiree Nielsen.
Other titles: Plant-based digestive health guide and
nourishing recipes for living well
Names: Nielsen, Desiree, author.
Identifiers: Canadiana (print) 20210211008 | Canadiana
(ebook) 20210211636 | ISBN 9780735240643 (softcover) |
ISBN 9780735240650 (EPUB)
Subjects: LCSH: Gastrointestinal system—Diseases—Diet
therapy—Recipes. | LCSH: Vegan cooking. | LCSH: Gastro-
intestinal system—Popular works. | LCGFT: Cookbooks.
Classification: LCC RC819.D5 N54 2022 | DDC 641.5/63—dc23

Cover and interior design by Andrew Roberts
Cover and interior photography by Janis Nicolay
Food and prop styling by Sophia MacKenzie

Printed in China

10 9 8 7 6 5 4 3 2 1

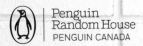

Penguin
Random House
PENGUIN CANADA

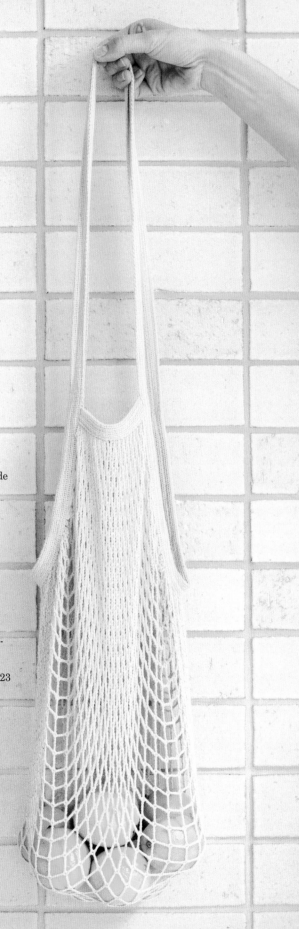

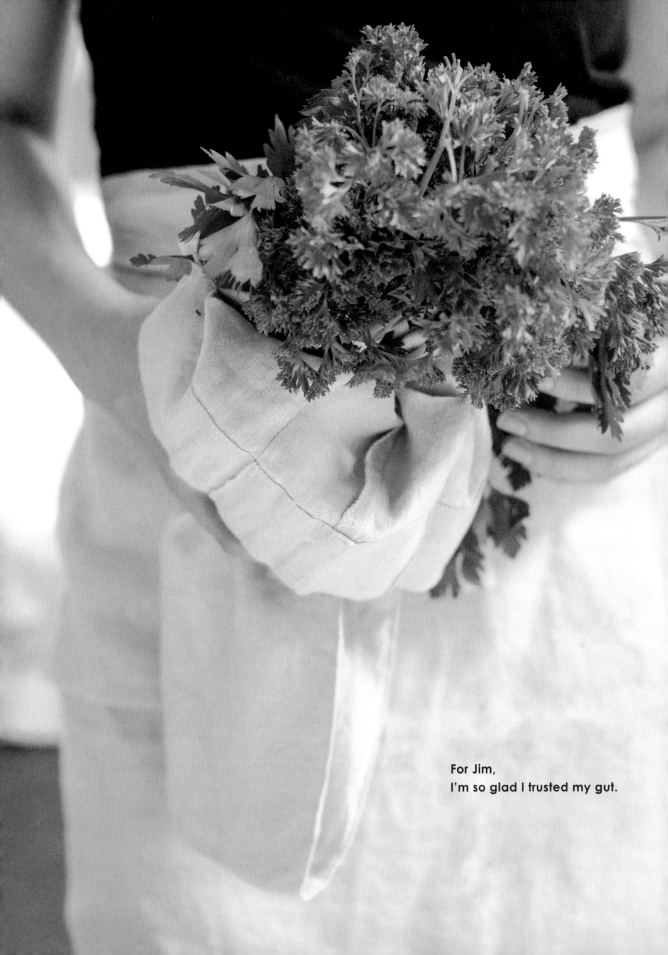

For Jim,
I'm so glad I trusted my gut.

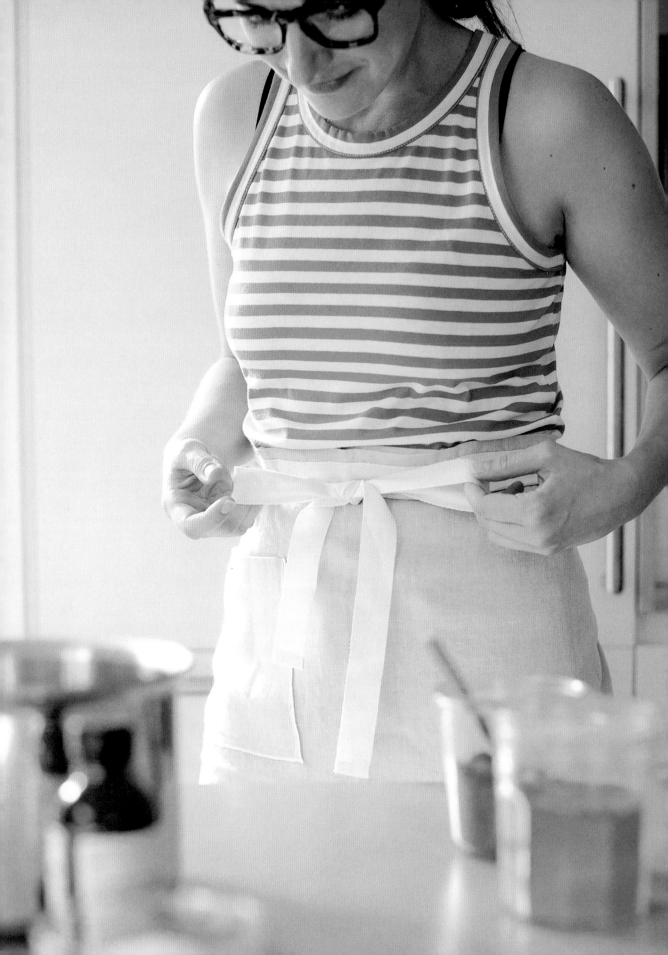

Contents

The Recipes

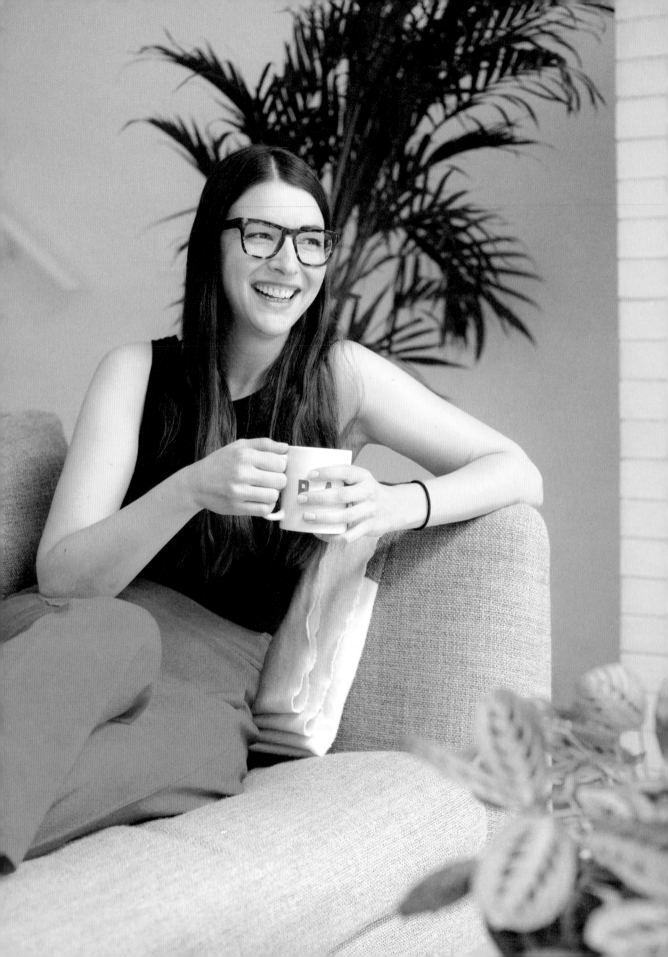

Introduction

Even with the surge of awareness around our digestive well-being, gut talk still feels a bit taboo. We talk around it all the time, citing regularity and balance, marvelling at the microbiome or admitting to a bit of bloating. But, we cringe a bit when talk about gas, constipation, poop, and perhaps the most dreaded word of them all, diarrhea.

In *Good for Your Gut*, we are going to get real to gain a true understanding of what is going on with our gut and the ways we can find healing when it goes off the rails. Whether you're just curious about your gut health as part of your self-care or you have something that needs fixing, it's time to set aside any hesitations that you might have about gut stuff. We are hardwired to think it's kind of icky, but it's natural and if we don't talk about it, we can't improve our well-being.

Not convinced it's a major issue? It is estimated that 16 percent of adults in the United States struggle with constipation. If that doesn't seem like a big number, when we do the math it's more than 50 million Americans who aren't pooping regularly.

If you're picking up this book, you either recognize that gut health is important or something is going on in your gut right now. Perhaps you have not said a word to your doctor for fear of embarrassment. I get it. It is one thing to talk about digestive health in general and quite another to admit to having digestive issues yourself.

So why don't I start? Digestive health was not my first love—it was inflammation. When I started learning about anti-inflammatory nutrition, the fact that inflammation is intertwined with gut health wasn't really on the radar.

However, I could not ignore that the vast majority of clients I was talking to on a daily basis had questions about their gut health. Whether it was finding a dietitian who understood celiac disease, why they couldn't find a gluten-free trail mix, or looking for answers about their digestive issues when their medical tests came back clear, people needed help. Since they weren't finding it elsewhere, I jumped into the void along with them.

As a dietitian, gaining a clear understanding of what was going on for my clients was tough at first. The microbiome wasn't a household term like it is now. Gut-brain connection? Way too out there. Even trickier, when I was starting out, I had just one clinical gold-standard diet at my disposal—the gluten-free diet for celiac disease. The only accepted evidence-based nutritional therapy for digestion at the time was meant just for those with celiac disease. Everyone else was left adrift in chat groups, blogs, and—if they were lucky—the office of an integrative practitioner looking for a path forward.

In the early days, even the low-FODMAP diet was considered controversial. It is now considered (close to) gold standard for those with irritable bowel syndrome (IBS). We'll do plenty of talking about FODMAPs in Chapter 6.

Why Gut Stuff Is Hard to Fix

Not having agreed-upon therapeutic diets is the first challenge of being a digestive health dietitian. It's up to me to piece together the latest research on food and digestion, to understand the ability of certain nutrients to alter digestive function or gut healing, and to navigate any issues my clients are having with actually digesting healthy foods.

To add another wrinkle, addressing digestive issues is tough because I can't see what's going on in your gut. You tell me you're bloated, but it might be difficult for me to determine if your belly is actually distended. Of course, just because I can't see it doesn't mean it isn't happening. A lot of digestive health—short of having a doctor place a camera inside your gut—is based on subjective experience. How do you feel? Where do you feel it? What does your poop look like to you?

Barriers like these are probably why it took so long for functional digestive issues like IBS to be taken seriously by the medical community. If you have IBS, on paper "nothing is wrong" with you except maybe you poop a lot and you feel pain or urgency. There is no lab test to diagnose your issue like there are for high cholesterol or blood sugars. We have diagnostic criteria, but IBS is also defined by subjective terms such as pain, which is tricky because we all have a different tolerance to pain. So, I did everything I could to understand what my clients were going through. Honestly, sometimes I was a bit skeptical of what I was hearing. I was still an outsider to their experience. And then I wasn't.

In my twenties, I never once thought about my gut health. I was lucky to be healthy and I took full advantage: eating veggie burgers and fries at 10 p.m. or dancing all night and going to school after four hours of sleep. I always felt pretty good, so other than generally eating well—I was studying to be a dietitian, after all—I didn't take any other steps to protect my health.

And then I got pregnant with my son. As a dietitian working in holistic health, I was super focused on creating a healthy environment for my baby. I ate my veggies, avoided coffee, went to yoga, and even took probiotics. I was now learning about the microbiome and wanted my own bacterial flora to be healthy so I could pass it on to him. However, nature had a little wrench to throw in the works.

My son was delivered early, just shy of thirty-six weeks. I had to give birth to him on an antibiotic drip because I had not yet done the routine thirty-seven-week screening to be sure I was free of a dangerous microbe called group B strep. I'm happy to report that he was born healthy. After that came the sleepless nights, constant takeout dinners, and the stress of caring for a new baby. Within a few months, I wasn't feeling as good as I used to. Exhausted, I chalked it up to new mom syndrome until the pain started—searing pain that made me feel like my gut was exploding. It made it almost impossible to sit down sometimes.

As a dietitian—and a skeptical one at that—I visited my physician more than once to ensure that I didn't have celiac disease or any other serious cause of my distress. My symptoms didn't suggest that I had something like Crohn's disease because I wasn't pooping all day long, but something was seriously up. This pain could not be normal. The fact that I had about thirty seconds between the urge to go and actually going was not normal. I found myself living in the world of "something's wrong, but the tests are clear," like so many of my clients.

Over the past ten years, I have tried many supplements, dietary strategies, and integrative therapies to try to get to the root cause of my digestive issues. Eventually, I found a set of solutions that has helped me feel healthier than I've ever been. One of the greatest gifts that this experience has given me is the ability to intuitively respond to what my body needs. However, this book isn't about just telling others to do what I did. Instead, I will draw on the latest research and my experience working with clients for over a decade to share the most effective strategies to support digestive well-being. I know that what works for one person may not work for another. I can have two clients with the same condition who respond to nutritional therapy quite differently.

What the Heck Is Wrong with Our Gut?

In North America, our digestive health is in the toilet. Literally. It is estimated that sixty to seventy million Americans and about twenty million Canadians have digestive issues. However, these statistics are not the same around the world. Most countries in Europe have far lower rates of IBS, despite the cheese, wine, and pasta. Inflammatory bowel disease (IBD) is less common in Africa and Asia, although rates in Asia are climbing alongside Western-style diets.

How is this possible? There are a number of potential reasons, and the real answer is probably a combination of culprits. Our hyper-sterilized environment is thought to lead to immune systems that overreact, which may contribute to allergy, autoimmunity, and perhaps digestive disease. It's known as the hygiene hypothesis because apparently you can be *too* clean. Some countries may not recognize or diagnose digestive issues—or its citizens may not have access to non-urgent medical care—as many of us do here in North America, although there is research to suggest that conditions such as celiac disease are more prevalent now than ever before.

In 2009, researchers were able to study blood samples taken fifty years earlier and compare them to blood samples from modern adults. What they found was that levels of the celiac disease antibody were four times higher in 2009 than in the late 1940s. Of course, our rate of celiac disease in North America is still only about 1 percent, which is a lot less than you might have guessed. In Italy, it's actually closer to 7 percent. Seems unfair, given how good the pasta is there. So why are health gurus telling us all to avoid gluten if perhaps only 1 percent of us need to? Let the scientific record show that gluten isn't evil and we don't all need to be avoiding it.

Low vitamin D levels could contribute to our risk, as we see more IBD in countries farther from the equator, but that doesn't explain what's going on in Asia, a continent with a hefty dose of tropical countries. It is thought that vitamin D may influence the way the body reacts to pathogens, which are disease-causing microbes. What's more, vitamin D insufficiency is rampant in IBD, perhaps affecting 60 to 70 percent of patients. Another study suggests that supplementing with just 2,000 IU of vitamin D3 daily helps to decrease inflammation in Crohn's disease. Vitamin D is an interesting nutrient, as it isn't readily available in our food supply—our body is designed to make it in our skin upon exposure to UV light. Living indoors and living in far northern and southern reaches may mean that we are more at risk of gut inflammation due to a lack of vitamin D.

Then there is the matter of the trillions of little critters living in our gut known as the microbiota. The word *microbiota* means "tiny life" and I'll use this term interchangeably with gut bacteria and gut flora, which are more popular terms. Our gut microbes—or microbiota—seem to be doing all manner of fascinating things in the darkest recesses of our colon. Here is just a sample:

- Fermenting our digestive leftovers to create short-chain fatty acids that decrease the pH of our gut. A slightly more acidic gut helps prevent the growth of disease-causing bacteria.
- Feeding our gut cells and calming inflammation through those same short-chain fatty acids.
- Producing vitamins, like anti-inflammatory vitamin K, that are absorbed into our body and help us absorb more calcium and iron.
- Improving the function of the gut barrier by increasing the thickness of the protective mucus layer that covers it. Sounds icky, but it's very important.
- Communicating with our gut—or enteric—nervous system and producing helpful little neurotransmitters like serotonin.
- Telling our immune system to calm unnecessary inflammatory responses.

Keeping these microbes happy is in our best interest and we're not doing a very good job of it. Pretty much 100 percent of all the gut problems we experience are connected to unhappy gut microbes. If you do not feed friendly gut bacteria the plant food they need, they might not grow well. What will grow to take their place? The wrong kind of gut bacteria that cause inflammation, wreck your gut, and mess up your bowel movements.

The Modern Gut Needs a Modern Solution

I strongly suspect, as you might once you learn more about how the gut works and what makes it malfunction, that our modern, always-on lifestyle, lack of exercise, and lack of fresh whole plant foods are primarily to blame for our gut woes.

Our body—more precisely, our gut—is designed to digest a lot of high-fibre plant food. Just how much fibre? It is estimated that paleolithic humans ate about 100 grams of fibre a day.

Paleolithic gut microbes must have been tough little soldiers, which is probably important since those early humans didn't have refrigeration and probably ate a lot of questionable raw wild game.

Today, the average American eats just 16 grams of fibre per day. This means that some people are eating a lot more than 16 grams of fibre, but the majority of people are probably eating *less*. It's not hard to avoid fibre in our modern food supply. Many of us eat packaged and hyper-processed foods that have had any real nutritional value stripped from them. We're not eating wheat berries, or black beans, or sunchokes. Instead, we're eating takeout pizza and drinking pumpkin spice lattes that don't have any actual pumpkin in them. Our bar for what qualifies as food is kind of skewed—it just has to be convenient and taste good—and it's definitely having an impact on our gut and on our gut bacteria.

In 2017, researchers set out to study how dietary changes, as well as urban versus rural locations, impact the gut microbiota of children. They studied groups of children in Burkina Faso, West Africa, living in both rural and urban environments and compared them to a group of children in urban Italy. What they noticed was that the children living in rural Burkina Faso, who had a diet that was relatively unprocessed and filled with high-fibre plants, had a distinct and favourable community of gut bacteria that was unique to them. Sort of like the terroir in winemaking, but in your gut. The children living in urban Burkina Faso, whose diet included more meat, fat, and sugar, had a gut microbiota that was less favourable and more similar to the kids living in urban Italy. The lesson here: eat more plants because it's good for your gut.

Feeding your gut bacteria all the dietary fibre they crave means that a healthy gut isn't just about going vegan. It's about eating a truly plant-based diet. Cookies and veggie dogs are fun once in a while, but they aren't going to get you the healthy gut you want. You need to incorporate more fibre into your diet. How much fibre are we talking about? About 25 grams a day for women and 38 grams a day for men is required for a healthy gut. The 16 grams of daily fibre the average adult American eats is barely sufficient for a two-year-old. This probably explains why constipation is nearing epidemic proportions.

What We Get Wrong About Gut Nutrition

Usually, when gut health and nutrition are mentioned in the same breath, what follows is a long list of what *not* to eat—gluten, dairy, soy, corn, sugar, alcohol, and lectins. This eliminate-everything approach is incredibly short-sighted. We're more likely to eliminate a healthy whole food because of a bit of lectin than ditch our hyper-processed food habit, which is far more detrimental to gut health. If you want to foster good gut health while your gut is still healthy, you won't accomplish it through eliminating foods that could set you up for deficiency, food intolerance, and suboptimal gut function. People on a gluten-free diet have a hard time getting enough fibre, and it's even worse if you avoid beans because someone put the fear of lectins into you.

Of course, getting into a groove with plant-based nutrition is about making some real changes. Eating kale twice a week will not be enough. Your gut is a creature of habit, so it's more about your overall dietary pattern than never eating another piece of birthday cake. If you're the average North American, you're probably eating way too much added sugar and fat, which is leading to inflammation and issues with your gut microbiome. So, yes, I want you to eat less added sugar, but sugar isn't dangerous or harmful if you have a little bit once in a while. Just eat more whole plant foods and naturally you'll eat less added sugar.

I would be remiss, though, if I didn't admit that elimination has its place. Research tells us that someone with IBS might benefit from six weeks of low-FODMAP living. (You'll learn what the FODMAPs are in Chapter 6.) And, yes, ditching gluten or dairy might help someone's gut calm down. Lots of my clients feel better on gluten-free diets. But it might not be the thing for *you*. For example, I can't eat a big gluten-free cinnamon bun and feel okay. The starch and sugar and lack of fibre in the bun make my stomach feel icky almost immediately. I can, however, eat less processed gluten-containing grains like wheat berries or 100 percent rye sourdough and feel good.

The more you eliminate, the harder you make it to properly nourish your digestive tract and immune system. What's more, a focus on food elimination can create an unhealthy relationship with food and take the joy out of eating. And no matter what's going on with your gut, food should still be joyful, which is why this book is packed with plant-based recipes to help you *love* what you eat.

About This Book

Good for Your Gut is different from many of the other gut health books available because it's grounded in plant-based nutrition and the idea that addition, not elimination, is the path to better digestion. I truly believe that eating more plants is the number one thing you can do to support digestion; this is supported by research.

Good gut health is not *just* about food. In this book, you will learn more than you ever could have imagined about how the gut works and just how complex the interactions are between the gut, the immune system, and the nervous system. Your gut is impacted by everything you do. In over a decade of practise, I have seen strategic nutrition change lives countless times. But I am not going to tell you that nutrition is 100 percent of the solution. How stressed you are, how much you exercise, even how you chew your food all contribute to optimal digestive health. We aren't just going to talk about food. Better digestion demands a *holistic* lifestyle approach.

Are You Ready to Get Started?

This book is a digestive healing guide with over 90 gut-friendly, plant-based recipes. As much as space will permit, I will share the breadth of knowledge, tools, and resources that I share with my clients in private practice. Of course, the reasons why you're reading this page may be different from those of other readers, so how you use the book depends on what you are hoping to learn and what, if anything, you're hoping to fix.

The first three chapters are the foundation of good gut health and are a great place for everyone to start. Chapter 1 teaches you how the gut works and Chapter 2 explains everyday gut issues such as constipation and reflux and how best to handle them. In Chapter 3, I explain my core nutrition philosophy and what the science says about how to eat to protect your gut.

The next three chapters go a bit deeper into therapeutic lifestyle and nutrition. Chapter 4 dives into the gut microbiome and gut-brain connection so you can understand how issues arise. Chapter 5 looks at IBS and small intestinal bacterial overgrowth as well as gastroesophageal reflux disease (GERD)—both incredibly common digestive conditions. Finally, I lay out the low-FODMAP diet for IBS, the research behind it, and how to put it into practise in Chapter 6.

If you have diverticulitis, celiac disease, or IBD, you can find disease-specific information on the Good for Your Gut website at www.desireerd.com.

Then, of course, we have the food. This book contains delicious plant-based recipes designed with digestive health in mind. You'll see that they are labelled as either Protect, Heal, or Soothe. While every single one is healthy and delicious even if you don't have any tummy troubles, I've created each recipe to address one of three core areas of digestive health:

> PROTECT: recipes high in fibre and/or fermentable FODMAPs to support elimination and a healthy microbiome

> HEAL: gluten-free and low-FODMAP recipes to support those with IBS, intense bloating, or gluten intolerance and celiac disease

> SOOTHE: gluten-free and easy-to-digest recipes for the most irritated guts, such as those with significant food intolerances, Crohn's disease, or newly diagnosed celiac disease; these recipes are great for building up tolerance to plant-based eating when it feels like everything irritates your gut

I have outlined seven-day meal plans at the back of the book that correspond with each of the three recipe categories. If you want to see how good you can feel, start following a meal plan right away while you read more about the why. Consider these meal plans as just the start of your new gut-healthy life. If you have IBS, you're going to need more than seven days of low-FODMAP living, but this meal plan will give you the tools to demystify your journey.

Good for Your Gut represents over a decade of experience in digestive health practice, and I am thrilled to be able to share it with you. I think it is so important that you understand how your gut works and what is actually happening when you experience digestive issues. All too often, I encounter clients who are given very little information about their conditions, which leaves them vulnerable to the misguided and sometimes dangerous information that can be found online. You'll get real, concrete solutions here as well as the science behind them. Because you can't act on theory alone. You need practical steps to help you heal your gut.

Our understanding of how our gut impacts our overall well-being has grown to the point that better digestive health is not just for those with digestive diseases. A well-functioning gut means a healthy body and a healthy life. If you want to be well, this book will help guide you toward a deeper understanding of what it means to be healthy. And whether you're serious about gut health or just serious about good food, each and every one of these recipes will help you create an eating plan that is delicious and as nourishing for the gut as it is for the soul.

NOTE: *the information in this book is for educational purposes only and is not meant to take the place of advice from your physician or dietitian. Always talk to your doctor before beginning any new dietary plan or supplement. Also, some of the Caucasian-centred language in this book, such as "Western-style" diet or binary terms such as men/women are used to maintain accuracy with what is reported in the scientific literature. I look forward to when we have non-binary alternatives to depict dietary guidance accurately.*

For a complete list of source references for this book, visit www.desireerd.com.

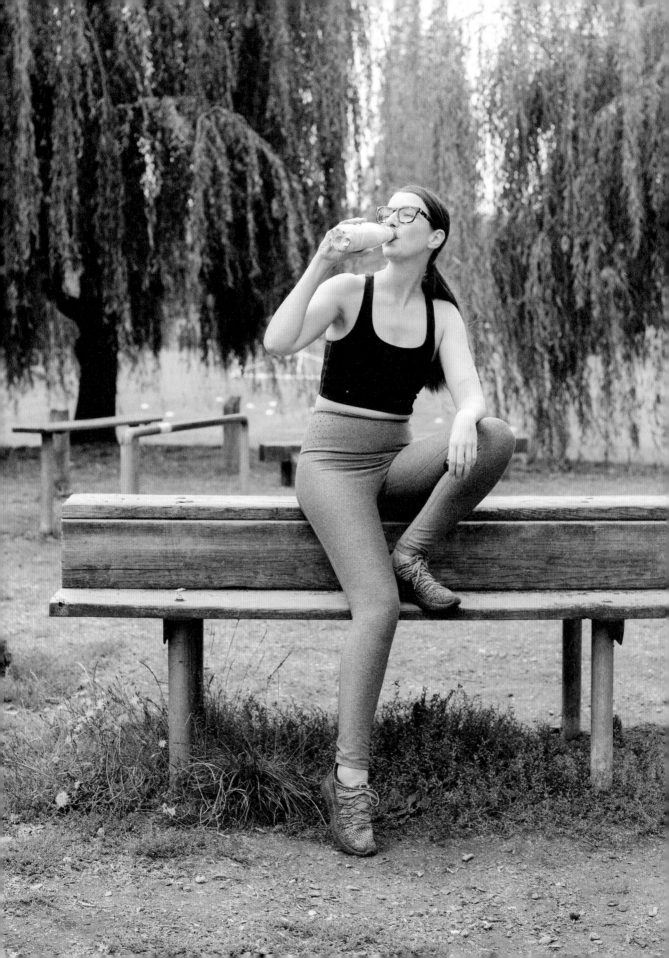

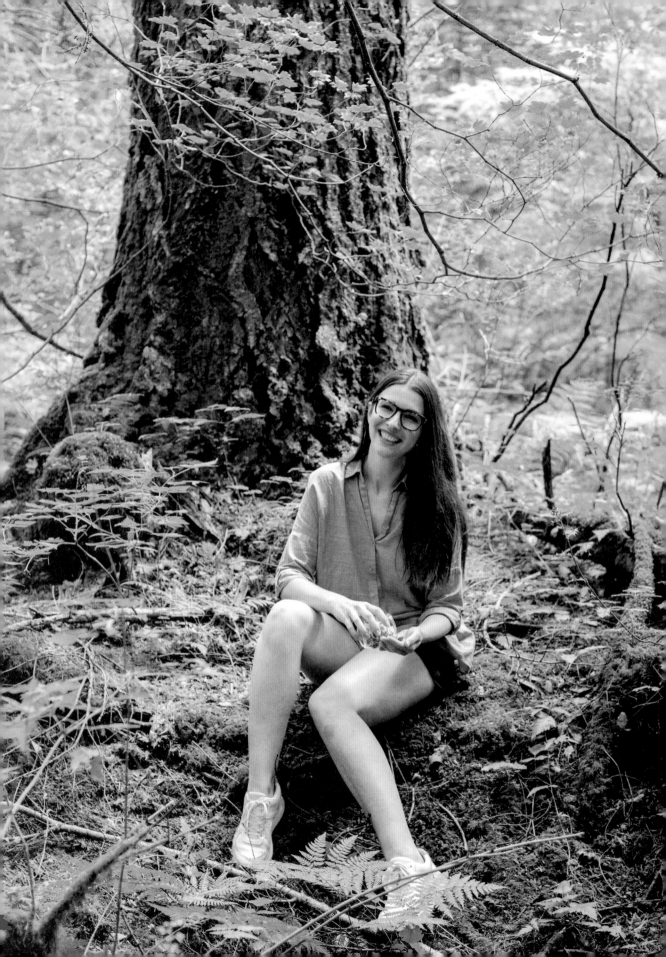

1

Say Hello to Your Second Brain

People don't usually talk enthusiastically about the beauty of the digestive tract—it's filled with poop after all—but your gut really is a marvel of biological design. I want you to fall in love with your gut and appreciate just how complex and amazing it is. Understanding how your gut works will help you understand what can go wrong in the gut and how best to fix it. There is so much fearmongering and half-truths out there about gut health, so let's get super nerdy and take a look at how the gut works, from a single gut cell to the long, winding path that makes up the digestive tract.

Imagine an area about the size of half a badminton court intricately folded over and over itself until it resembles a lush, velvety carpet in some spots. Now, roll it into a tube and then delicately assemble it into an area about the size of a shoebox. Even a contortionist couldn't manage that kind of feat, but that's exactly what's going on in your belly. Your digestive tract is about 30 feet (9 metres) long from mouth to rectum, and it has a lot of different specialized zones for digestion, absorption and, you know, pooping. Your mouth is more about physical digestion like chewing, your stomach offers chemical and physical digestion through stomach acid and mixing, and your small intestine houses the machinery of absorption. Let's dive in.

A Closer Look at the Digestive Tract

Lining the gut tube is a single layer of cells, known as the *epithelium*. The outer layer of your skin is called an epithelium too, which gives you a hint that there might be some similarities between the two. Just like your skin, your gut epithelium is in constant renewal, with new cells continuously pushing themselves through to the surface so that you have a completely new gut lining every three to five days. Your skin is a slacker by comparison; its renewal cycle is weeks long.

In the small intestine, the gut tube is highly folded, which is how it can cram such a huge surface area into such a confined space. To increase that surface area even more, gut epithelium cells have finger-like projections on them known as *villi*, and those villi are again covered in tiny projections called *microvilli*.

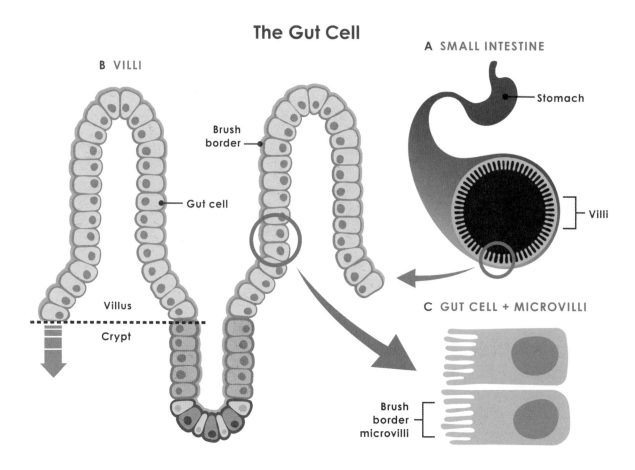

The Gut Cell

B VILLI

A SMALL INTESTINE

Brush border

Gut cell

Villus

Crypt

Stomach

Villi

C GUT CELL + MICROVILLI

Brush border microvilli

Your gut cells are held together at points called tight junctions. Think of tight junctions like little zippers that keep everything tightly organized—unless they get unzipped. We generally don't want unzipping to occur, because just like our skin epithelium, our gut epithelium is an important barrier between us and the outside world. If the gut cells aren't zipped tight, that barrier function might falter, resulting in what is called leaky gut. We'll talk more about leaky gut in Chapter 5.

This unzipping is what happens in celiac disease, where gluten in our food triggers a molecule called *zonulin* that unzips those tight junctions, causing inflammation and damage to our gut lining. However, it does happen a little bit over the course of everyday eating and living; some nutrients are absorbed in between the gut cells, for example. Alcohol can also cause a bit of short-term leakiness too. When the gut is working well, small changes in barrier function fix themselves quickly. This is going to be an important theme here—our gut is adaptable, constantly renewing, and built to heal. So let's look at what makes this complex tube tick.

The gut tube is more than just a single cell covering—it would be pretty flimsy otherwise. In fact, that single-cell epithelium we just learned about is actually part of a thicker layer called the *mucosal layer*. The epithelium covers a layer of connective tissue (for structure), blood vessels (for circulation), and immune tissues (we'll talk more about this in Chapter 4) known as the *lamina propria*. Completing the mucosal layer is a thin wrapping of smooth muscle to hold it all in.

The Layers of the Gut

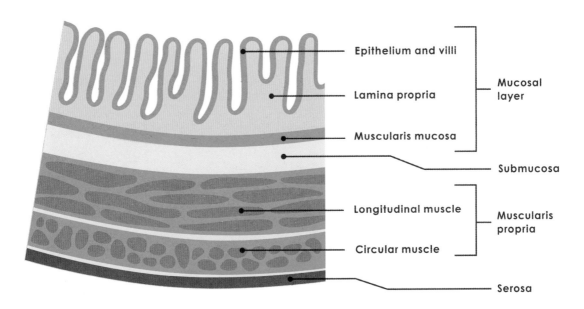

Epithelium and villi
Lamina propria
Muscularis mucosa
Mucosal layer
Submucosa
Longitudinal muscle
Circular muscle
Muscularis propria
Serosa

Under the mucosa is the *submucosa* (sub means under), which has more structural connective tissue, immune tissue, and nerves. Those nerves are super important, and they are why the gut is called the second brain. The submucosal layer is covered in a double layer of smooth muscle known as the *muscularis propria*, which is how the gut moves. Yes, your gut is a muscle. Gravity isn't enough to help food move through your gut; you need a lot of muscle to squeeze it along. This rhythmic, coordinated muscle movement is called *peristalsis*. Sometimes, that muscle can seemingly have a mind of its own, as anyone with irritable bowel syndrome (IBS) can attest to. Too fast, too slow, too unpredictable—how your nervous system coordinates that muscle movement is super important.

There is one last layer to tell you about to complete our deep dive into the structure of the gut. The muscularis propria is covered in a bit more connective tissue to make it even tougher, with some nerves, blood vessels, and immune cells to complete the layer called the *adventitia*.

I started this chapter with some detailed facts about the gut, but understanding the basic structure of the gut is important and will help you understand all of the things that can go wrong with your gut and how we can start to fix them. So let's take that weird, folded, muscular tube we just described, put some food in it, and talk about what happens when you eat.

The Digestive System

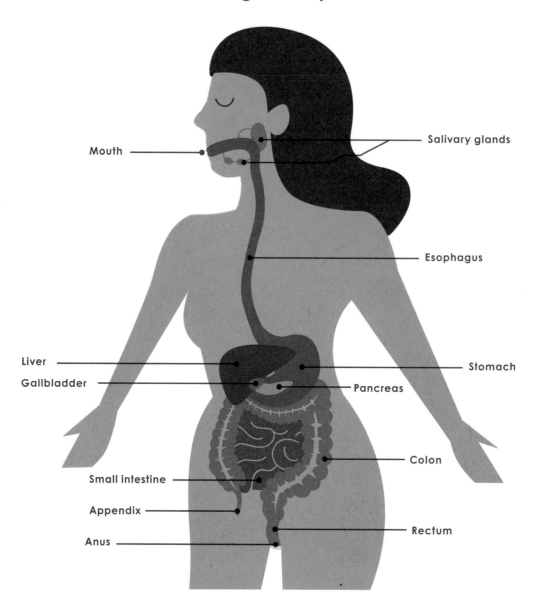

The Phases of Digestion

There are three phases of digestion and the first phase starts before you even put a bite of food in your mouth.

Seeing, smelling, and just thinking about food is enough to turn on the digestive process. This is called the *cephalic* (means head) phase of digestion. Think about biting into a juicy, sour lemon. Did your mouth just water? That's your brain talking to your gut to get it ready for a tart treat.

When you put a bite of food into your mouth, glands underneath your tongue release more saliva, which contains enzymes known as *amylase* that break down carbohydrates like sugars and starches.

Your teeth are designed to physically tear and grind your food down to a pulp, which gets mixed with saliva by your tongue. Saliva lubricates food, making it easier to swallow. Chewing increases the surface area of food particles, which helps acids and enzymes attach to food and work their magic. So, if you don't chew your food well, it won't digest well.

When you finally swallow that well-chewed mass, the rhythmic movement of your gut muscle takes over and ushers the food down your esophagus toward your stomach. Before it gets there, it passes a trap door called the lower esophageal sphincter (LES). The LES is important because there is a lot of acid in your stomach sometimes. When the LES doesn't work well, acid can splash back up into your esophagus, which causes pain. It's called reflux or heartburn. Now, you're officially in the *gastric*, or stomach, phase of digestion.

Once food reaches the stomach, it activates receptors in the gut lining that trigger two things: the secretion of stomach acid and protein enzymes from *parietal cells* in the stomach, and lots of contraction in the smooth muscle layers that line the stomach. Essentially, your stomach becomes a big mixing bag of acid-laced mush.

The acid is important because it begins to unfold proteins—close up, proteins look like twisted up little knots—so that *protease* (protein-digesting) enzymes can start to digest them. The stomach is all about digestion. Not much is absorbed here, except for a bit of alcohol.

As you get older, those parietal cells may release less acid, making digestion more sluggish. What's more, along with the acid, the parietal cells release a substance called *intrinsic factor*. Intrinsic factor is important for absorbing vitamin B12, which is why people over the age of 50 need to take a supplement, even if they eat vitamin B12-containing animal foods.

Typically, food will be held in the stomach for twenty to thirty minutes before it starts to slip through the trap door to the small intestine. However, the length of time food stays in the stomach depends on several factors, including:

- **Size of the meal. The more food in your stomach, the slower the emptying.**
- **How much fat and protein are in the food. Increased amounts will slow stomach emptying.**
- **How much fibre is in the food. Fibre triggers stretch receptors in the stomach to slow down stomach emptying.**
- **Acidity of the food. pH also affects stomach emptying.**

Once the food—now called *chyme*—starts to enter the small intestine, the small intestine has ways of controlling the rate of stomach emptying to optimize digestion and absorption.

The Long and Winding Road of the Small Intestine

As mentioned, the small intestine actually has a way of talking to the stomach to slow down its emptying, if needed. This is your *enteric* (gut) nervous system at work. You are now in the *intestinal* phase of digestion.

This communication is important because digestion and absorption is a tightly coordinated dance. Too fast, and your body won't have enough time to fully absorb all the nutrients from the food you eat. Too slow, and it can cause discomfort or even damage to the gut. This is all coordinated by your enteric nervous system acting on the muscular layers surrounding your gut to move things along. Remember, this coordinated movement is called peristalsis.

The small intestine is the main event where both digestion and absorption take place. As soon as the acidic chyme from the stomach empties into the small intestine, your pancreas and gall bladder release digestive juices that are quite alkaline, helping to neutralize the acid to create the right pH for all of the digestive enzymes to do their work. There are bile salts to emulsify fats, and enzymes for fats (lipases), proteins (proteases), and carbohydrates (amylases) here. Their job is to chop larger nutrients into their tiny, absorbable, components such as fatty acids, amino acids, and single sugars. There are also enzymes across the tops of the folds on your gut cells, known as the brush border.

Digestion, Absorption, and Food Intolerance

Your body wants nutrients in their most basic form for absorption. For example, you don't absorb dietary fats; instead, they are broken down into the fatty acids and glycerol backbone that hold fats together. Same goes for sugar. We tend to think of sugars as one thing because we eat a food called sugar, but in fact there are many different sugar molecules. Lactose, the sugar naturally found in milk, is a two-sugar molecule made from one glucose and one galactose stuck together. In order to digest and absorb it, you need the *lactase* enzyme found on the brush border of the gut cell. We all make this in differing amounts based on our genetics, but age or damage to the gut lining can also reduce brush border enzymes like lactase.

This is why people with celiac disease, who have a lot of flattening of their villi folds due to inflammation, often become intolerant to lactose, at least until they've fully healed their gut. Eat more lactose than you have the ability to digest, and that lactose will float through your gut, drawing water to it and getting fermented by bacteria, creating the telltale gas and diarrhea of lactose intolerance.

Once the digestive enzymes have done their job, absorption can take place. Some nutrients flow easily right across the gut lining. Others need little transporters to shuttle them across. Yet others flow in between (temporarily) unzipped gut cells. The small intestine is about 20 feet (6 metres) long and divided into three sections: the *duodenum, jejunum,* and *ileum.* Most of the absorption happens in the duodenum and jejunum. However, the ileum (pronounced *ill-lee-um*) is the site of an interesting recycling loop you'll want to know more about.

In the small intestine, along with your digestive juices, you will also find bile. Bile is made from cholesterol by the liver and stored in the gall bladder. You need bile for emulsifying fats in the watery environment of the gut so the fat enzymes can get at them. When the bile has done its job, it travels along to the ileum, where it is reabsorbed into the bloodstream. However, if you eat a lot of fibre, particularly the gel-like soluble fibre found in oatmeal, it can bind the bile and carry it out of the body. Why might this be a good thing? It forces your liver to pull cholesterol out of your blood to make more bile, effectively lowering your blood cholesterol.

Bile isn't the only thing your gut recycles. In fact, alongside the water in your food and drink, all of these secretions are pretty wet. If you lost that much fluid every day, drinking water would become your full-time job. Luckily, by the end of the small intestine, about 90 percent of the water that existed in the gut is reabsorbed. Unless it isn't. For example, if you don't digest lactose, it draws water to itself for the journey though the gut, which can loosen up your stools. And when things are rough, such as when you get food poisoning, the body can actually dump more water into the small intestine to try to get those bad bugs out, leading to diarrhea.

The End of the Line: The Large Intestine

Your small intestine is an action-packed ride. By the time you reach the end of it, it's been about six to eight hours since you ate and, when the gut is working well, 80 to 95 percent of everything you ate and drank will have been absorbed. What's left as we leave the small intestine? Mostly—we hope—lots of fibre, maybe a bit of fat or protein, and some water. This passes through the ileocecal valve, designed like a digestive door attendant to prevent the backflow of waste and bacteria into the small intestine. It goes into the cecum where the waste is mixed with mucus to lubricate it for the very slow journey across your abdomen through your colon. This mixture passes through the ascending colon, which climbs up the right side of your abdomen from the bottom to just under your rib cage. You can think of this first part of the colon as a bit of a bioreactor. Here is where trillions of bacteria, along with viruses and yeasts, ferment whatever you send them. Your trash, their treasure.

It takes about twelve to twenty-four hours (longer if you don't get your fibre) to take the rather short journey from the small intestine to the end zone. This pace is important, as it allows for adequate fermentation of the fibres and reabsorption of water. A few vitamins are absorbed here too. If it sounds boring in comparison to the wild digestive ride that's passed, it kind of is. Except that the bacteria that live in your colon are, in my opinion, the most exciting thing that actually happens in your gut. We'll talk more about your gut microbiota in Chapter 4.

Once that bacterial fermentation is complete, the vitamins and water absorbed, we're ready for the final phase: *elimination.* You have two trap doors, or *sphincters*, controlling the excretion of feces, AKA the poop party. You don't have control over the inner anal sphincter; when stool passes the inner door, you will feel the sensation of needing to go. That last door is the one *you* control. Sometimes, you just can't go to the bathroom when you want to, and we are designed to deal with it. However, if you can avoid holding in your stool, it's a good thing to heed the call.

The digestive tract is quite the wild ride, isn't it? I hope that this chapter has helped you appreciate just how complex, powerful, and unique your gut is. All too often, people are not aware of how their gut actually works, which can really trip them up if something goes wrong. Knowledge is power, and it will help you make better decisions on how to keep your gut healthy.

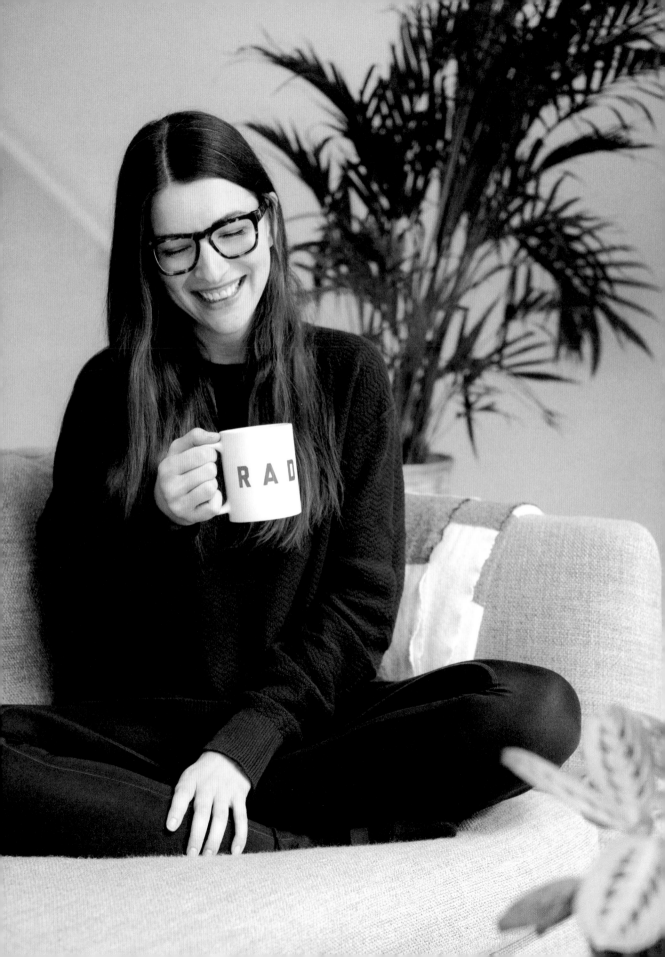

2

Everyday Gut Stuff

Now that we have discussed how our gut works, we can explore what normal variations in digestive function look like. It is a bit of a tricky subject because what passes for normal can be very different these days. The reason for this is that it is quite *normal* to be unwell. Never before have so many people struggled with chronic diseases, and that includes the digestive ones. The National Institutes of Health (NIH) in the United States suggests that sixty to seventy million Americans are affected by poor gut health. Unwell *is* the new normal. But it doesn't mean that it is the normal, or *natural,* state for your body.

On the other end of the spectrum is the borderline obsession with perfect digestive health we see in some wellness circles. You can't expect to have a textbook perfect poop every day or to never get bloated or noticeably gassy. Gas is a fact. So for that reason, we are going to call what happens a lot *common* and what should happen *normal.* For example, it's exceedingly common to be chronically constipated; however, anything beyond occasional constipation is not normal for the body.

In this chapter, we are going to take a look at normal, healthy digestive function and what kind of things can go wrong on an everyday basis. We'll cover the basics of gas, bloating, reflux, constipation, and diarrhea that are all part of normal variations in gut health, but also potential indicators that something more serious is happening. You'll learn how to tackle these everyday annoyances with food and lifestyle approaches and when it's time to seek help from your doctor.

The Gas You Pass

As much as we would all like to think that we don't pass gas, the average human passes litres of gas a day. In fact, you may toot up to twenty times in a single day. And much of that happens when you sleep because your body is in a non-compressed position, making it easier for the gas to release. Hours after your last meal, strong muscular waves help sweep gut contents through the digestive tract. In addition, you're not consciously trying to hold it in like you would be when you're in a meeting with your boss.

Gas is 100 percent normal and critical to your digestive function. But what is gas and where does it come from? Intestinal gas is made up of swallowed oxygen, nitrogen, and carbon dioxide along with the hydrogen, methane, and perhaps hydrogen sulfide gases created by gut microbes. You may also be surprised to learn that it's actually only hydrogen sulfide that smells bad. We'll talk more about that below. Intestinal gas is caused by the following:

- Gas you swallow, for example, while chewing gum, when sipping through a straw and swallowing air, and when drinking carbonated beverages. This makes up more of the gas in your gut than you might think.
- Gas produced when the acidic contents of the stomach get neutralized by the alkaline secretions in the small intestine.
- Gas that infuses into the gut from the bloodstream.
- Fermentation by the trillions of microbes living in your gut. When some microbes ferment fibre, they produce gas that becomes your gas.

BUGS AND THEIR BUBBLES

Fermentation is the process of microbes eating the foodstuff they find in your gut, transforming that into end products like gases and short-chain fatty acids. Some types of bacteria favour short-chain fatty acid production, while others favour gas production. And some bacteria eat the gas produced by other bacteria. Yes, some bacteria eat the farts of other bacteria, which makes your farts in the process.

Remember, 80 to 95 percent of everything you eat and drink will get absorbed. So that means those trillions of industrious critters are making something out of almost nothing. When gut microbes ferment your dinner leftovers, it has the potential to improve not just your digestion, but your nervous system, your immune system, and the health of your entire body.

Of course, if there is gas in the gut, it has to go somewhere and it is better out than in. Interestingly, when gas is in the digestive tract, some of it can actually diffuse across the gut wall and enter the bloodstream, so not all gas that makes its way into the gut turns into either a fart or a burp. It might be an exhale or it might get gobbled up by gas-eating bacteria, but a lot is going to become a fart. So it's time to make peace with the idea that gas is a fact and something you actually want in your healthy life.

As a plant-based dietitian, I cannot tell you how many times people have told me that they don't eat a certain food, such as tofu, chickpeas, or barley, because it makes them gassy. If this is you, I suspect that your current diet might be low in fibre and perhaps even in protein, and your gut just isn't used to eating those things. You may also have some digestive issues to deal with that this book will help you uncover, for example, that feeding a lot of chickpeas to someone in an irritable bowel syndrome (IBS) flare is going to cause some distress. However, for the rest of us, it's a signal that it's time to work on flexing our fibre muscle. Of course, you can't expect to go from a diet high in pasta, cheese, and chicken to a diet rich in lentils and cauliflower overnight and not feel super gassy. You are going to need to train your gut for life as a fibre champ the same way you would train your body to be a CrossFit champ— slowly and consistently over time. For example, start with steel-cut oats today, then add chickpeas to your diet next week. Chapter 3 will help you adopt a higher-fibre diet with ease, as will the Protect recipes in this book.

Given that we've firmly established that gas is good, it's time to acknowledge that sometimes it doesn't feel so good. Maybe all too often it's loud or smelly. Or, maybe it doesn't seem to move and it makes us feel bloated, or the bloating hurts.

Intestinal gas is rarely considered abnormal or harmful on its own. You will also want to allow for some natural variation; for example, it's not unusual to have some smelly gas if you've just devoured half a head of roasted cauliflower or to have a bit of bloating if you've been chained to your desk for a ten-hour day in tight-fitting pants. But what if it isn't just natural variation? If intestinal gas is accompanied by any of the following issues, you should talk to your doctor:

- **Diarrhea lasting more than three days**
- **Constipation lasting more than three months**
- **Chronic abdominal pain**
- **Chronic joint pain**

In theory, we should all be happily passing relatively scent-free farts in peace. But what if your toots are troublesome on a daily basis?

SMELLY GAS

Smelly farts definitely get in the way of you passing them without reproach. The first thing to check is whether or not you need to have a bowel movement. Gas that slips by a bowel movement picks up some of its smell. So making sure you are regular and giving yourself the opportunity for a bowel movement when the sensation arises are ways to help lessen smelly gas. And if moving your bowels daily is an issue for you, read on for how to deal with constipation.

If your toots have more of an eggy smell, that's hydrogen sulfide gas. While hydrogen sulfide typically makes up less than 1 percent of the gas you pass, we are keenly attuned to its smell. However, there are a few things you should know about these hydrogen sulfide–producing bacteria. The first is that women tend to have more of them than men. The second is that a diet high in animal protein, which is high in sulfur-based amino acids, may also encourage the production of hydrogen sulfide gas. This is an important point because of the associations between a meat-heavy diet and the risk for colon cancer and inflammatory bowel disease (IBD). It is thought that excessive exposure to hydrogen sulfide gas may increase inflammatory damage to the gut cells. In contrast, eating a high-fermentable-fibre diet, like the foods in the Protect recipes in this book, may actually decrease hydrogen sulfide production in the gut. So while eating a lot of cruciferous veggies like cauliflower and broccoli can increase the sulfur smell, I am less concerned about that from a health perspective.

TOO MUCH GAS

If you are dealing with more farts than you can get away with passing in an open-plan office, there might be a dietary trigger to blame. Some foods, such as beans and lentils, or cruciferous veggies, like broccoli, are known gas producers. That doesn't mean you shouldn't eat them. On the contrary, you simply need to mind your portion as your body gets used to eating them consistently.

Other ingredients, such as lactose in dairy, or fructose, a common sweetener in hyper-processed foods, are also poorly digested, leading to increased fermentation. Lactose and fructose are part of the FODMAP family of poorly absorbed, fermentable carbohydrates that can cause an issue for people with IBS. More on how to know if they are an issue for you in Chapter 6. It could also be that in your enthusiasm for living that high-fibre life, you simply went too big too soon. Cut back, sticking to one high-fibre meal a day, and wait for symptoms to subside before you add more fibre to your diet. Consistency is key to adaptation.

You also may have developed a set of bacteria that is highly gas producing. While we have little evidence to guide us here, early research suggests that consistently eating foods with prebiotic and fermentable fibres may help drive the growth of bacteria that produce less gas to balance things out again.

PAINFUL GAS

Painful gas is likely to be connected to one of two issues. The first is slow motility (gut movement) that leads to bloating or constipation. (Read the bloating and constipation sections in this chapter for more information.) The second is a hypersensitive gut (enteric) nervous system. In certain conditions, including IBS, the nervous system can become hypersensitive, so the receptors in the gut label the normal stretch of the intestine as severely painful. We'll talk more about this in Chapter 5.

When the Gas Won't Pass, You've Got Bloating

Bloating is super common and occurs in about 30 percent of adults. It can be tricky to investigate because it is a relatively subjective symptom and can have multiple causes. Bloating can include the physical, measurable distention of the abdomen or it also can be a feeling without any visible distention. It can occur right after eating or take a few hours before causing discomfort. It might build up over the course of the day or, less commonly, you might wake up bloated. The bloating may disappear when you pass gas or it may be constant. You might assume that bloating means you have extra gas in your gut, but research suggests that actually isn't the case. Hang on tight to your waistband; bloating is way more complex than you can imagine.

Simple Fixes for Troublesome Gas

If you don't have any of the warning signs we talked about earlier (if you do, see your doctor), you are ready to tackle troublesome gas using good old-fashioned nutrition and lifestyle approaches. Ideally, you would try each of these strategies one at a time for a period of time so you can isolate which ones are effective and worth continuing. Try five things at once and you'll never know which of the five is actually working.

1. **REDUCE SWALLOWED AIR.** Swallowing gas puts more gas into your gut to pass. Here's how to reduce it:

   - Avoid chewing gum and drinking fizzy drinks.
   - Avoid using drinking straws; sip beverages slowly.
   - Breathe through your nose.
   - Chew with your mouth closed and avoid slurping.
   - Avoid talking with your mouth full.

2. **CHEW THOROUGHLY AND SLOWLY.** You want to avoid the urge to swallow until the food feels thoroughly mushed. This sounds too simple to be effective, but it works in the following ways:

   - It decreases the swallowing of air.
   - It improves surface area to maximize digestion and absorption, reducing the amount of undigested foodstuff that can be fermented in the colon.
   - It calms the nervous system and helps to support effective movement of the gut (peristalsis).

3. **TRY GAS-REDUCING FOODS, TEAS, AND SUPPLEMENTS.** Many traditional remedies exist for gas, some of them with modern scientific evidence and some without. While it is safe to try these remedies in food form, remember that effective doses of these herbs may not be safe in pregnancy or certain chronic diseases. So before you try anything stronger than a bit of fresh or dried herbs in your cooking, consult your doctor. Consider trying:

   Ginger: Ginger is traditionally used to reduce reflux, nausea, and flatulence. It is known to be prokinetic, meaning that it helps facilitate the movement of the gut. Ginger is particularly good for improving stomach emptying and evidence-based for reducing nausea, while its effects on flatulence are not well studied.

   Try eating crystallized or pickled ginger, drinking ginger tea, or adding fresh ginger to smoothies, juices, and other recipes.

Fennel Seed: Fennel seed is a traditional remedy for gas and bloating. If you visit an Indian restaurant, you may receive little candy-coated fennel seeds at the end of the meal. Fennel is thought to be antispasmodic, helping to reduce intestinal spasms. There isn't a great deal of clinical research confirming these effects. However, fennel is a common ingredient in infant colic remedies, where some evidence suggests benefit.

Try chewing four or five fennel seeds or drinking fennel tea.

Digestive Bitters: Digestive bitters are traditional tinctures that contain a combination of bitter herbs, such as angelica, gentian, and dandelion. They have long been used to stimulate digestive secretions, ease indigestion, and reduce gas, but have not been well studied for efficacy.

Try using bitters as directed before or after a meal to soothe the stomach. They are an herbal medication (and often contain alcohol) and should not be used while pregnant. Check with your doctor if you have a pre-existing health condition.

4. **KEEP A FOOD JOURNAL.** For two weeks, write down everything you eat and drink along with your physical activity and stress level. Notice any potential patterns you see. Perhaps you are overdoing it with high-fibre foods. If so, ease off and then work your way up slowly over two to three months. Perhaps you'll notice some very clear reactions to certain foods. If so, consult your doctor to confirm whether more serious gastrointestinal issues such as IBS or celiac disease might be causing them. Once you have the all-clear, consider working with a registered dietitian to test elimination of the potential trigger foods and help you create a long-term dietary plan to ease your gas.

What Causes Bloating?

Here are several causes of bloating that might help explain what's going on inside.

1. **ABDOMINAL WALL WEAKNESS.** Women often report more bloating than men. Our digestive tract is far more twisty and turny than a man's, and this contributes to bloating. In addition, women tend to have weaker abdominal walls, particularly if we've been pregnant or aren't as active as we used to be. That means that when food or gas fills the gut, our abdominal muscles don't push back as hard and we feel bloated.

2. **ABDOMINAL WALL DYSREGULATION.** When a volume of food expands the gut space, the abdominal wall is supposed to contract to provide structure and movement. But in some people, the abdominal wall may actually relax in response to food in the gut. This may lead to an almost instant bloating upon eating any meal, which is not often talked about but an important root cause of bloating that should not be overlooked. Instant bloating is considered a sign of small intestinal bacterial overgrowth (SIBO). It is important to rule out abdominal wall dysregulation so you don't undergo SIBO treatment unnecessarily.

3. **FERMENTATION.** If you eat fibre, you'll make gas. However, if you are malabsorbing a carbohydrate like lactose, fructose, or other FODMAPs, it could cause excessive fermentation when you eat those foods and way more gas and bloating than normal. Or, if there is an imbalance in good to bad bacteria, known as dysbiosis, there also could be increased gas production in the gut, leading to bloating.

4. **INFLAMMATION.** Inflammation can contribute to bloating in a number of ways, including water retention, or create a gut microbe imbalance that alters the sensitivity and movement of the enteric nervous system. We'll talk more about this in Chapter 4.

5. **PHYSICAL SPACE.** If you eat a big meal, it will take up space in your gut. And fermentation by microbes will add to it. It is normal to be bloated after a big feast. If you typically eat a large volume of food, you will feel it take up space in your gut, versus someone who eats small food portions. What's more, if you have a small body size, eating just a regular meal may increase the size of your belly in a completely normal way.

6. **SLOW OR ALTERED MOTILITY.** A gut that moves more slowly will feel fuller longer. Since food moves through the small intestine fairly quickly and then through the large intestine rather slowly, each meal you eat compounds that slow movement, fermentation, and fullness effect in your gut. Think of it like cruising down the open highway and then finding yourself in gridlock. If you aren't moving your bowels once a day, this could be the primary reason for your bloating, particularly if your gut gets visibly distended.

7. **VISCERAL HYPERSENSITIVITY.** This is where the feeling of bloating but not the distention comes from. It's a gut-brain thing. When the gut space expands a normal amount due to eating food or fermentation, the dysregulated nervous system in the gut can send a hyper-reactive pain signal to your brain. If this is common for you, you can become more consciously aware of the feeling of food expanding your gut, leading to the perception of bloating when digestive function is otherwise normal.

How to Banish the Bloat

If someone tells you that the key to banishing the bloat is avoiding gluten, lectins, or sugar, run away as quickly as you can. Given the complexities of bloating, it's important to know that no one fix will work for everyone. Perhaps you need a combination of strategies to get it under control. I recommend that you evaluate things one at a time so you can discern what does and doesn't work for you.

Something else important to discuss is that certain solutions can help reduce your bloating, but they can also be band-aid solutions that don't address the root cause. For example, perhaps your love of plant-based eating has you feeling super bloated all the time. When you eat high-fibre foods like chickpeas and broccoli, you become bloated, but after eating low-fibre foods like white pasta or tofu, the bloat goes away. This leads you to believe that high-fibre foods are bad for you. Not so fast. While they may lead to less bloating in the moment, they certainly aren't the best for your long-term gut health. Similarly, digestive enzyme supplements are a popular fix for gas and bloating. Digestive enzymes help fully break down the foodstuff so you absorb its content instead of it getting fermented, which also starves your gut bacteria. Digestive enzymes are fine for an occasional quick fix, but I'm not a fan of their regular use.

NUTRITION FIXES FOR BLOATED BELLIES

Meal Spacing

If eating a meal makes you feel bloated, it does not make sense to eat something else an hour later. However, in our hyper-snacking society, this is often what we do. Instead of our traditional three-meals-a-day pattern, we may eat six to ten times a day. If this feels healthy to you and your gut, that's great. But if you're dealing with gut issues, eating multiple times a day can cause havoc in your gut.

There are a couple of meal-spacing options to explore. The first is the interval between meals. For example, try enjoying a balanced and large enough meal to keep you full for four hours. Spacing eating opportunities four hours apart gives you time for the migrating motor complex to sweep your gut in between meals. If you find yourself hungry between meals, by all means eat. But keep those snacks light, just enough to get you to the next meal, like an apple or a small handful of nuts.

If this doesn't feel good to you or work for your schedule, another option is to extend the overnight fast. For example, if you finish eating dinner by 7 p.m. and then wait until 7 a.m. to eat breakfast, you just gave yourself a twelve-hour overnight fast. This may help your gut feel calm and less bloated in the morning. I know that intermittent fasting is very popular, but for digestive health, I don't typically recommend going more than twelve hours without food. In addition, I don't recommend intermittent fasting for anyone with a history of disordered or restrictive eating; anyone who is pregnant or looking to become pregnant; or anyone with type 1 diabetes or using insulin to control diabetes.

Fat Content of Your Meals

I love healthy fats because they keep you feeling full and satisfied. Healthy fats slow blood sugar rise and help you absorb more fat-soluble vitamins and phytochemicals from your food. However, if you are someone who lays it on quite thick, eating a lot of coconut, nut butters, and avocado, you may find it causes gas and bloating. Evidence suggests that since fat slows stomach emptying, it may also slow down intestinal transit, meaning that any gas in the intestines will move slower too. Don't skip eating these healthy fats, just try eating smaller portions to see if it helps. For example, if you usually eat a whole avocado at one sitting, try scaling it back to half a fruit.

Low-FODMAP Diet

We are going to talk a lot more about the FODMAPs in Chapter 6, so I won't go into detail here, but it's helpful to know that decreasing fermentable FODMAP carbohydrates means less fermentation and gas. However, it's not a long-term solution. If nothing else is helping with your bloating, it might be worth a two- to three-week trial. During that time, focus on pro-gut strategies such as getting more active, moving toward a high-fibre diet, and meal spacing to help you adapt successfully post-FODMAP elimination. I highly recommend you do this with the help of a dietitian.

Three Meals a Day Versus Four to Six Small Meals a Day

I believe that you are the best judge of whether or not a certain food or habit is healthy for you. There is no one right way to eat. However, figuring this out means tuning into how habits make you feel and then acting accordingly. Some people feel best eating three meals a day with minimal snacking. I am one of those people now. My body—no doubt influenced by my age and irritable gut—simply doesn't like being given food constantly. Others feel sluggish, bloated, and awful after a big meal and feel much better eating four to six mini meals a day. That also used to be me.

What is most important here is that you eat when you are physically hungry and you keep yourself well nourished. So if you are going to eat three square meals a day, ensure that the meal is well balanced (high fibre, plenty of vegetables, protein, and a bit of fat) to keep you going until your next meal. If you are going to eat multiple times a day, make sure it is mostly whole foods and not a constant stream of hyper-processed packaged food without a single vegetable in sight.

Figuring this out means getting quiet and listening to your body. Someone with reflux may not want to overfill their stomach, so smaller meals will feel better. However, someone with bloating and constipation may want to take advantage of activating the migrating motor complex and ensure plenty of time between meals. This is the time to get mindful. If it helps, keep a food journal to help clarify that connection.

HERBAL REMEDIES AND SUPPLEMENTS FOR BLOATING

There are a lot of digestive health supplements available, but that doesn't mean they all work. Here are two supplements that often work to reduce bloating.

Enteric-Coated Peppermint Oil

Peppermint oil is an antispasmodic, meaning it helps to ease intestinal spasms, which might ease bloating pain. But watch out if you have reflux, as it can make your lower esophageal sphincter (LES) more reflux-y.

> HOW TO USE: Take 200 mg of enteric-coated peppermint oil before each meal as prevention or on an as-needed basis. Enteric-coated peppermint oil is different than the peppermint essential oil you might have in your home. Do not take essential oils internally.

> ALTERNATIVE: Try brewing double-strength peppermint tea. Use two teabags per cup, steep for the recommended time, and then carefully squeeze the teabags to get as much peppermint extractives into the cup as possible.

Probiotics

In theory, if you have an imbalance of gas-producing gut bacteria, a probiotic may help you right that balance and find a calmer gut. There are several probiotics on the market that have shown decreased gas and bloating in clinical trials. There are also a lot of ineffective and well-marketed products on the shelves. We'll talk more about that in Chapter 4. My favourite tool for deciding which probiotic to take is the Clinical Guide to Probiotics. (The Canadian version can be found at www.probioticchart.ca and the US version at www.usprobioticguide.com.) This guide is curated by a clinical pharmacist and outlines the evidence available for the probiotics currently on store shelves. Ideally, stick to the products that have Level I evidence. This means that manufacturers have done at least one clinical trial in humans. Trust science, not marketing.

When you try a probiotic, particularly a clinical strength one, you may actually see an increase in gas and bloating for the first three to four days. This is common and typically a sign that the probiotic is doing its job. Continue taking the probiotic for twelve weeks to truly assess benefit. What does benefit look like? If you are trying to reduce gas and bloating, you should have less gas and bloating after three months. If not, stop using the probiotic or try a different one. Seems like common sense, but all too often I see clients spending their money taking a probiotic for years that has done nothing to improve their symptoms. If a probiotic is working for you, you will feel it.

Lifestyle and Other Therapies

Gut health isn't always about what you eat. Here are a few holistic approaches that might help banish the bloat without having to fuss with your diet too much.

1. **STRENGTHEN THE ABDOMINAL WALL WITH CORE EXERCISES LIKE PILATES AND YOGA.** This is a simple solution, but having strong abs helps hold your gut in. I notice how my Pilates-based workout lessens distention for the forty-eight hours post-workout that my abdominal muscles are at their strongest.

2. **BE MORE ACTIVE IN GENERAL.** Exercise helps enormously. Movement enables movement. It also helps minimize stress, which can have a negative impact on gut function. In addition, it can get the gas out. If you're sedentary, adopting even a twenty-minute daily walk after lunch or dinner can have a positive effect. Some people call it a fart walk. Find your favourite sports or workouts and enjoy them as often as possible.

   Build more movement into your life by turning coffee dates into walking dates, parking far away from the store entrance, and enjoying more active play with the kids. If you find that your bloating builds up over the workday, you may need more movement breaks. Try setting a timer for every thirty minutes to do either a simple torso twist or a stretch at your desk or to get up to fill your water glass.

3. **WEAR LOOSE-FITTING CLOTHING (particularly around the waistband).** If you sit at a desk all day in clothes with a tight waistband, it can limit the movement of gas through the abdomen. If you feel like you are going to bust through your pants by 5 p.m., this might be a culprit along with needing more movement. Buy bigger-sized pants or consider skirts or dresses in softer fabrics or without a waistband.

4. **BIOFEEDBACK.** Biofeedback has been shown to help regulate abdominal wall contractions and ease bloating. Find a local biofeedback practitioner in your area. For a home alternative, try doing deep diaphragmatic breathing for five to ten minutes a day. There are plenty of breathwork tutorials online to help you learn this technique.

5. **MASSAGE YOUR GUT.** Massages greatly assist gut movement and elimination. Here is how to do a simple five-minute self-massage:

   - Lie down somewhere comfortable while wearing lightweight clothing.
   - Gently sweep your palms from the bottom of your pelvis up to the rib cage ten times; this is known as sweeping and prepares your abdomen for a deeper massage.
   - Place your palms on the small of your back and then sweep them over your hip bones and down toward the front of your groin to stimulate the nerve that regulates elimination.
   - Next, start moving the contents of your colon: with a fist, push the contents through by starting at the bottom of your abdomen on the right side, slowly moving up toward your rib cage, then across your rib cage and down your left side. Do this for about one minute.

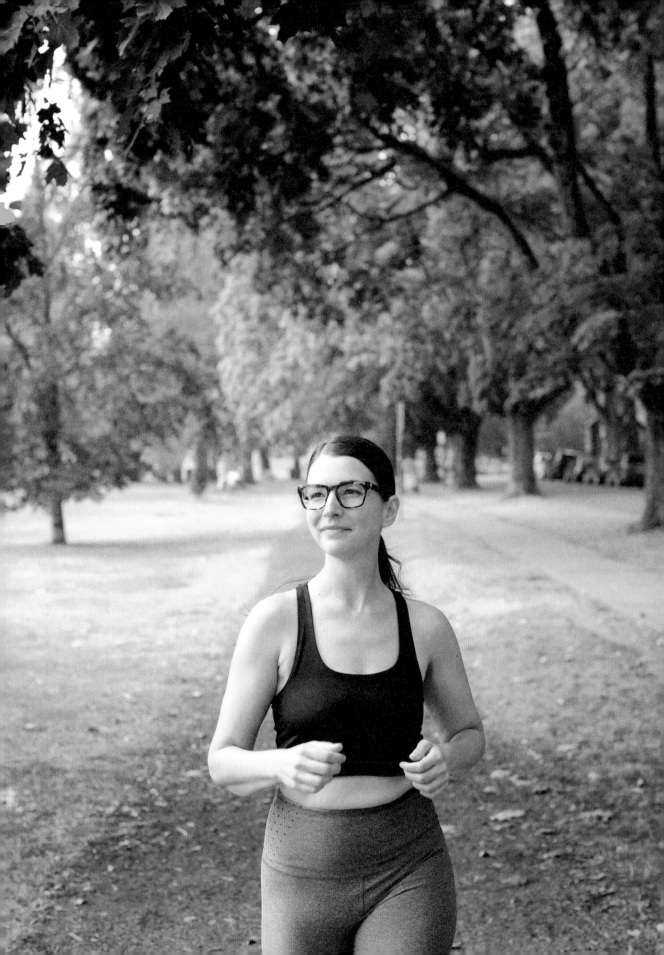

- Finally, spend a minute or two kneading your colon in small circles with your fist. This time, start at the left rib cage and knead toward the groin. Then begin at the bottom of your abdomen on the right side, move up toward your rib cage and then across to where you started. Repeat for one minute.

WHEN TO TALK TO YOUR DOCTOR

Bloating is not always benign and should not be ignored. It can be associated with a number of disease states from celiac disease to diabetes to ovarian cancer, so if significant bloating is a daily issue for you beyond one to two months and the dietary changes and simple fixes described here have had zero impact, you should head to the doctor. A doctor can also talk to you about pharmaceutical options, such as special antibiotics, that may be of help in tackling the root cause of the issue.

You should also speak to your doctor right away if bloating is excessive on a daily basis or accompanied by any of the following symptoms:

- **Weight loss**
- **Severe abdominal pain**
- **Chronic diarrhea**
- **Blood in stool**
- **Fever**

Heartburn (Reflux)

Much like a case of the toots, burps happen. Eat too fast, drink a fizzy beer—your mouth is essentially a rapid-escape hatch for too much gas in the stomach. Of course, sometimes what repeats is the contents of your stomach, not gas. So we're going to talk about heartburn; what it is and when you should take it more seriously.

Heartburn, also known as reflux, is when the contents of the stomach move back up into the esophagus or throat, causing symptoms like burning or pain. Essentially, it's like giving your esophagus an acid bath. If you are wondering why I bothered with that major anatomy lesson back in Chapter 1, it's because I want you to understand how the contents of your stomach can find their way back into your throat. Because when you understand the physiology of what's going on, it might impact the way you choose to address it.

Remember how you have a little trap door between the esophagus and the stomach called the lower esophageal sphincter (LES)? That little door is generally intended to be one way only. Your muscles slowly squeeze the contents of your esophagus toward your stomach; the trap door opens and then digestion begins in the stomach. This is important because all of those acids that get released in your stomach to digest food aren't meant to be in contact with your esophagus. It hurts when they come back up. In fact, your LES is what we call *acid labile*, meaning that when it feels things getting more acidic in your stomach, it's supposed to snap shut even tighter. However, sometimes there is a malfunction and the LES lets the acidic contents back up. There are a few potential culprits discussed on the next page.

INCREASED PRESSURE IN THE STOMACH

We've been talking a lot about stomach emptying, and it is important here too, although the degree to which it's important is a bit controversial in the research. Your stomach is a storage sack, and the body has intricate hormonal feedback to ensure that the stomach empties into the small intestine at just the right rate for good absorption. If the stomach is filling quickly yet emptying slowly—which could happen if you have slow motility (movement) or if you eat a really big, high-fat meal—then the contents of the stomach could start to put pressure on your little trap door and it might fail. Having more weight around the middle or pregnancy can also put physical pressure on the stomach contents.

DECREASED PRESSURE IN THE LES

Other foods and substances, such as alcohol, caffeine, or fat, can affect how tightly the LES snaps shut. Even something as simple as peppermint or cinnamon can relax the gut muscles. Love peppermint gum? You might want to cool it if you're dealing with heartburn. Getting older can also mean less pressure in the sphincter muscles. I probably never thought twice about doing a cartwheel post dinner in my teens, but now, I occasionally have trouble loading the bottom rack of the dishwasher after a big meal.

DECREASED ACID IN THE STOMACH

You don't often hear people talking about too little acid. We are typically focused on too much. When you have less acid in the stomach, as with the use of some medications or with age, the LES gets less chemical feedback to snap shut. This is why older people, who have decreased sensitivity in their nervous system, may not even realize they have reflux because their lower acid stomach contents don't cause the same burn.

DIETARY TRIGGERS

Many people feel that dietary triggers are behind their heartburn. It's possible, but there are still some questions in the research as to how big a role food actually plays. This is just a short list of common dietary triggers (and not all triggers will affect all people):

- Chocolate
- Spicy foods
- Fatty and fried foods
- Acidic foods (citrus, tomatoes, soda, coffee)
- Allium vegetables (garlic, onions)
- Alcohol
- Carminatives (cinnamon, peppermint)
- Caffeinated drinks

WHAT TO DO IF HEARTBURN STRIKES

Heartburn is typically a one-off event, so you could just ride it out if it's not too bothersome. For relief, a few options include the following:

- Chew (non-cinnamon and non-mint) gum, which may help dilute the acid.
- Mix a half teaspoon of baking soda into a glass of water and sip slowly. The baking soda is a base that will help neutralize the acid.
- Eat a couple of pieces of black licorice or take deglycyrrhizinated licorice (DGL), which may soothe things. Don't take DGL without a doctor's approval, as it can interact with some conditions or medications such as those for high blood pressure.
- Drink a glass of soy milk. Calcium is another acid neutralizer and the creamy texture may help coat your esophagus and calm it down.

WHEN TO TALK TO YOUR DOCTOR

The occasional bit of heartburn is totally normal. Perhaps you had a big feast and didn't wait long enough to go to yoga class and downward dog hits you like a fire in your chest. Or you chased down Friday night nachos with a second pint of beer. If it happens once in a while, don't worry about it.

It's also exceedingly common to have heartburn all the time, but that isn't normal. It's called gastro-esophageal reflux disease (GERD) and we are going to talk about it more in Chapter 5. Here is when to talk to your doctor:

- If you are having heartburn consistently more than twice a week
- If your symptoms don't respond to the usual at-home remedies or antacids
- If you are having difficulty swallowing
- If you are nauseous regularly

If you find that heartburn is happening more regularly, it would be worthwhile to keep a food and symptoms journal for two weeks to share with your doctor and your dietitian. It could help them uncover your triggers and create a long-term plan to help you soothe the fire.

Constipation

It happens to all of us occasionally, but you might not realize that chronic constipation is a common issue. On average, about 14 percent of us are chronically constipated, although the numbers in the research range anywhere from 2 percent to a whopping 40 percent. You might also be surprised that a diagnosis of constipation is possible even if you are pooping every day. In fact, a diagnosis of constipation requires just two (or more) of the following symptoms over the past three to six months:

- Straining for at least 25 percent of your bowel movements
- Having hard and lumpy bowel movements more than 25 percent of the time

- Feeling like your bowel movements aren't complete at least 25 percent of the time
- Feeling like your gut is kind of blocked at least 25 percent of the time
- Requiring manual assistance (yes, your finger) to poop at least 25 percent of the time
- Having a bowel movement less than three times a week

That was probably more than you thought you wanted to know about constipation, but knowledge is power. These symptoms aren't easy to talk about, and feeling constipated can be kind of subjective. Knowing what constipation is or isn't helps you get really clear on what is going on for you. It's also going to make it easier to find the solution you need. The key takeaway here is that if either you're not going or going is really difficult, you are probably constipated.

How Often Should You Poop?

In the wellness world, there are a lot of opinions about what makes the perfect pooping schedule. In the medical world, as long as you are pooping a few times a week, you're good. So what's normal?

What you need to understand is that everybody is different. So good health won't look exactly the same for all of us. However, pooping is also kind of important. I believe, based on the fact that it fits within normal transit time and that you are eliminating waste, that you don't really want poop hanging around longer than it should. A daily poop is in order for most of us. If you have one poop daily and it's not super tough to pass, I think you're doing okay.

Normal could be anywhere from one to three poops a day. If it's more like four or more a day, particularly with any other symptoms, I would get concerned that maybe something else is going on that you want to check out.

Staying Regular

Fibre, water, and moving your body will help you maintain regular bowel movements. These three simple requirements aren't a lot to ask, but the majority of people aren't meeting them most of the time. We move less, don't eat enough fibre, and some of us won't consider drinking water unless it's infused with coffee or sugar. The good news is that you don't have to suffer from constipation with these simple solutions at hand.

1. **FIBRE.** Fibre does a couple of things: it bulks up the stool to help gravity and peristalsis (muscle movement) do their job and it keeps the stool hydrated so it's easy to pass. Given that so many of us aren't eating enough fibre, our stool may move more slowly through the colon. The recipes in this book will help you get more fibre. Just be sure to take it slowly, as the combination of constipation and too much fibre too soon could spell bloating disaster.

2. **WATER.** In order to have hydrated stools, you need to drink water. If you don't, your body goes into water conservation mode, which includes robbing it from your stool, making stool super hard and difficult to pass. Besides all that digestion and fermentation, your gut actually reabsorbs a lot of water from the gut contents. If you are dehydrated, the colon will take even more water from your poop. So try drinking more water. How much water? Hydration is ever-changing and completely individualized based on:

   - Your body size and activity level
   - The temperature and humidity
   - Your diet—whether you eat a lot of high-in-water foods like fruit and vegetables or eat a lot of low-in-water foods like cookies, protein bars, and bread
   - How much caffeine and alcohol you drink, which can increase your water losses

   With so many variables, the best way to know if you are drinking enough water is to check your urine. If your urine is pale yellow or clear and you're urinating every couple of hours, you're drinking enough water. Now, a few things can change your urine colour, like how B vitamins turn it neon yellow, but in general, this observation method works.

   Get serious about drinking water in whatever form works for you—hot, cold, or with some lemon or cucumber slices. Make herbal tea, add a tiny splash of fruit juice, whatever you need to encourage yourself to drink it. Ideally, drink a big glass of water as soon as you wake up in the morning (before coffee) to help initiate that morning gastrocolic reflex.

3. **MOVEMENT.** Gravity definitely helps move the gut a bit, but the more you move, the better your gut moves. If you are sedentary, your gut isn't going to move as well as if you work on your feet or you go for a daily power walk.

   Start moving your body more. You don't have to become a gym rat, just do whatever movement (living room dance parties, soccer, or your favourite workout class) feels good to you. If you are currently sedentary, even a daily twenty- to thirty-minute walk will work wonders.

EVERYDAY WAYS WE GET IN OUR GUT'S WAY

Beyond the basic three requirements for regular bowel movements discussed above, there are a whole host of ways we can mess with our elimination habits. Some common culprits include:

- Not going to the washroom when you need to
- Changes to your routine, such as travel, different time zones, and eating different foods
- Medications and supplements that can cause constipation (ask your doctor)
- Stress
- Too much dairy or meat

BONUS STRATEGIES TO HELP YOU GO

While you're on the path to a higher-fibre, better-hydrated, more-active life, there are a few things you can try to help speed up your recovery and make it easier to poop. You can also try these strategies if you feel that you need a little extra help once you've mastered the basics. When a gut has been sluggish for a long time, it needs a little TLC and patience to really get moving again.

Psyllium

Psyllium is a soluble fibre that is not super fermentable. This means that it isn't irritating to the gut, it doesn't cause a lot of gas or bloating, and it has the dual purpose of hydrating stool and making it easier to pass while gelling gut contents together, lessening loose stools. Psyllium husk is found at health food stores and sold under a few brand names, such as Metamucil, at the pharmacy too. I recommend people use psyllium as follows:

- Start with a 1-teaspoon (5 mL) daily dose mixed into the food or beverage of your choice. Do this consistently for four or five days and ensure that you drink at least one extra glass of water daily.
- If this feels good but you don't have relief, increase the dose by 1 teaspoon (5 mL) daily for the next four or five days as above. You can go as high as a 1-tablespoon (15 mL) daily dose, but you'll probably want to divide it into two or three doses, as that is a lot of psyllium to swallow in one go.
- If extra symptoms arise, stop and go back to the previous dose until they subside. And if you are at the 1-tablespoon (15 mL) daily dose and drinking enough water and things don't get moving in a couple of weeks, then it's not for you.

Prunes

Grandmas everywhere can't be wrong. Prunes work. Try eating four or five prunes a day, perhaps chopped with some nuts like a trail mix. Don't like prunes? Try eating two kiwis a day, which may also help.

Create a Better Bathroom Routine

Your gut loves a good routine, so let's build one. I'm not talking about rising before sunrise for hours of meditation; instead, try something incredibly simple. For example, wake up fifteen minutes earlier so you aren't rushed in the morning. Head to the kitchen and drink one or two large glasses of water while you make your morning coffee or tea to help stimulate the gastrocolic reflex. Then, go and sit on the toilet for ten minutes. Set a timer. Do not strain or worry about whether the bowel movement will happen. If it doesn't happen, get up and go about your day. This is about telling your nervous system that now is the time to go. After a couple of weeks, it may help.

Rethink Your Seat

For some people, something as simple as getting a "squatty potty" can work wonders. Your body will do a better job of eliminating if it's in the squat position—countless countries outside of North America have squat toilets for a reason. So you can buy a little stool that fits with your toilet to elevate your knees to a more physiologically correct pooping position.

Meal Spacing

Picture this: You haven't pooped in two days. You have a meal. In six to eight hours, undigested leftovers will be added to the slow twelve- to twenty-four-hour journey through the colon. In other words, with just three meals a day, your small intestine could outrun your colon's capacity to clear itself, which will become glaringly apparent after two days of not going. Review the section on bloating on page 26 for more on meal spacing.

Magnesium

Magnesium citrate is a mineral that works as an osmotic laxative, meaning that it draws water into the bowel to stimulate a bowel movement. Grandma's Milk of Magnesia is actually made of magnesium. No clinical trials have been done to date, but taking 1 to 2 teaspoons (5 to 10 mL) of a magnesium citrate powder may help as a rescue remedy when you really need to go.

Probiotics

Some research has found that the gut microbiota in people with constipation is different than in those with a healthy gut, although it's unknown whether the microbiota changes are the cause of constipation or vice versa. However, people with constipation may have higher levels of methane-producing microbes, which results in slow transit time.

There is some evidence to suggest that a few probiotic strains may actually increase transit time and decrease symptoms of constipation, but they are not my first line of defence.

If your constipation isn't too intense and you are free of any other symptoms, you are probably good to work through all of these natural solutions on your own. Don't just brush off constipation as no big deal; you want your gut working properly so you feel your best, but also because constipation can cause issues like hemorrhoids, diverticulitis, or incontinence. Do the work, make those poops happen.

Constipation is often simple in scope, but it can be quite difficult to treat. We're going to talk about this more in Chapter 5, but know that constipation also can be caused by more complex issues like thyroid function, the type of microbes in your gut, or wonky gut-brain communication.

Constipation also can be a symptom of more serious diseases such as diabetes, autoimmunity, or even cancer. If you have any of the following symptoms, see your doctor right away:

- **Persistent abdominal pain beyond the discomfort of being overly full**
- **Significant and persistent bloating**
- **Nausea or vomiting**
- **Blood in the stool**

Diarrhea

Diarrhea is the worst. There is no other way to put it. It's always a sign that something is up, although not always something worrisome. It is typically defined as loose or watery stools. Diarrhea can happen every once in a while in a healthy life for a variety of reasons, including:

- **Eating a lot more fructose or lactose than you're used to, like a 3-scoop ice cream sundae on your birthday; fructose and lactose are poorly absorbed sugars that draw water to them in the gut, loosening up the stools**
- **Eating large quantities of fruit and vegetables with osmotic sugars or stimulatory compounds, such as collard greens, kiwis, or prunes**
- **Having a gut infection, like food poisoning or antibiotic-associated diarrhea**
- **Taking medications or supplements, such as magnesium citrate or certain medications (hundreds of them in fact), such as proton pump inhibitors (PPIs) for GERD**
- **Having anxiety and stress, which can cause increased intestinal transit**
- **Having hormonal shifts—if you've ever had diarrhea during your period, blame the hormonal flux; it's thought that prostaglandins, hormones released before your period to encourage your uterus to contract and shed its lining, also influence contractions and movements in your gastrointestinal tract**
- **Running long distance—we're not exactly sure why, but the combination of movement, altered blood flow, and brain-gut stuff all probably contribute to the well-known runner's diarrhea or the trots**

If you've been hit with a bout of diarrhea without any other symptoms, you needn't panic. Instead, take some basic steps to help calm your gut:

- Drink Plenty of Water. **Diarrhea means that you are losing more water than normal, so you need to replenish it. Soups with a bit of salt and potassium-rich vegetables are great to help with electrolyte balance, as are watered-down fresh juices.**
- Take a Probiotic. **If you suspect that diarrhea is from food poisoning or antibiotic use, a clinical-strength probiotic can help fight off the bad bugs so you can bounce back faster. See Chapter 4 for probiotic guidance.**
- Consider Psyllium. **If diarrhea lasts for more than two days, consider taking psyllium, which can help bind stools to lessen gut irritation. See page 36 for more information on how to use psyllium.**
- Avoid Dairy and High-Fructose Foods. **This will reduce the amount of osmotic sugars that can draw water into the bowel, making things worse. Try the low-FODMAP Heal or Soothe recipes in this book.**

While a day or two of diarrhea probably isn't an issue in an otherwise healthy body, if it comes with any alarming symptoms, such as severe pain, fever, or blood in the stool, see a doctor *immediately*. Yes, don't wait. Go now. Otherwise, if it lasts longer than seven days, and probiotics or psyllium don't seem to be working, you probably want to see your doctor because it could be:

- Lactose or fructose intolerance
- Post-antibiotic infection such as *Clostridioides difficile*
- Bile acid diarrhea
- Irritable bowel syndrome with diarrhea (IBS-D)
- Inflammatory bowel disease (IBD)
- Celiac disease

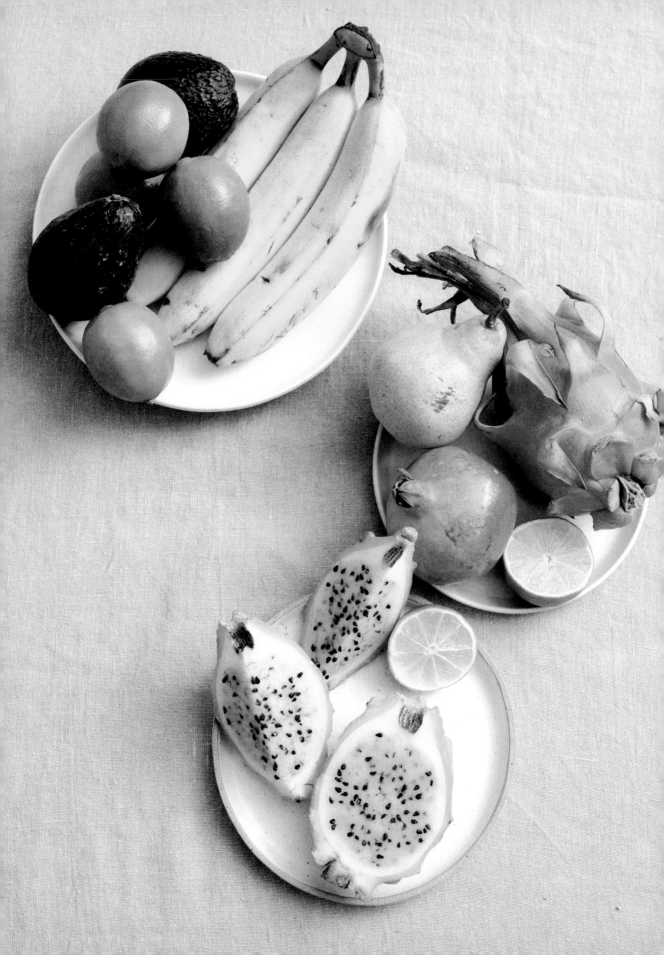

3

How to Feed Your Gut for Life

Let's talk plants. There's a lot of scientific truth to the statement "You are what you eat." Your body is built of the nutrients—the amino acids, glucose, fats, vitamins, and minerals—that your gut digests and absorbs from food. Lentils are high in iron, but your red blood cells will have to wait until your gut cracks those lentils open and releases the iron from its fibrous cage. You owe your health to your gut, so you need to feed it right so it can thrive. That's what this chapter is about: how to feed your gut now, even when it seems to be working (mostly) fine, to help optimize *its* function so you can optimize *yours*.

If you have irritable bowel syndrome (IBS), celiac disease, or inflammatory bowel disease (IBD), consider the advice in this chapter the foundation of what will come next. The goal is always to eat as much high-fibre, anti-inflammatory, and plant-based foods as you can tolerate. However, you'll probably have to modify your eating plan to suit where your gut function is at right now, and you'll find that advice in Chapter 5. I'd also encourage you to enjoy the Soothe recipes for irritated guts. What you eat to thrive when things are well won't always look the same as what will help you heal when things aren't.

Way too often, when people think of healthy eating, they think of restriction. We think of how we need to stop eating our favourite foods, or how we *shouldn't* eat certain foods (or entire food groups). This approach kind of dooms you from the start because it associates health with a sense of loss, and it robs you of the joy of healthy eating. And joy is a healing state.

I prefer what I call a positive approach to nutrition. When you focus on what to eat more of, your mind doesn't get into that anxious, restrictive place. And let's be honest, with very few exceptions (avoiding gluten if you have celiac disease comes to mind), your health is created by what you *do* eat, not by what you avoid.

If you've done my online wellness challenges, you already know the Daily 3: beans, greens, and omega-3-rich seeds. The Daily 3 has become a fan favourite because it creates a simple structure to organize your healthy eating efforts. In addition, it's truly transformative to eat these three foods daily. All plants are good plants, but these three are especially important. As you're reading through the book, why not experiment with the Daily 3? It's simple. For example:

- Eat 2 to 3 tablespoons (30 to 45 mL) of omega-3-rich seeds (hemp, ground flax, or chia) daily
- Eat 2 cups (500 mL) of leafy green veggies (spinach, kale, broccoli, etc.) daily
- Eat ¼ to ¾ cup (60 to 175 mL) of beans or lentils daily. Start with ¼ cup (60 mL) if you don't usually eat them, then every few weeks or so, add another ¼ (60 mL) cup to your portion. Trust me on going slowly. You want to feel better, not more bloated, and it takes your body a while to acclimate to the plant power in beans and lentils

You could easily get all of these foods into a lunchtime salad bowl if you want or sprinkle them into your eating throughout your day. And if you want to get a bit wild, try my Chocolate Cherry Rebuilder Smoothie (page 132) that sneaks in chickpeas.

Eating More Plants Is Good for Your Gut

Eat more plants isn't just a tagline for me, it's how I live. In my opinion, a plant-based, anti-inflammatory diet is the ultimate foundation for better digestive health and optimal well-being. I talk a lot about anti-inflammatory nutrition in my book *Eat More Plants*, but let's take a quick peek at the basics of how a more whole-foods, plant-based diet affects your gut.

An anti-inflammatory diet is really about eating as many whole plant foods as possible. I'm talking fruit, vegetables, grains, legumes, nuts, and seeds. It's that simple. We are part of the natural world and have survived this long by eating what we find in nature. So when we ditch the fad diets and drop hyper-processed foods, we don't need to worry as much about the minutiae of nutrition. When you eat mostly whole plant foods, you are automatically eating in a way that:

- **Improves blood sugar balance by reducing high-glycemic and pro-inflammatory processed foods like white flour and added sugars**
- **Improves the quality of fats consumed: less saturated fats and more unsaturated fats**
- **Increases your intake of antioxidant and anti-inflammatory compounds**
- **Provides ample fibre and fermentable carbohydrates to encourage regular elimination and to feed your gut microbes well**

Eat more plants is easy to say, but our collective habit of eating out of boxes and bags is so deep that sometimes our brain has a hard time processing the change. We associate snacks with packaged snack foods so intensely that simply grabbing some almonds or a peach seems odd. Or we'll scour the ingredients lists of every granola bar and cracker on the shelf looking for the healthiest one instead of buying some hummus and carrots.

It's so easy to eat plants, but I also get that it can be a challenge if you're not in the habit yet. If your typical breakfast is a coffee shop breakfast sandwich and a latte or if you snack on packaged protein bars instead of fruit, this way of eating might feel foreign to you. It will also feel like an energy revolution, which is really exciting for me as a dietitian because I know how good you'll feel eating this way.

More often than not, eating a plant-based diet is about shifting mindsets and habits instead of eating in a drastically different way. Making change can feel overwhelming, but it doesn't have to be when you realize that it doesn't need to happen overnight. Just keep tweaking your habits until all of a sudden you realize that you are rocking plant life. Here are some simple ways to shift to eating more plants:

- **Buy enough fruit and vegetables at the grocery store (we're talking pounds of them) to get more onto your plate. If all you buy is a couple of bananas, a few apples, and a head of broccoli, it won't get you through a week of plant-full eating.**
- **Double the fruit and vegetables in your favourite recipes or add beans to them.**
- **Cook with what's in your fridge, as opposed to on a whim, to ensure that produce gets eaten, not wasted. Vegetable waste is always a big concern for clients, and it leads them to skimp on buying plants at the store.**
- **Always order a side of vegetables at a restaurant if your main isn't plant-y enough.**
- **Snack on whole foods, not packaged foods.**

Remember that *all plants are good plants*. Choose the foods that fit into your budget. Buy what's on sale and make a plan to use it up. Don't underestimate the power of frozen fruit and veggies. You can usually adjust my recipes to use up what is on hand instead of creating waste.

Many plant foods, like bulk dried beans and grains, are much more cost-effective than typical groceries. Other foods (like cashews) and super foods (such as goji berries and spirulina) are more expensive. Luckily, they are also not mandatory for a healthy life. Financial stress, like all stress, is bad for the gut. Choose what works within your budget.

You might be worried that the way you currently eat is wrong or fearful that the only way to be healthy is to go vegan overnight, and that sparks some anxiety for you. But, remember, it's a marathon, not a sprint. This is about consistent, gentle, daily effort toward a healthier you.

The best place to start is to choose a habit or two to focus on until it becomes automatic. It could be a green smoothie for breakfast or some fruit mid-afternoon instead of a candy bar. The good news is that drinking a glass of wine or eating a piece of cake on Friday night doesn't magically erase your healthy habits.

The magic is that the more you eat plants, free of any restrictive or good/bad mindsets, the more you'll begin to crave them naturally, and you just might find that you want a bowl of pasta with a big helping of roasted broccoli or garlic-sautéed white beans on the side. Sometimes, you won't and that's fine too. Your relationship with food, just like your relationship with your body, is an important part of this whole wellness equation.

How Eating More Plants Helps Your Gut

I like it when nutrition advice is simple—just eat more plants—but the science behind why plants are so good for you is really quite complex.

Let's start with the most science-y reason to go plant-based: good bugs like plants. You see, the kind of bacteria you want in your gut need fermentable fibres and carbohydrates that you will find only in plant foods. These are the good bacteria that fight off the gut-wrecking bugs, create plenty of short-chain fatty acids to feed gut cells, calm inflammation, and support the integrity of your gut barrier. Bacteria are kind of amazing, and they are starting to get the credit they deserve.

In the research, we see a lot of evidence that plant-based diets boost the microbiome. For example, people who follow vegetarian or vegan diets tend to have a more anti-inflammatory ratio of *Bacteroidetes* to *Firmicutes* bacteria. Vegans tend to have increased levels of *Faecalibacterium prausnitzii,* a species of bacteria with anti-inflammatory and gut-protecting effects.

Now, before you get all excited that eating vegan cake and cookies all day is going to help you live your healthiest life, it's important to know that how many *actual plants* you eat matters. For example, a study that compared omnivores, vegetarians, and vegans against a "healthy plant-based diet index" found that those who ate an unhealthy plant-based diet had much higher cardiovascular disease risk than those who ate a healthy plant-based diet, even if they ate some animal products. That's why the amount of plants you eat is key. As much as I love vegan candy, I know it's not building me a better microbiome.

A Healthier Gut Starts in the Supermarket

The power of a smart weekly shop shouldn't be underestimated. The more plants you buy, the more you can put on your plate. Let's take a look at what I hope will make it into your cart on a weekly basis so you can power up on plants.

PRODUCE

- All veggies are good, but make sure you always put some brassicas and greens into your cart, like broccoli, parsley, bok choy, kale, and cauliflower.
- Make extra space for anti-inflammatory aromatics such as onions, garlic, ginger, and turmeric.
- When you can, focus on higher-fibre and temperate fruit most often, such as apples, pears, and berries. Bananas, kiwis, and pineapple are excellent for their gut-soothing properties, and peaches and watermelon for their bacteria-boosting FODMAPs.
- Don't forget about frozen fruit and veggies. They are healthy and budget-friendly.

NUTS AND SEEDS

- Nuts and seeds are packed with fibre, minerals, and healthy fats. Always have two or three types on hand, such as cashews, almonds, pistachios, hemp hearts, and pumpkin seeds. Avoid sweetened trail mixes that are more candy than they are nuts.

WHOLE GRAINS

- Whole, intact grains are tops for gut health. I find the high-chew grains, such as wheat berries, spelt, and barley, the most satisfying, but they contain gluten so they aren't for everyone. For gluten-free options, try buckwheat, gluten-free oats, and millet.
- Keep it 100 when it comes to prepared grains, such as 100 percent sprouted grain breads, 100 percent whole-grain traditionally fermented sourdough breads, and 100 percent whole-grain crisp breads; 100 percent whole-grain pastas (cooked al dente) also fit the bill.

BEANS AND LEGUMES

- Plant protein is essential for a happy gut. Always have two or three legume options in your kitchen, such as chickpeas, tempeh, and lentils. Canned (no salt added) is convenient. Dried is more economical and typically has a nicer texture.
- Smoked tofu is a great ready-to-eat option, and pre-marinated tempeh saves time in the kitchen while boosting flavour.
- Chickpea flour is a great way to incorporate more protein and fibre into baked goods and is also an alternative for eggs.

- Whole-grain or sprouted-grain flours for baking.
- Calcium-rich dairy alternatives like oat, cashew, or soy milk.
- Fermented foods such as kombucha, miso, or kimchi (more about fermented foods in Chapter 4).
- Canned goods such as no-salt-added tomatoes.
- Healthy oils such as olive oil.
- Spices and condiments.

The Many Facets of Fibre

If we're going to hang our hat on plants being good for our gut microbiome, we have to talk about fibre. Many people have heard of soluble and insoluble fibres, but perhaps aren't really sure how they're different or why both are important. Insoluble fibres like cellulose are typically found in the cell walls of plant foods and act like a broom to help sweep the gut clear. Insoluble fibres speed up elimination by adding bulk to your stools, discouraging the attachment of harmful bacteria to your gut wall, and encouraging cell turnover in the gut as they brush past to help keep that gut running smoothly. Soluble fibres are different, more of a gel-like sponge that holds water to hydrate stools in addition to having the potential to bind substances like cholesterol or bile salts and carry them out of the body. In addition, soluble fibres tend to slow down elimination a bit.

However, soluble or insoluble isn't the only factor here. We need to talk about microbiota-accessible carbohydrates (MACs). MACs are carbohydrates that gut bacteria can ferment. Some MACs are fibres, like hemicellulose; others are prebiotic fructans like inulin or even resistant starches in unripe bananas or cooked and cooled potatoes.

If you want to have a healthy and resilient gut microbiota, you need to feed your gut bacteria. This means you need to feed *yourself* plants.

Phytochemicals Mean More Plant Power

Plant foods contain naturally occurring substances called *phytochemicals*, many of which produce anti-oxidant and anti-inflammatory activity in the body. Since these phytochemicals come into direct contact with the digestive tract, you might wonder if they're good for the gut. Yes, they are very good for the gut.

Research suggests that people who consume more of a specific type of phytochemical called *polyphenols* have a healthier microbiome. Why? Well, not everything we eat is so easy to digest and absorb. Fibre is a classic example: we don't absorb it into our body, but it does a world of good as it passes on through the gut. Polyphenols have been perplexing researchers for some time because they perform well in lab studies but they aren't that well absorbed in the body. And a lot of them need to be activated by enzymes first so they're more bioavailable.

How Much Fibre Do You Need in a Day?

Dietary fibre is perhaps one of the most important factors in living an anti-inflammatory, gut-friendly lifestyle. So how much is enough? Official recommendations are for adult women to consume 25 grams daily; women over fifty years of age need 21 grams. Adult men need 38 grams of fibre a day, decreasing to 30 grams at the age of fifty. That's a lot of fibre. But it's fairly easy to get the fibre you need, even for smaller appetites, as long as you know your high-fibre swaps.

A HEALTHY BUT LOWER-FIBRE DAY

Breakfast: 1 cup (250 mL) Cheerios (3.2 g) with ½ cup (125 mL) blueberries (2 g), ½ cup (125 mL) unsweetened almond milk, and coffee

Lunch: sandwich on 100% whole wheat bread (4 g) with sliced tomato (0.9 g), sprouts, and vegan cream cheese

Snack: ¾ cup (175 mL) non-dairy unsweetened yogurt and an orange (2.3 g)

Dinner: 2 cups (500 mL) spinach salad (1.4 g) with 1 tablespoon (15 mL) dried cranberries (0.4 g), a 3-ounce (85 g) piece of grilled tofu (3 g), and croutons

TOTAL FIBRE = JUST OVER 17 GRAMS

A HIGH-FIBRE, ANTI-INFLAMMATORY DAY

Breakfast: smoothie with 1 tablespoon (15 mL) ground flaxseed (1.9 g), 1 cup (250 mL) kale (1.7 g), ½ cup (125 mL) blackberries (4 g), 1 cup (250 mL) unsweetened almond milk, and 2 tablespoons (30 mL) protein powder

Lunch: sandwich on 100% sprouted grain bread (12 g) with ½ cup (125 mL) chickpea salad (4 g), ½ cup (125 mL) spinach, and 2 tablespoons (30 mL) pickled carrots (0.5 g)

Snack: ¼ cup (60 mL) raw almonds (3.6 g) and an apple (4 g)

Dinner: ½ cup (125 mL) wheat berries (4 g), 1 cup (250 mL) roasted broccoli (4 g), and a 3-ounce (85 g) piece of grilled tofu (3 g)

TOTAL FIBRE = JUST OVER 42 GRAMS

Enter your tiny plant munchers. Approximately 90 percent of the polyphenols we eat end up in our large intestine, and they appear to have some direct antioxidant effects on the gut tissues. However, what's really significant is that polyphenols and other phytochemicals are interacting with our gut microbiota.

Our gut microbes have the power to activate many of these polyphenols into a more absorbable state. In turn, polyphenols alter the gut microbiota in a couple of ways. They may have a direct prebiotic effect, and some, like ellagitannins, help kill off more harmful bacteria. If you need even more proof that whole foods are beneficial, it appears that a high-fibre diet—plenty of plants—may alter the microbiota in such a way that they get even better at transforming polyphenols.

Most plants contain polyphenols, but gram for gram, spices like cloves and cumin typically have the most. However, we don't eat spices in large quantities like we do fruit and vegetables. Consume spices daily, as well as these high-polyphenol foods:

- Berries
- Cocoa and dark chocolate
- Coffee and tea
- Hazelnuts and almonds
- Spinach and broccoli
- Soybeans and soy milk
- Whole wheat and rye flours
- White and black beans

More Plants Means Fewer Gut Busters

I'm not one to focus on negatives, but it's true that eating a more plant-based, anti-inflammatory diet means you won't be eating as much of a few things that can be detrimental to your gut health long term.

As a dietitian, my goal is to never demonize foods or encourage you to be rigid in your dietary choices. Yes, I want you to eat as many whole plant foods as you can, but I don't want you to stress over eating something that isn't. For example, I love olive oil, which isn't technically a whole food. But it is healthy and it makes food taste really good. I also like pasta. I even like chips and cake and ice cream. If you're generally well, flexibility and ease are *part* of a healthy diet and a healthy relationship with food. Rigid mindsets about eating or old school good/bad labels will actually make you less healthy. So with that in mind, let's talk about the things that your gut doesn't want you eating in huge amounts.

GUT BUSTER ONE: TOO MUCH SALT

We generally eat too much salt, even if we don't use a salt shaker. The vast majority of the sodium in our North American diet comes from packaged and prepared foods like fast food, condiments, and baked goods. These types of foods are high in sodium, but standard supermarket versions are also low in the electrolytes magnesium, calcium, and potassium that help moderate the effects of sodium on our body.

Too much salt can harm your gut, which might surprise you. High-salt diets are associated with pro-inflammatory states that can affect the gut; high-salt intake also has been shown to harm the gut microbiota itself, decreasing beneficial *Lactobacillus* species and lowering levels of short-chain fatty acids in lab trials.

Consuming less sodium is important, and plant foods will help you get there. But it doesn't mean you have to go salt-free (unless your doctor recommends it). Salt makes whole foods taste delicious. And pleasure is an important part of a healthy lifestyle. I use iodized salt in all of my cooking. While iodized salt has fallen out of fashion, it's a critical source of thyroid-supportive iodine in a plant-based diet, as plant foods have little to no iodine. Once you're eating less hyper-processed foods, you won't have to worry about a little salt. I cook with no-salt-added, whole food ingredients like fresh vegetables, canned beans, and canned tomatoes so I have room in my sodium budget to season my meals properly so they taste amazing.

GUT BUSTER TWO: TOO MANY ADDED SUGARS

Our hyper-processed food supply is literally drowning in added sugars—everything from actual table sugar to high-fructose corn syrup to fruit juice concentrates. We consume a lot of sugar and it's not good for fighting inflammation or for our gut. However, I want to clear up a myth. A bit of sugar isn't going to cause bacterial overgrowth or a leaky gut. So go ahead and have a slice of birthday cake or put a teaspoon of sugar in your salad dressing.

If that sounds radical for a gut-health book, it's because a lot of gut-health "gurus" are still locked in diet-culture traps like food demonization and fear. Our modern food system is making us sick and I certainly don't want you consuming a lot of sugar, but a small amount of sugar is not going to be detrimental to your health.

The research on diet and microbiota typically focuses on high (saturated)-fat, high-sugar, and low-fibre diets as a dietary pattern. I have yet to see a nutrition study that looks at the effect of a healthy, high-fibre diet that includes some added sugars. So, yes, the current evidence suggests that this high-fat, high-sugar, low-fibre dietary pattern is awful for our gut microbiota. Here's why:

- **A diet that is low in fibre and high in absorbable sugars robs the healthy gut microbiome in the colon of their primary fuel, lowering healthy diversity.**
- **Fewer short-chain fatty acid producers mean that your gut barrier might not falter and you might be exposed to bacterial endotoxins that cause inflammation.**
- **A high intake of fermentable sugars such as fructose and lactose can cause IBS symptoms in people who malabsorb them or can feed gut bacteria that have already overgrown.**
- **High-sugar diets can stoke chronic inflammation and that can have its own impact on the microbiota.**

If you consume a lot of added sugar every day, it's not great. But what's too much? According to the American Heart Association, *too much* works out to anything more than 6 teaspoons (25 g) of added sugar a day for women and 9 teaspoons (36 g) of added sugar a day for men. I really wouldn't advise eating more sugar if you already eat less, but these numbers show that in the context of a healthy diet, you've got some wiggle room for a bit of juice or the occasional ice cream. Where we go off the rails is when a caramel coffee Frappuccino has 62 g of sugar or a bottle of cola has 52 g of sugar and we consider it a reasonable daily food. We call those "sometimes" foods in our house.

The Difference Between Sugars and Added Sugars

There are a whole bunch of different sugars: single sugars like glucose, double sugars like sucrose (table sugar), and even biological sugars that are made by our body. Our body is designed to run on glucose; let that be a reminder that carbs are part of our biological destiny.

Our digestive system disassembles all digestible carbohydrates into single sugars so they can be absorbed. Steel-cut oats? Slowly, but surely, they will be broken down into glucose, once your gut breaks down those tough cell walls. The only carbs that bypass digestion are ones like fibre or any fermentable sugars like lactose that we lack adequate enzymes to break down.

WHAT ARE ADDED SUGARS?

When talking about avoiding added sugars, I mean any sugar that is *not* naturally occurring in a food. Don't avoid fruit. Their natural sugars are locked behind cell walls that take time to release. They're also incredibly nutrient dense—full of vitamins, fibre, and anti-inflammatory phytochemicals—and part of a healthy diet. If you have poorly controlled diabetes, you might want to watch the portion size of fruit, but you can enjoy ½ cup (125 mL) of berries with your breakfast or a small apple with peanut butter for a snack.

Added sugars are different, and they have many names:

- Date syrup, coconut sugar, coconut nectar
- Fruit juice, fruit juice concentrate, fruit purée
- Glucose-fructose, high-fructose corn syrup
- Maple syrup, honey
- Sugar, cane sugar, corn syrup

It's the added sugars we want to minimize. They are nearly pure sugar, devoid of a complex structure or nutritional profile that make it easy to overdo them and tip the balance of sugars in our diet.

ARE NATURAL SWEETENERS HEALTHIER?

My favourite sweeteners are the natural kind, like maple syrup and dates. They are flavourful, contain small amounts of nutrients, and are part of a healthy diet, but they're still sugar so we want to be mindful of how much we are eating. Yes, dates are prebiotic, but a single Medjool date is the equivalent of 3 to 4 teaspoons (15 to 20 mL) of sugar. It is okay to enjoy sweets sometimes. I just want you to be aware, so you aren't eating a cup of dates a day thinking it's no big deal.

WHAT ABOUT ZERO-CALORIE SWEETENERS?

Since a high-sugar diet isn't great for your gut, you might be tempted to try zero-calorie sweeteners. I'm not a fan of these sweeteners, and you definitely want to avoid artificial sweeteners at all costs. They aren't really that delicious, and there's a chance they might mess up your appetite circuitry and your microbiome. But what about natural sweeteners like stevia, monkfruit, and xylitol? While they are better, I would much rather you use real sugars, just less of them. Especially for those with IBS, sugar alcohols are a big, gassy no-no (they're a FODMAP). I think it's more important to wean your sweet tooth a bit than to reinforce a die-hard love of sugar with zero-calorie sweeteners.

GUT BUSTER THREE: TOO MUCH SATURATED FAT

The media has been back and forth on saturated fat. It blamed it for heart disease in the 90s. Then fat was back and fans of keto and paleo diets started claiming it was a health food. What does the science say now? Let's take a look.

As was the story with sugar, few studies have looked specifically at high-saturated-fat diets and the gut. Research usually looks at Western dietary patterns (high fat, high sugar, high salt and low fibre) or high-fat, high-sugar diets. However, we have some lab research and a bit of human data that suggest that saturated fat alone isn't great for our gut in excessive amounts. High-saturated-fat diets are associated with the following:

- **Detrimental changes in the gut microbiota, including more bile-tolerant, sulfate-reducing bacteria and less diversity overall**
- **Chronic inflammation and decreased mucus barrier in the gut**
- **Increased translocation of lipopolysaccharides (LPS) across the gut wall, which promotes chronic inflammation**

As with all things, the amount you eat matters. You actually need some saturated fat in your life. If you're plant based, a little coconut (in all the various forms) is helpful. It's when you go overboard that it's not a good idea, which we are so good at doing. So eat more plants and you'll naturally lower your saturated-fat intake found in dairy and meat. If you make monounsaturated, anti-inflammatory extra-virgin olive oil your go-to oil, you won't consume too much coconut oil.

GUT BUSTER FOUR: TOO MUCH HAEM IRON

When I first learned about iron, I was taught that haem iron—the kind from animals—was the best kind and that plant-based iron was inadequate. This idea originated from the biological fact that haem iron is well absorbed. However, what I was not taught is that excess haem iron is a gut irritant. Haem iron is associated with negative changes in the microbiota as well as increased inflammation in the gut and is even a risk for colon cancer. So, yes, I'm good with plants.

If you eat red meat, I recommend keeping it to one small portion a week while you explore putting more beans, tofu, and tempeh on your plate.

How You Eat Matters as Much as What You Eat

Eating well is as much about the *how* as it is about the *what*. Let's start by talking about how you chew your food. As mentioned in Chapter 2, chewing is more important than you might think. For example, it's your only chance to optimize digestion by physically grinding the food into a pulp. Chewing creates more surface area so the acids and enzymes in your gut can do their job better. Do carrots hurt your stomach? It could be that you aren't chewing this dense vegetable well enough.

The act of chewing also primes the stomach to release stomach acid in preparation for the arrival of food. What's more, the very act of chewing is thought to be calming. So, it's probably more effective to stress-eat carrot sticks than it is chips. Think of eating really high-chew foods and chewing them properly as a mini meditation for your nervous system. Chewing well also slows down the rate at which you eat, giving your body more time for the satiety hormones to kick in and tell you that you're full.

So chew slowly and thoroughly. Try noticing how your teeth grind the food—it will improve your digestion. Also, grandma was right: don't chew with your mouth open. You'll swallow more air.

REACH FOR HIGH-CHEW CARBOHYDRATES

Since we're talking about chewing, let's talk about a sneaky little trick I use to make healthier choices. You want to reach for carbs that I call high chew. For example, a wheat berry instead of couscous or sprouted grain bread instead of soft wheat bread. Foods that require a lot of chewing have a lot of structure, like dense cell walls and fibre. The more you have to chew, the slower the nutrients will reach your bloodstream, leading to more stable energy levels and appetite.

There is a small body of literature evolving around the detrimental nature of acellular carbohydrates on health. Acellular carbohydrate are those that are refined, like table sugar and white flour. Despite what carb-haters say, a carb is not just a carb. Refining carbohydrates—removing them from their cellular structures—changes how your body interacts with them. And it matters. An orange and a glass of orange juice are not the same thing. The first takes time to digest and leaves behind microbe-accessible carbohydrates (MACs) to feed your gut bacteria. The second is rapidly absorbed with almost no leftovers to fuel your microbes.

CREATE LITTLE ROUTINES IN YOUR DAY

Want to keep your gut happy? Keep your routines consistent and your gut will love it. Ideally, your gut wants you to wake up, go to sleep, and eat meals at the same time every day. Also, it would appreciate it if you work out every day, have consistent periods of eating and not eating, and not be too stressed.

Well, that can be a challenge in the modern world, but creating some routine in your day-to-day schedule will go a long way to having a happy, healthy gut. Consider waking up at the same time every day and drinking a big glass of water before you do anything else. Or always having a cup of chamomile tea at 9 p.m. and putting away your phone. These micro-routines can really do a lot.

It's worth noting that erratic eating habits and schedules like shift work are associated with functional dyspepsia and other issues. So if this is you, be sure to read Chapter 5 for more information on how to deal with these concerns.

ENSURE MOVEMENT AND MENTAL WELL-BEING

Exercise is critical for gut health. I'm not saying you have to become a marathoner, but if your body is able to move, get moving. Exercise supports your gut in multiple ways. The more you move, the better your gut moves. It's that simple. Gravity can take your gut only so far, and if you're sedentary, it is more challenging for your gut to move well. Exercise is also anti-inflammatory and exceptionally good for reducing stress and increasing mental well-being, which support the gut-brain aspect of whatever you have going on in your gut. There is a deep connection between mental and digestive well-being, so if you find yourself dealing with severe stress, depression, or anxiety, addressing it can help support your gut function too.

GET SOME SLEEP

Many of us spend a lot of money on wellness to heal and de-stress, but our sleep quality is poor. Taking a truly holistic approach to wellness means talking about root causes. If we aren't sleeping, it's like trying to patch up a boat with chewing gum as we sink into the ocean. Sleep is a time of repair and fasting, so it's critical for proper immune function and an important part of the circadian rhythm of our microbiome. In addition, being well rested improves our energy levels and our motivation for healthy habits.

Make it a priority to get seven to nine hours of sleep a night, unless you have a wee one literally waking you up. I've been there. It's a phase you just have to power through, but for the rest of us, go to bed and get your required sleep. You might be amazed at how much better you feel once you simply start sleeping.

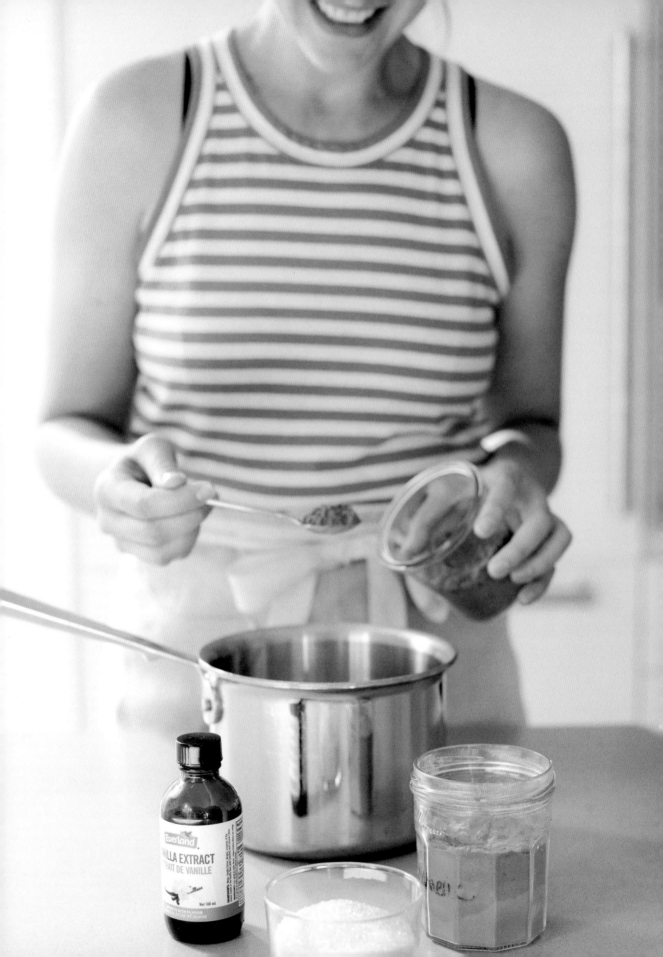

4

Gut-Health Connection to Your Brain and Immune System

In Chapter 1, you got in touch with the wild, winding, and complicated genius that is your digestive tract. Now, we're going to dive deeper into how your gut aligns with your immune system and nervous system—and what the heck those bacteria are doing in there. It's all connected. Fixing your gut isn't about just going grain-free or taking an antacid, it's about taking a step back and realizing just how much is influencing how you feel at this very moment.

When we learn about the body in school, it's typically in *systems* such as the immune system, the digestive system, and the cardiovascular system. Because we tend to think about these systems in compartmentalized ways, it can be easy to see them all as distinct and independent of one another. But actually, there isn't a cell in your body that exists without constant interaction with its environment. What happens in one part of your body, or system of your body, can impact what happens in another. And sometimes, that interaction is *a lot closer* than you might expect. So we are going to start doing some intermingling here. First, we'll describe the nervous system in the gut, then we'll pay a visit to your microbes, followed by a peek at the immune system in the gut. For the grand finale, we'll connect all the dots between the gut-brain-immune connection.

The Gut-Brain Connection

Let's start by talking about why the gut-brain connection is so important. We know that the enteric nervous system is responsible for contracting the gut muscle in rhythmic waves we call peristalsis. It's pretty important that food moves through your gut properly. If you've ever been constipated, you know just *how* important. But that's just the beginning. Your enteric nervous system does a lot of communicating with your brain about what's happening inside your gut. In fact, it is thought that 90 percent of that communication comes from the gut to the brain and not the other way around.

For example, when you eat a big meal, particularly one high in fibre with some protein and fat, the receptors in your stomach sense both the physical stretching of the stomach and its chemical contents. Those receptors attach to your nervous system and help moderate how quickly your stomach empties to optimize digestion. Receptors also send messages to your brain that tell you that you are getting full and to slow down your eating. This is why we can eat a big bag of potato chips and not feel full. Potato chips take up almost no space in the stomach and they bypass that normal stretch-receptor response.

Your brain, of course, also can tell your gut what to do. If you've ever needed to go to the bathroom during a road trip, you can thank your brain for helping you hold it until the next rest stop. That's helpful, but sometimes the brain-gut connection can feel less helpful. For example, when you're stressed, your irritable bowel syndrome (IBS) or ulcerative colitis can get way worse.

This feedback loop of organs sensing the environment, talking to the brain, and the brain telling them what to do is pretty normal. It's how most of the body works. Your enteric nervous system, however, is a bit of an overachiever. In fact, there are more nerve cells (neurons) in your gut than there are in your spinal cord. The nervous system in the gut can even operate semi-independently of the brain and can sense what's happening in one part of the gut and tell another part of the gut—all without the brain getting involved. In fact, if you cut the connection between the gut and the brain, the gut will continue moving, secreting, and doing its thing all by itself. So you see, your second brain really does have a mind (well, at least an independent nervous system) of its own.

The Feel-Good Chemical

Given the complexity of the nervous system and the way that messages travel along nerve cells, it's interesting that those nerve cells aren't technically connected. Instead, messages travel from one nerve cell to the next thanks to neurotransmitters. You can think of neurotransmitters as chemical messengers that either boost, supress, or alter the signal from one nerve cell to the next. It's like a giant game of telephone, but your nervous system is way better at it than a group of seven-year-olds.

Probably the most famous neurotransmitter of them all is serotonin. We typically call serotonin the "feel-good neurotransmitter" because it is associated with positive mental well-being. For people with depression, a medication called a selective serotonin reuptake inhibitor (SSRI) may be prescribed. The way that medication works is to increase the amount of serotonin between nerve cells.

You might be surprised to learn that serotonin is the primary regulator of gut peristalsis. That's one big gut-brain connection right there. In fact, about 95 percent of the serotonin in your body is produced in

Vagus, not Vegas

Because of how connected our gut is to our immune system and nervous system, what happens in the gut can reverberate throughout the body. I'm always saying that your gut is not Vegas: what happens there doesn't stay there.

The vagus nerve is the largest of the cranial nerves. It travels from the brain through the spinal cord to the rest of the body. It takes quite the meandering path through the body, which is how it got its name. Vagus means *wanderer,* and wander it does, from tensing the jaw to regulating heart rate and even digestion.

The vagus nerve is the major nerve servicing the gut, and it is also the main cranial nerve of the parasympathetic nervous system, which we call the "rest and digest" nervous system. That moniker is not an accident: activating the parasympathetic nervous system helps you chill out. In fact, many of our most popular de-stressing practices activate the vagus nerve, from meditation to yoga to deep breathing. It's also essential for optimizing your digestion. If you're super stressed (in your fight-or-flight response) when you quickly eat your lunch, it's probably not going to digest well, and you'll feel very gassy afterward.

If you are interested in the brain-gut connection, get to know the vagus nerve. We have a lot more to learn about the complexities of this communication because we can see the effects of these connections in the research. For example, the majority of our clients with gut-health issues also have challenges with their mental well-being. These observations are confirmed in the clinical research: according to one recent meta-analysis, people with IBS have a threefold increased risk of depression or anxiety compared to those without it. Whether it's the gut or the brain driving the changes remains to be seen; however, in one Australian trial, it was estimated that two-thirds of the time it was gut changes like IBS that preceded changes in mental health.

your gut's nervous system. Most of the gut's serotonin is in enterochromaffin (EC) cells that are nestled into your gut lining.

Here's where the brain-gut connection really starts to come together: changes in serotonin levels can alter digestive function.

Large increases in serotonin can cause diarrhea, nausea, or vomiting. In fact, this is a potential side effect of taking SSRI medications. It is also what happens if you get food poisoning: your EC cells release a lot of serotonin, which causes the diarrhea or vomiting (or both if you're unlucky). What's more, having depression or getting a gut infection like food poisoning can result in you developing IBS down the road, which is also associated with serotonin messing with your gut motility. It is thought that people with IBS-D (a type of IBS that causes increased diarrhea) may have increased serotonin production and decreased serotonin reuptake transporters (SERTs), meaning that extra serotonin is causing those urgent, loose bowel movements.

In addition to its function in the gut and nervous system, serotonin may act as both a pro-inflammatory and an anti-inflammatory molecule in the gut. Dr. Michael Gershon, who popularized the term "second brain," or the brain in our gut, says that serotonin can act as "both the sword and the shield" when it comes to immune function. As serotonin affects the immune system, so too can the immune system alter serotonin levels in the gut. If you've ever wondered why it's so hard to treat gut issues, by now you should be starting to see why.

How Stress Messes with Your Gut

Do you ever eat your lunch way too fast while working to meet a deadline and then realize that your stomach is in knots an hour later? Yes, you're probably not chewing properly, but also, you're stressed. The stress response, coordinated by your sympathetic nervous system, is at direct odds with optimal digestion, coordinated by your parasympathetic nervous system. When you're preparing for fight or flight, rest and digest goes in the dumpster. We'll cover stress and the gut a bit more in Chapter 5.

Ideally, we would not eat at our desk, on our commute, or while we work—but life happens. So what do you do?

First, give your gut a fighting chance and take a minute to calm down. I encourage my clients to close their eyes and do one minute of "square breathing" before they take their first bite. If you need extra calming, make your exhales longer than your inhales. It's super easy to do. Follow these steps:

1. Inhale for a count of four.
2. Hold the inhale for a count of four.
3. Exhale for a count of four.
4. Hold the exhale for a count of four.

Next, do not force yourself to quickly eat your entire lunch at once if you're really stressed. Instead, give your stomach a smaller task. For example, if you're hungry, perhaps take five minutes, breathe, and then eat just a quarter of your lunch. Then in half an hour, do the same thing. Breathe then eat. It should help keep bloating to a minimum.

Sniffles, Joint Aches, and Tummy Trouble

Your gut is pretty amazing and complex. So let's embrace that complexity and talk about the immune system in the gut. Approximately 70 percent of all your body's immune function is centred in and around your digestive tract. This means that your gut is perhaps the single most important part of your body when it comes to your immune system. How well your body heals, and how well it fights off infection, is impacted by what is happening in your gut.

Inflammation, Sleep, and the Microbiome

Spending over a decade in private practice means being exposed to many questions and unique situations that really drive home how everything is connected. For example, I had a client with severe small intestinal bacterial overgrowth (SIBO; discussed in more detail in Chapter 5) who also had insomnia. She was convinced the inflammation was contributing to her insomnia, and when I looked into it, I found that there is some evidence to support the connection between inflammation and insomnia.

In SIBO, there is significant gut barrier dysfunction that will incite chronic inflammatory responses and allow for the leaking of bacterial fragments known as endotoxins into the circulation—driving inflammation further. In the research, there is an association between sleep disturbances and inflammation. It is often assumed that sleep disturbances drive the inflammatory response, but there also is some evidence that chronic inflammation and perhaps bacterial endotoxins cause sleep disturbances as well.

In fact, some pro-inflammatory messengers called cytokines also have direct sleep regulatory functions. It is well documented that rheumatoid arthritis and inflammatory bowel disease (IBD), two conditions with marked inflammation, are associated with sleep disturbances.

A DELICATE BALANCE

It seems like your gut and your immune system would make pretty unlikely roommates, until you remember that your gut lining is a critical barrier between you and the outside world. If you've never thought of your gut as being outside of your body, consider this: while it is surrounded by your body, in reality, from entrance through exit your gut is actually continuous with the outside world. Any number of weird, toxic, or disease-causing things could hitch a ride on your fork, so it's important that your gut helps keep them out. In addition, your gut houses trillions of bacteria that, while beneficial if they stay in the gut, could cause a massive infection if they made it into your bloodstream. Since there is just a single cell layer standing between you and the outside world, you'd better have a strong backup plan.

Luckily, your amazing body has placed a powerful defence system at its most delicate border. The acidic stomach is a strong chemical barrier to infection; most microbes will die when exposed to the rapid pH shift from the very acidic stomach to the more alkaline small intestine. The gut barrier is an important physical component of your gut-immune system. Specialized cells secrete a thick mucus over the gut epithelium cells to make it harder for gut bacteria to directly interact with gut cells. And cells within the gut wall itself secrete antimicrobial substances to kill bugs off before they make contact. Should microbes actually make it past this barrier and come into contact with the epithelium layer, the gut cells release chemical messengers that send a distress signal to your immune system.

The local immune force in the gut is layered into the gut in three places: in between the gut cells themselves, within that middle *lamina propria* layer we talked about before, and in the gut-associated lymphoid tissues (GALT). GALT is comprised of specialized cells nestled under the gut layers. Some of those cells can sample what's going on inside the gut space with little probes, looking for anything that is amiss. When signals are detected, your immune machinery processes the messages it receives from the immune patrols and decides on the appropriate response. The term *appropriate* is key here; it is the immune system's job to know when to be tolerant and when to take action. If it loses that balance between tolerance and action, that's when chronic inflammation takes over from normal immune response.

THE INNER ECOSYSTEM

It's time to explore how our gut-immune system communicates with our gut microbiota, especially since at first glance, it doesn't quite make sense how an immune system designed to protect us from germs doesn't just kill them all.

Your presumably boring colon is home to trillions of bacteria, along with archaea, viruses (sometimes referred to as the *virome*), and yeasts (mycobiome). In fact, there are more bacteria in your gut than there are stars in the Milky Way Galaxy. It's a digestive after-party that's stacked to the rafters. But these bacteria are not just digestive freeloaders scooping up whatever table scraps they can get their tiny microbe "hands" on. The bacteria that make up our microbiome are super important to the health of our gut and our entire body. We exist in a mutually beneficial relationship, one that begins at birth and continues to evolve throughout our entire lives.

Bacteria are found along the entire digestive tract—they are responsible for your bad breath and they're what you floss out of your teeth at night. You find bacteria in the stomach in tiny amounts, and a few of them live in your small intestine where pH shifts and the more rapid movement of the gut usually prevents them from overgrowing (sometimes). However, the main event is absolutely the bacterial party in your large intestine, or colon.

In the colon, the slow transit time, lower oxygen levels, and higher pH allow for a more stable population of hardy, fermenting microbes that turn your trash into treasure. Remember, you've already absorbed 80 to 95 percent of everything you've eaten. There isn't much left of value to you once it gets to the colon. And yet, these castoffs support a remarkable diversity of species in the human gut, and these industrious little microbes impact your health in more ways than you might expect. Think of those colon bacteria as the ultimate upcyclers. Here is what they can do:

- Produce vitamins such as vitamin K and some B vitamins that we can absorb
- Decrease the pH of the gut slightly so we can better absorb minerals like calcium and iron
- Digest hard-to-digest food components such as fibre or lactose into absorbable components that may provide up to 10 percent of our daily caloric intake
- Activate dietary polyphenols from berries, cocoa, and other plant foods for better absorption and anti-inflammatory activity
- Improve gut-cell health through production of short-chain fatty acids that are used as fuel by the gut cells
- Help to discourage the growth of more harmful species such as *Clostridium difficile* or *Escherichia coli* through both passive and active means
- Communicate with our immune system and modulate immune response
- Interact with the gut nervous system and endocannabinoid system
- Help to preserve the barrier function of the gut lining

I believe that our gut microbiota just might be the single most important new discovery in developing a clear understanding of—and potential therapeutic approaches for—human health. In fact, many consider the microbiota to be another organ, like the heart or the lungs. Sound like a bold claim? It is and it's 100 percent supported by science. What you'll learn over the coming pages will show you just how influential those tiny bacteria are. As a dietitian with an integrative approach to nutrition, the biggest surprise of my career has been just how foundational the health and function of our digestive tract is to our overall health. If our gut health is off, it likely isn't the only issue. Like I said, everything is connected.

SORTING GOOD BACTERIA FROM BAD BACTERIA

Given that you have trillions of bacteria in your gut, and your immune system is designed to kill off bacteria, how is it not firing 24/7? Well, your beneficial gut bacteria generally stay far away from the gut barrier, so they don't cause a stir. They also have ways of communicating with your immune system to ensure tolerance. That's right, your gut bacteria can actually alter your immune response to ensure their survival. And that's not the only way they support your immune system.

Your gut microbiome, by physically taking up space and fermenting your leftovers, compete with potentially harmful bacteria to ensure that they don't have the space or nutrients they need to survive. The short-chain fatty acids that come from fermentation actually lower the pH of the gut, making it less hospitable to other microbes. And if that is still not enough, they send out little interspecies antibiotics like bacteriocins and hydrogen peroxide that kill off nasty bugs. That is what happens when your gut microbiome is healthy, diverse, and working well. We are going to talk a lot in this book about what happens when it isn't, because an imbalance in the microbiome, known as *dysbiosis,* is a major factor in many digestive issues. More on that later.

Short-chain fatty acids (SCFAs) are exactly as they sound. Tiny, little fats. Created by bacteria via fermentation, SCFAs have a few important functions in the gut. The first is that they are absorbed by the gut cells and used as fuel to feed your gut bacteria. It always amazes me that the connection between a healthy gut and gut bacteria is so deep that your gut bacteria literally feed your gut. *Pre*biotic (fermentable) foods feed your *pro*biotic bacteria and create *post*biotic party favours like butyrate.

But that isn't the only reason why SCFAs are important. SCFAs, specifically one called butyrate, appear to have beneficial effects on human health. According to research, butyrate:

- Supports gut barrier function and a healthy mucus layer, which reduces bacterial translocation and immune activation
- Lowers the pH of the gut, making it less homey to pro-inflammatory critters such as those from the species *Escherichia coli*
- Plays a role in regulating cell growth and development, and may protect against colon cancer
- Helps to calm chronic inflammatory responses, interacting directly with the immune system and pro-inflammatory compounds

All this, despite the fact that butyrate is actually the least abundant short-chain fatty acid in the gut, making up perhaps only 15 percent of the total SCFAs your gut bacteria produce. Total overachiever.

Should You Try a Probiotic?

Depending on what you read, either probiotics are the answer to pretty much every single health concern under the sun or they're well marketed, overpriced, and ineffective. Increasingly, some physicians are discouraging the use of probiotics in their patients. In 2020, the American Gastroenterological Association recommended that people with Crohn's disease, ulcerative colitis, and even IBS should consider *stopping* their probiotics altogether.

However, I disagree. I have been recommending probiotics to my clients and reading the research on them for over a decade. Perhaps probiotics are neither a snake oil nor a miracle cure. Couldn't the correct answer be somewhere in the middle? I think so. Probiotics are an almost 70 billion dollar industry, and many of them have zero research behind them, making them a waste of money. However, there are some manufacturers creating products that have human clinical trials to prove their efficacy for a handful of concerns; those are the ones with real potential to help improve your gut.

Probiotics are pricey, but be wary of ones that seem too inexpensive. If they don't fit the budget, don't take them. I would rather you work on eating more fibre-rich plant foods like chickpeas than bust your budget on probiotics.

If your budget allows for probiotics, then consider the following:

1. **Are you already doing everything you can to heal your gut and foster a healthy microbiota, such as getting adequate sleep, managing stress, and eating lots of plants? If the answer is no, start there.**

2. **Do you have severely compromised immunity, like in HIV, or take immunosuppressive drugs, such as post-transplant medications? If so, do not consider probiotics until you talk to your doctor.**

3. **Is there a probiotic with specific research for your condition? Go to www.probioticchart.ca (Canadian version) or www.usprobioticguide.com (US version) to find out. If yes, try it for twelve weeks to know for sure. If no, how comfortable are you rolling the dice to see if one helps? Does your dietitian or doctor have a history of success using probiotics in a case like yours? If you're comfortable, give an evidence-based probiotic twelve weeks to prove its worth.**
   - **Are your symptoms improved after twelve weeks? If so, keep going or try stepping down your probiotic to see if you can maintain benefit.**
   - **If you have seen no improvement after twelve weeks, stop taking the probiotic. Maybe it was a great probiotic for someone else, but it's just not right for you. Remember that our microbiomes are all unique—you can't expect a probiotic to be a perfect match for everyone.**

Wondering if there is enough evidence for using probiotics in IBS, constipation, or ulcerative colitis? You'll find more information in the specific sections of this book for each condition.

What About Prebiotics?

Prebiotics are substances that feed the growth of beneficial bacteria in the gut. The best-researched prebiotic is a FODMAP called *inulin*, which is naturally found in chicory and sunchokes. By increasing the growth of bacteria like *Bifidobacterium,* which favour short-chain fatty acid production rather than gas production, you may improve gut balance. In fact, there are a few trials that suggest that taking prebiotics may improve gas tolerance. There also are trials that suggest that prebiotic fermentable fibres such as inulin and fructooligosaccharides (FOS) may help decrease the production of hydrogen sulfide gas in the gut.

I typically recommend you go the whole-food route; the reason for this is that whole plant foods contain a spectrum of bacteria to boost carbs like resistant starch in addition to classic prebiotics. In fact, data from the American Gut Project suggest that people who consume more than thirty different plant foods a week have more robust and diverse gut microbiomes than people who consume fewer than ten.

It is diversity of plant foods that matter more to the microbiome than whether you are vegan or paleo or what have you. Just eat more plants, right? But, if you're interested in prebiotic powders, *start slowly*. Your gut bacteria are going to ferment these prebiotics, and you might get gassier at first. Take a low dose, like 1 tsp (5 mL), and take it consistently until it no longer causes any noticeable symptoms. Only then should you increase the dosage. Also, I do not recommend that you take a prebiotic supplement if you have IBS or any other condition with hypersensitivity and digestive pain like ulcerative colitis. Prebiotics may cause even more distress.

Where Do Fermented Foods Fit In?

Fermentation is a way of preserving fresh foods because their acidity, combined with the growth of beneficial microbes, discourages the growth of bugs that can make you sick. Many traditional food cultures consume fermented foods in one form or another, whether it's kefir or kimchi or kombucha. Despite the fact that fermented foods have been around for hundreds of years, our love of gut health has made fermented foods the darlings of whole-food nutrition, so it's important that we understand what they are and what they aren't. Fermentation transforms foods in a few different ways:

- Since they are made from healthy foods like cabbage or tea, fermented foods can improve the bioavailability of some of their nutrients, such as flavonoids.
- Fermentation can increase some vitamins and antioxidants in foods, such as vitamin K and gamma aminobutyric acid (GABA).
- Fermentation breaks down food nutrients into new goodies, such as short-chain fatty acids from fibre or peptides from proteins.
- Fermentation increases the number of potentially beneficial microbes—exposing your microbiota to other friendly microbes is always a good thing.

Note that I said *potentially beneficial*. Most fermented foods don't have detailed information on which microbes they contain, so we can't be sure what—and how much—is in them. In addition, what's in them can vary from batch to batch and brand to brand, so we can't guarantee that kefir x is as beneficial as kefir y.

In the controversy surrounding probiotics, many practitioners in one breath are discouraging their use due to lack of evidence and then are suggesting fermented foods in the next breath. This doesn't make a lot of sense, because fermented foods have very limited human research to confirm they do anything probiotic-wise. Kombucha? Zero clinical trials at time of writing. In lab studies, fermented foods may have anti-inflammatory, antimicrobial, and even anticancer properties, which is super exciting. But in real live humans? There are only a handful of trials, mostly for kefir and kimchi.

Fermented foods are delicious and I totally think they belong in a gut-friendly diet. One thing to watch: some of them, like sauerkraut, miso, and kimchi, can be really high in salt, so think of them as a condiment, not as a salad.

Connecting the Gut-Brain-Immune Dots

Now that we have a good handle on how the nervous system and immune system operate in the gut, we can begin to knit together all of these little nuggets of knowledge to see how your gut is affected when life throws a wrench into the works.

Let's say that you're on deadline for a big project at work. That stress has been sending a bunch of erratic messages to your gut and you've been a bit more bloated and gassy than normal. Because you're stressed and not feeling so great, you're reaching for a lot of convenient comfort foods like chips, coffee shop muffins, and frozen lasagna that tend to be low in fibre and high in sugar and fat. All of a sudden, you've gone from gassy and bloated to full-on constipated. That slow motility, coupled with the effects of stress on your nervous system, has increased the pain and discomfort you feel, so you're really tired and maybe not so into working out.

Over time, the lack of fibre and increase in sugar are starving out your beneficial gut bacteria, and perhaps your gut barrier falters just a little bit, fanning the flames of inflammation. Now those bacteria living in your gut that love an inflamed environment have the opportunity to grow and perhaps cause even more inflammation and digestive distress. Your immune system senses these troublemakers and starts becoming a little less tolerant.

You may notice your mood is taking a nosedive, so you skip your usual workouts altogether and you enjoy a bit more end-of-day wine to take the edge off. You're tired, but all that stress also has you wired, so you find yourself endlessly scrolling until late at night and not getting enough sleep. It's starting to feel like a phase has become a new normal. And it doesn't feel good.

Sound familiar? This has probably been you at one time or another. It's definitely been me on multiple occasions in my past. And if this is a period of two or three weeks a couple of times a year and you return to your usual healthy self once it's over, it is probably no big deal. Your body is designed to heal, repair, and restore balance, so as soon as you start working out and eating high-fibre plants, that constipation will ease. Drink less, and the gut barrier leakiness will knit itself back together. Once it does, your energy will return and your sleep may improve. That will help restore your motivation for healthy habits, which help you process that stress, give your body what it needs to repair your gut barrier, and allow your immune system to calm down.

However, should these symptoms not pass, this book is meant to help. What happens when balance is lost for a long time? I'm here to tell you that when that balance is lost, it can be restored. Someone with Crohn's disease may never have the gut health of someone without it, but their gut can feel a lot closer to healthy and normal than you might expect. Reflux can become an occasional annoyance rather than a daily hardship. We are all on unique paths, but we can find *our* better.

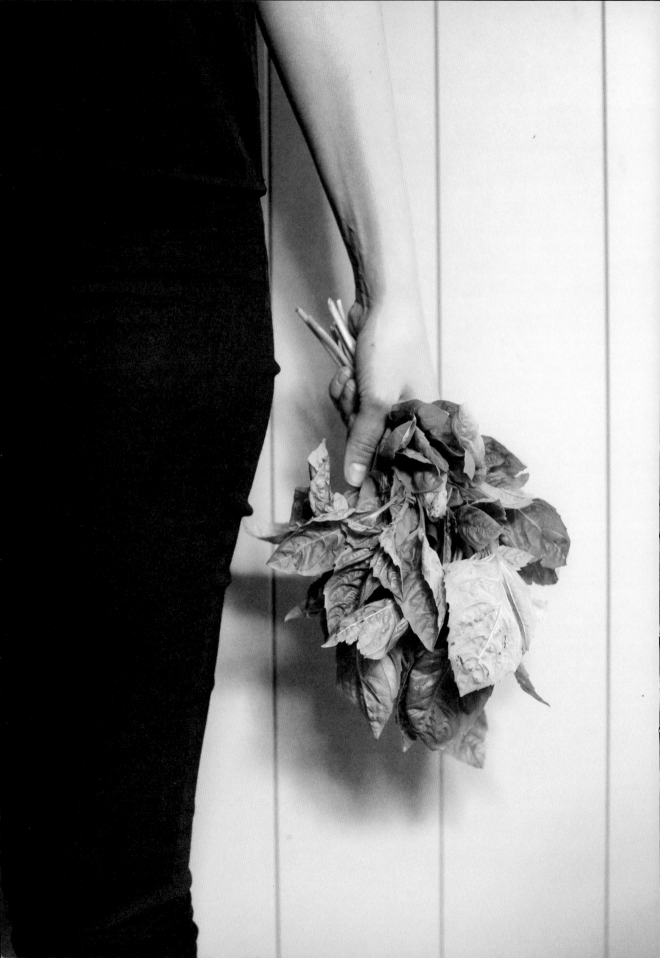

5

When Your Gut Has a Mind of Its Own

I remember what it was like to have a chill gut, but that's not my life now. I know that when something goes wrong with your gut, it can feel like your body is betraying you a little bit. Or a lot, if we're honest. It can create doubt, fear, and confusion on top of feeling sick.

Why is this happening? I don't claim to know all of the answers, but I don't doubt for a second that what is going on with our guts is a symptom of the ills of modern society. We're overworked and over-screened, overfed, undernourished, and not moving our bodies enough. Our bodies are trying to adapt to a new reality that they were simply not designed for.

It's important to remember that there is usually more than one root cause when it comes to gut issues. Healing your gut requires taking a holistic view of your lifestyle and doing everything you can to foster a healing environment. In this chapter, we're going to do just that for a few conditions: gastroesophageal reflux disease (GERD), irritable bowel syndrome (IBS), and small intestinal bacterial overgrowth (SIBO). To understand these conditions more deeply, we'll be revisiting two core issues with digestive health: altered motility and dysbiosis. And then in Chapter 6, we'll dive deep into the low-FODMAP diet, along with lifestyle approaches to get you back on a healthier path.

When Reflux Goes Chronic: GERD and Functional Dyspepsia

When your dinner hits your stomach, it's not really supposed to come back up. But for some of us, it happens a lot. It's called gastroesophageal reflux disease. GERD is related to reflux, which we talked about in Chapter 2. It's reflux, but all the time—continuous burning and burp-back. GERD is very common and is a frequent reason for a visit to the doctor. If it sounds like it's not a big deal, consider this: people with GERD often report that it impacts their quality of life as much as someone with IBS.

We won't dive as deep into the physiology here since we've covered it, except to remind you that you have a little trap door known as the lower esophageal sphincter (LES) that isn't snapping shut as tightly as it should. There are a lot of reasons why that might happen, including physical pressure due to weight, weaker muscular contraction as you get older, and even lower levels of stomach acid.

This is also the perfect time to tell you about functional dyspepsia (FD) because GERD and FD have overlapping symptoms. Let's start by looking at why your LES is misbehaving and what exactly is going on.

Beyond something understandable—like you just ate a three-course meal and then tried to load the dishwasher—there are many reasons why food might come back up.

- **Physical Pressure on the Lower Esophageal Sphincter.** Fat stores around the middle—or a baby—can apply upward pressure on the stomach, making it harder for the LES to keep things down. You can also have a hiatal hernia, where the top part of your stomach squeezes above the diaphragm muscles, which is going to make you super reflux-y.
- **Lower Levels of Stomach Acid.** This is something that is more widely accepted in integrative medicine and is a bit controversial in conventional medicine. The idea here is that the LES is acid-sensing, so that when the stomach contents are acidic, it snaps shut tighter. So if acid levels are lower—from chronic dieting and undernutrition or even from proton pump inhibitor (PPI) medications for GERD—it might make the LES floppier. It can also alter the microbiome in the stomach or small intestine, which can have a deleterious impact on symptoms.
- **Low Muscle Tone in the LES.** As we get older, muscle tone can wane, making our LES as floppy as our triceps.
- **Low-Grade Inflammation.** Inflammation, particularly in the small intestine, is discussed in Chapter 4.
- **Bacterial Dysbiosis.** An imbalance of the microbiota can influence everything from inflammatory status to motility, via the interaction of the microbiota with the nervous system and immune system as well as barrier function.
- **Slow Motility and Slow Stomach Emptying.** If your stomach empties slowly, there will be more pressure on the LES as your stomach fills up. Gastroparesis is the most pronounced form of slow stomach emptying but, again, PPI medications can slow motility as can a host of other factors, such as stress.
- **Use of Some Medications.** Many pharmaceuticals, such as nonsteroidal anti-inflammatory drugs (NSAIDs) or angiotensin-converting enzyme (ACE) inhibitors, can impact the gastrointestinal environment, altering motility or causing irritation and inflammation.
- **Stress and Anxiety.** Anxiety is strongly associated with dyspepsia symptoms.

Wait, isn't reflux just too much acid? We have to work with our doctors to make sure that we dig into all potential causes. GERD is treated like such a cut-and-dried issue, yet I've had clients who were on PPIs for a decade and still suffering from their GERD symptoms.

Women are more likely to suffer from GERD than men—and it is certainly more common in all of us as we age. As mentioned in Chapter 2, it's normal to have occasional heartburn. But if you have chronic reflux or dyspepsia, you need to talk to your doctor so you can get the help you need. In case that doesn't motivate you, know that dyspepsia and reflux can be signs of a more serious concern, such as *Helicobacter pylori* infection, gastroparesis, or even some cancers. That goes double if you have any bleeding, unintentional weight loss, difficulty swallowing, or vomiting.

Is It GERD or FD?

GERD is a chronic refluxing of acidic contents back into the esophagus or even the throat, which causes the telltale heartburn. However, FD is a bit different; it's defined by Rome IV criteria (a group of disorders classified by gastrointestinal symptoms), which look at four core symptoms:

1. **Epigastric (stomach) pain** *or*
2. **Epigastric burning** *and*
3. **Early satiety (you get full from a small volume of food)** *or*
4. **Postprandial fullness (feeling really full after a normal meal)**

These symptoms are intense, occurring at least three days a week in the last three months. As you can see, doctors have a monumental task when it comes to diagnosing digestive disorders. Reading about this does not replace a full diagnostic work-up with your physician.

Setting It Right Naturally

If you have GERD or FD, it's time to start paying attention to what triggers your symptoms and what makes you feel better. This is going to look a bit different for everyone. Keeping a food and symptoms journal in a notebook or on your phone will help you see any patterns of what triggers your symptoms. And if journalling doesn't provide any clarity for you, it will probably help any dietitian you choose to work with understand more about your condition.

It's worth noting that obesity, particularly having abdominal fat, is a risk factor for GERD, and weight loss is associated with decreased symptoms. However, the research isn't clear on how much of that association is related to diet and activity or to the abdominal fat stores causing pressure. So my advice is not to embark on a torturously restrictive fad diet. Instead focus on bringing more gut-friendly meals into your life and consider specific trigger foods. The more you focus on adding positive behaviours, the better you will feel.

Understanding Triggers

Most people feel that certain foods trigger their symptoms. Unlike the dietary patterns that lead to digestive disorders, a dietary trigger is a food that produces immediate results, like what happens when you drink peppermint tea or chew peppermint gum. Peppermint is a carminative that relaxes muscle tone and can make you more reflux-y. But peppermint may be beneficial if you have FD. You can see how getting a proper diagnosis really helps you do the nutrition work. Common triggers include:

- Chocolate
- Spicy foods
- Acidic foods (citrus, tomatoes, pop, coffee)
- Alliums (garlic, onions, leeks)
- High-fat meals
- Alcohol

A few of these are worth talking about in more detail. Let's start with alcohol. Alcohol decreases LES pressure, slows gastric emptying, and increases acid release. Sounds like a perfect reflux situation. Fat is another nutrient with a complicated effect on the stomach. Eating healthy fat is important for overall health, but eating a lot of fat slows stomach emptying. Fats trigger the release of a messenger hormone called cholecystokinin (CCK). CCK is great in that it helps you to feel full and satisfied, but it also slows motility down so that you have ample time to properly digest those fats. More stomach holding time means more exposure to acid; fat may also decrease pressure in the LES. We still need a bit more research here to confirm, though—especially because in one trial, a low-carbohydrate diet improved reflux in those with obesity.

Pattern Versus Plate

While I'm always saying how pattern matters more than plate for overall health, reflux is a bit different because some nutrients can cause an immediate reaction. It's important to know your triggers and adjust your diet accordingly.

However, I still think it's worth talking about how dietary patterns affect reflux and dyspepsia. There is surprisingly little evidence with respect to dietary patterns in reflux but there are a couple of trials to guide us. In 2017, researchers compared a 90 percent plant-based, Mediterranean-style diet to proton pump medications and found that diet might be a reasonable alternative to medication. In one Italian trial, lower adherence to a Mediterranean dietary pattern was associated with increased functional dyspepsia in young people. This means the standard Western dietary pattern of high fat, high sugar, and low fibre isn't doing you any favours. Work toward a more anti-inflammatory, high-fibre diet to support your overall digestive health and your gut will likely benefit.

Now, we're going to get into some interesting territory with nutrition and functional dyspepsia. A bit of evidence suggests that a dietary pattern that includes wheat might be associated with FD. Remember that wheat can impact you in a few ways. We need to look at FODMAPs, the highly refined ways we eat wheat (24/7 white flour), and gluten. Evidence from one 2020 trial suggests that a subset of patients with FD might actually have non-celiac gluten intolerance. It's not a ton to go on, but it's something. We'll talk more about the controversy of non-celiac gluten intolerance versus FODMAP intolerance in Chapter 6.

Not Too Fast, Not Too Slow

Stomach emptying is probably top of the list of things you never thought you cared about, but when it comes to GERD, it's important. Not overfilling the stomach and encouraging quicker stomach emptying should help with reducing your symptoms. It's important to eat slowly and chew foods well to optimize digestion and minimize holding time. The general guidance on meals is that smaller, lower-fat meals may help make you less reflux-y, so it is well worth trying. Eating this way could reduce stomach holding time, although it also means that you may need to eat more frequently.

You can also encourage appropriate stomach emptying with prokinetics. Ginger is a classic prokinetic food that has been shown to reduce inflammation, improve motility, and decrease nausea, but it hasn't been well researched specifically in GERD or FD. Luckily it's food, so there is no harm in trying it! You could chew on a couple of pieces of candied ginger after a meal or sip strong ginger tea and see how it goes.

There is also an herbal tincture called Iberogast that has a small evidence base to support its use in a few different conditions, including FD and IBS—we'll talk about it more in Chapter 6. Finally, this one might surprise you, but there are two trials that suggest melatonin can improve motility. Serotonin gets all the gut-brain spotlight but melatonin is also made in the enterochromaffin cells in the gut. Yes, we are talking about the same melatonin you take to fight jet lag. Melatonin is thought to have an impact on motility, but in the research, it would appear that small amounts increase it and large amounts slow it down. We don't have a ton of research here, but I will give it a go when my first line of tools isn't enough for a client. It's especially handy if you have trouble sleeping because of your gut issues. Talk to your doctor or pharmacist to see if it's right for you.

Living a Low-Reflux Life

What we eat is important, but remember that how we eat and how we live matter too. Stress is a primary factor for GERD and FD.

Stress and anxiety are strongly associated with symptoms of functional dyspepsia. Remember that stress can increase sensitivity in the nervous system, making pain worse. It can also increase acid release in the stomach, which is a red flag for anyone refluxing on the regular. Stress reduction and management have to be a big part of getting better. We'll talk about some very practical, doable strategies for stress management in Chapter 6.

Movement helps; exercise is thought to strengthen the musculature around the diaphragm. Although exercise definitely helps with stress, you don't want to do a vigorous workout after a meal. That can cause reflux. It's better to take a gentle walk to facilitate movement or do more vigorous workouts at another time of the day. As much as you can, you want to avoid lying down after a meal. Avoid things like bending over to the fill the dishwasher. Finish eating at least two hours before bedtime; you may find that elevating the head of your bed helps too.

IBS: The Black Hole of Gut-Brain Communication

You could say that I have some skin in the digestive health game since I have IBS. The better I get at caring for the condition, the more it helps me feel better too. IBS is annoying at best and absolutely awful at worst. I've been lucky in that I've lived in that awful stage for only about a tenth of my tenure with the condition, mostly at the very beginning.

I also feel pretty lucky because there is so much research and physician recognition of the condition now. IBS is one of those things that twenty-five years ago probably would have been dismissed as being "all in your head" because there is no specific medical test to confirm the condition. Even a colonoscopy (an exam using a camera in the colon) does not reveal much—hearing "the tests are all clear" is not a lot of comfort if your gut is in agony.

IBS is known as a functional gastrointestinal disorder, which is equal parts vague and fairly descriptive. Unlike a disease that has a defined trigger (gluten) and changes to your physiology (autoimmune reaction in the gut) like celiac disease, IBS is a change to the *function* of the gut. Your gut will look fine. Your basic blood work will look fine. But your symptoms will be anything but fine. In fact, in one study, *people with IBS were willing to accept a 10 percent chance of death if a medication could promise a 99 percent chance of eliminating symptoms.* That's just how seriously IBS can affect people.

The studies on how common IBS is vary greatly; on average, 10 percent of the population has IBS and more women than men are affected. Trials using the new Rome IV diagnostic criteria so far have a lower prevalence rate; however, IBS is still way more common at this point than celiac disease or inflammatory bowel disease (IBD), so I suspect that a lot of folks reading this book have IBS just like me.

New thinking on IBS explains it as a group of symptoms with a spectrum of underlying causes. So for you, it might be your gut bacteria messing things up. For me, it's definitely stress. And this realization is changing how we think of IBS: the Rome Foundation (it created the Rome IV diagnostic criteria) declared that it is more accurate to call IBS a "disorder of gut-brain communication." Our gut-brain discussion in Chapter 4 laid the groundwork for understanding why your gut is so irritable.

Early on in the research, two things became fairly clear: there's altered motility (movement) in the gut and a hypersensitivity to both normal sensations and pain—all thanks to your nervous system. And here is where everything starts to get complex: there is a big overlap between depression, anxiety, and IBS. So your nervous system isn't just messing with your gut, it trickles up to your brain too. Irritable bowel syndrome can alter mood—no surprise when your gut hurts all the time—but mood can also alter your experience of symptoms. Stress makes pain worse. In addition, stress can also make leaky gut worse, so it's important to recognize that stress is causing real, physical changes in your body. So, no, it's not all in your head. Your nervous system is causing very real symptoms.

How IBS Is Diagnosed

The big thing with IBS is that its symptoms can look a lot like other diseases, so your doctor is always going to first check to make sure you don't have something like celiac disease or ulcerative colitis. If you get the all-clear on those diseases, there are the Rome IV diagnostic criteria for IBS that involve recurrent abdominal pain associated with two or more of the following:

1. **Defecation (pooping)**
2. **A change in stool frequency**
3. **A change in stool form**

The symptoms must have been present at least once a week for the last three months, with the onset of symptoms being six months ago. In reality, my clients usually experience these issues every single day. You might also be experiencing other symptoms, such as dyspepsia, nausea, or even chronic pain. This is why a thorough checkup is so critical. Definitely do not go it alone.

In addition to IBS having a spectrum of causes, it also presents differently. There are three types of IBS:

- **Diarrhea-predominant (IBS-D)**
- **Constipation-predominant (IBS-C)**
- **Diarrhea/constipation mixed (IBS-M)**

There are a few commonly recognized risk factors for IBS, which include early life stressors, previous gut infection or antibiotic use, and food intolerance. But lifestyle factors weigh heavily here, so that is what we're focusing on.

It's also not just your nervous system. You now know how interconnected your gut, your immune system, and your nervous system are, so it's no surprise that one influences the other. For example, inflammation can increase visceral sensitivity in the digestive tract and alter your gut microbes.

This information is a big leap forward—IBS is typically not considered an "inflammatory" issue. However, increased cellular markers of inflammation like mast cells and lymphocytes have been discovered in the colons of people with IBS. So while there isn't overt inflammatory damage like we see in celiac disease or ulcerative colitis, there is low-grade inflammation present, at least for some. And inflammation can cause, or be caused by, dysbiosis—an imbalance of harmful, pro-inflammatory bacteria—that is also present for many with IBS.

Irritable bowel syndrome has mostly been considered a large intestine issue, but that may change. One 2018 trial suggests that gut barrier dysfunction (leaky gut) in the small intestine might be present in a subset of people with IBS-D. This is important news because leaky gut increases inflammatory markers, which would confirm the fact that low-grade inflammation is present in this group and may be driving the nervous system changes.

Is It IBS or Is It BAD?

Another, less-recognized, cause of IBS-like symptoms is bile acid diarrhea (BAD), which is probably the most accurate acronym in all of digestive health. Bile acids are made in the liver and stored in the gallbladder; their purpose is to help you digest fats. Fats don't like the watery environment of the gut, and bile acids have a fat-seeking head and a water-loving tail that emulsifies the fats so the digestive enzymes can do their work.

About 95 percent of bile acids are reabsorbed and recycled in the ileum portion of the small intestine, but a few things can hinder that reabsorption, such as binding by soluble fibre. That's a good thing, because you'll remember that bile is made from cholesterol. So if fibre takes bile salts for a swim down the colon, your liver will have to pull more cholesterol from the blood to make bile. This is why your morning bowl of (soluble fibre-rich) porridge can help lower your cholesterol.

However, if for some reason bile acids aren't being bound or reabsorbed properly, they can draw water to them and cause diarrhea. It is thought that those with BAD might be making too many bile acids and overwhelming the recycling system, but there are medications that can bind up those bile salts and help with this.

We don't talk enough about bile, but it is critical to proper digestion, and it's an issue for those of us walking around without a gallbladder. Be sure to discuss this possibility with your doctor; it is estimated that as many as 30 percent of those with IBS-D may actually have BAD.

Food intolerance is something else we should talk about. Many people with IBS feel that food intolerance makes their symptoms. However, that is not the same as saying that food intolerance *causes* IBS. This is a big leap for most people. We are so quick to blame food for our ills that realizing that our health condition might actually alter how we respond to food is a bit of a shift. Apples and lentils didn't cause your IBS, but once you have IBS, they may trigger symptoms. If you need further proof, early studies suggest the microbiota might hold the key to whether you respond to a low-FODMAP diet. This makes a lot of sense, as you'll see in Chapter 6.

IBS, the Microbiome, and Probiotics

The research suggests that the microbiota in IBS is different from a healthy microbiota, but there's a catch: the degree of difference, and exactly which microbes are different, varies between studies.

- Some studies found fewer *Lactobacillus* and *Bifidobacterium* species (the good guys).
- Others found fewer of the bugs that make the important short-chain fatty acid butyrate. Definitely not what you want.
- There even appears to be more methanogens—the bugs that make methane—in IBS-C but fewer in IBS-D. Methane is anti-inflammatory but it can also slow transit time.

What might be more surprising is that your microbiota may also be an important contributing factor in anxiety—there's that gut-brain connection again. The gut microbiota can secrete a whole bunch of chemical messengers that influence your nervous system function, such as:

- Gamma aminobutyric acid (GABA), the "chill out" neurotransmitter
- Short-chain fatty acids like butyrate
- Precursors of serotonin—the "feel good" neurotransmitter
- Oh, and they can also stimulate serotonin production in your gut's nervous system

This serotonin piece is a biggie: motility changes are likely linked to serotonin—higher levels of serotonin have been found in patients with IBS-D. It may also dictate the sensitivity of your nervous system: as many as 90 percent of IBS sufferers have visceral hypersensitivity to normal stimuli.

The role of bacteria in IBS makes even more sense because there is a well-documented post-infectious IBS presentation. For example, you go to a wonderful tropical island, pick up some bug, and spend the last four days of your trip on the toilet looking out the window at all of the fun you're missing. Then, once you get home, your gut goes haywire for the next six months. That's probably post-infectious IBS. So if bacteria can cause the problem, perhaps they also can fix it?

There is research to suggest that both antibiotics and probiotics can improve symptoms in IBS; however, probiotics are a hotly contested topic. There are probiotics on the market that have clinical trials to support their use in IBS; you can find them on the Probiotic Guide website (www.probioticchart.ca for Canada or www.usprobioticguide.com for the US). There is also research to show that they don't work, which is why the controversy exists. Remember that studies confirming one type of probiotic works doesn't mean that another probiotic will too, because every probiotic is different. Of course, the opposite should also be true: if one probiotic doesn't work, it doesn't mean all probiotics won't. In the research, there is a body of evidence to suggest that probiotics may help with a range of symptoms and underlying causes, such as:

- Consistency of bowel movements
- Frequency of bowel movements
- Gas and bloating
- Hypersensitivity
- Inflammation

In my opinion, there is enough research on probiotics to make them a part of my toolkit. I've seen probiotics do remarkable things for some clients, but that doesn't mean that every probiotic will work for every person. Make an evidence-based choice with your health professional, give it a twelve-week trial, and see if it works *for you*.

Here Is What to Do If You Have IBS

IBS is a spectrum of root causes and symptoms, so the approach needed to find relief isn't going to look the same for everyone. And it's not an overnight fix. I know how much it might suck to read that, especially if you are in the grips of really awful symptoms right now. So let me follow it up with this: you will not be here forever. You can feel better, even if not exactly like you did before. After over a decade in practice, I know you can figure it out with the right support because *almost every single one* of my clients has. It's all about exploring options and listening to your body's response. I highly recommend you do this with a dietitian, but if that isn't available to you, keeping a food and symptoms (and feelings) journal will be highly beneficial for this process.

Chapter 6 is going to get into the details of diet, supplements, and stress management, but I want to share a few thoughts with you right now.

FIGURE OUT THE DIETARY APPROACH THAT WORKS FOR YOU

The research supports that food—and breakdown products of food—can affect pretty much everything that happens in your gut, including motility and sensitivity, permeability, the microbiome, brain-gut communication, and immune and nervous function. Food matters and it definitely needs to be a part of the solution. But it has to be *your* solution.

The low-FODMAP diet is as close to an evidence-based solution for IBS as we have. Particularly if you have IBS-D, it's worth a try. I won't describe it in detail here as it really needs its own chapter. However, I will say that it doesn't work for 100 percent of people and it's not always my first line of defence, which might surprise you.

To be clear, I use the low-FODMAP diet a lot in practice. However, some clients find it too overwhelming or complicated to work with their lifestyle. Here is where science meets practice: the best, most evidence-based diet is useless if you can't afford it or don't have the skills or the capacity to follow it. So we find another way.

Sometimes, when I meet a client and read their food history, I suspect that just changing their diet might work wonders. And sometimes it really does. So we work together to create an eating plan that is packed with whole plant foods (like the recipes in this book). If clients react specifically to some foods, like beans, we keep those foods at a low-FODMAP serving size so as not to make symptoms worse while we work toward making them better.

If your diet looks a lot more like fries and boxed cereal than steel-cut oats, lentils, and vegetables, I suggest that you start working through the dietary recommendations in Chapter 3 for a month or two and see how you do. The least restrictive path is always the healthiest. You have to find your own unique way forward. The one thing I can guarantee is that eating more (tolerated) plants is an important part of that path.

FOCUS ON STRESS TO HELP YOUR GUT

We are so used to living high-intensity lives that many of us don't think we're stressed out when we really are. That definitely applies to me and many of my clients. You might think that working sixty hours a week and renovating your kitchen at the same time isn't stressful, but you can't fool your nervous system. Stress can influence motility and sensitivity, permeability, immune response, and even the type of bacteria living in your gut. Better get working on processing all that stress and taking some time to chill.

Most of us can't eliminate our responsibilities, so we need to manage the *effects* of stress. We can do this in multiple ways, such as breathwork, meditation, journalling, movement, and time in nature. It is critical that you find twenty to thirty minutes daily to do something to support your nervous system. If you think you don't have time, it might be worthwhile to document how you use your time each day. You probably spent twenty minutes on social media without realizing that you could have been in a bubble bath instead. You could be listening to a free, guided meditation on the bus. I've got affordable and practical ideas on how to bust stress in Chapter 6.

Small Intestinal Bacterial Overgrowth

Now that we've dug into IBS, we have to wade through the swamp of small intestinal bacterial overgrowth (SIBO). It's a swamp because there are a ton of unknowns, from how best to diagnose to how best to treat SIBO. Some practitioners don't recognize its existence, despite its presence in peer-reviewed literature. As mentioned above, there are questions about whether functional dyspepsia is associated with small intestinal dysbiosis; however, there are also questions about how much of IBS is actually SIBO. As I said, it's a big, murky, swampy mess. Forget wading, let's dive in.

When I talk about the trillions of bacteria in your gut, I'm mostly talking about your colon, or large intestine. Your colon moves slowly, there aren't many nutrients there to speak of, and the pH is relatively stable compared to the acid-alkaline rollercoaster that is the journey between your stomach and small intestine. So nice bugs can get really cozy without going overboard. Most of the bacteria in your colon are a type called Gram-negative bacteria, and they thrive in a low- or no-oxygen environment.

Candida Overgrowth

When I worked in a health food store, people were always on a Candida cleanse, meaning they were pretty much eating greens and chicken breasts and not much else. I was skeptical, to say the least.

Candida is a genus of yeasts that are commonly found in the human gut microbiome and are kept in check by a healthy microbiome and a strong gut barrier defence. Yes, that means that healthy people have Candida—just like healthy people have *Clostridioides difficile* in their gut. It's all about whether your gut microbiome is strong enough to keep it from overgrowing. These types of microbes are called opportunistic pathogens, meaning that given the opportunity, they'll overgrow and wreak havoc. They just don't usually get the opportunity.

The opportunity arises when immune defences, the microbiome, or the gut barrier is significantly disturbed. Thrush is a good example of this, as are vaginal yeast infections. These are very clear indicators that you've got a Candida situation. They're also common after a strong round of antibiotics. Wipe out the good, the bad crash the party. Left unchecked in someone with compromised defences, Candida can cause a serious infectious disease known as invasive candidiasis, which occurs when the yeasts leak through a weakened gut barrier and gain access to the circulatory system. Invasive candidiasis can lead to dangerous inflammation of the organs, including the brain. It's not something you're walking around with.

So, yes, Candida overgrowth is real. But if a naturopath suggests that you have intestinal Candida overgrowth, it's a bit different than invasive candidiasis. It's dysbiosis, but with Candida overgrowing instead of bacteria. What to do about it, however, is very poorly researched and there is a lot of debate about how common it truly is. We know it can occur in Crohn's disease, for example. But in someone who is generally healthy? Not so sure. So if you're going to go down this path, take care with overly restrictive diets, which can weaken your immune defences further and make it harder to heal. Restrictive diets can also starve out the very bacteria that are essential for fighting off Candida. Remember, the least restrictive path is always best, and you have to address the underlying issues that allow overgrowth to occur because once you're tired of starving, the overgrowth will return.

Your small intestine is totally different: it's awash in nutrients multiple times a day and it moves a lot faster than the colon. As a result, it has relatively few bacteria along its length, less than 1,000 bacteria per millilitre (about 0.03 fluid ounces). The bacteria living there are different too—mostly Gram-positive and looking for an oxygen party. Of course, the small intestine is pretty long, so the bacterial population closer to the stomach isn't the same as the one closer to the colon.

We still lack a gold standard set of diagnostic criteria in SIBO; however, it's typically when bacterial numbers reach over 100,000–1,000,000 bacteria per millilitre. When we get to these kinds of numbers, we have a real problem because there is plenty of food to feed them in the small intestine, so the bacteria party can really get out of hand. It's like the difference between treating wedding guests and treating an entire university campus population to an open bar.

Overgrowth Happens, But How?

Now here is the million-dollar question: how do bacteria defy basic chemistry and physiology to set up shop where they're not supposed to be? We have a lot more to learn, but what seems clear at this point is that the small intestine isn't moving as quickly as it should. Whoomp. We're back at the motility discussion again. Poor motility can occur for many reasons, from hypothyroidism to diabetes, gut surgery (including gastric bypass), low-fibre or high-fat intake, or an overgrowth of methane-producing microbes that can cause constipation. When motility is slow, bacteria in the small intestine are not swept clear and may be more likely to overgrow. It is thought that this slow motility may allow colon bacteria to grow up the small intestine as opposed to the small intestinal bacteria overgrowing, but again, we need a lot more research to know for sure.

We've seen how proper motility ensures timely digestion and elimination, but it also controls the bacterial population. When it comes to caring for SIBO, one of my priorities is to ensure we support the migrating motor complex (MMC)—think of it like a cleansing cycle your gut runs after you've finished digesting a meal. The strongest cleansing MMC waves occur perhaps every 90 to 120 minutes when you are in the fasted state; how long it takes to "turn on" post-meal is going to differ between individuals. These waves sweep from stomach though the small intestine, ushering food remnants and the bacteria that munch on them into the colon. When the moment is just right, intestinal cells release a hormone called motilin, which triggers the strong phase-three MMC waves in addition to a sensation of hunger. Encouraging the MMC waves means not eating constantly; you need time in between meals for the waves to initiate.

Other potential contributing causes of SIBO include:

- Frequent antibiotic use
- Low stomach acid, including from PPI use
- Digestive surgery, particularly loss of the ileocecal valve
  (between the small and large intestine) due to a resection

- Digestive diseases, such as celiac disease or irritable bowel syndrome
- Regular alcohol consumption
- A high-sugar, refined-starch diet
- Age
- Other disease states, such as diabetes, renal failure, or hypothyroidism

How Do You Know If It Is SIBO?

The symptoms of small intestinal bacterial overgrowth are fairly non-specific and have a lot of overlap with other conditions. SIBO is expected to result in gut barrier dysfunction and inflammation in the gut, leading to:

- Abdominal pain/discomfort
- Bloating and abdominal distention
- Diarrhea (more common)
- Constipation (less common)
- Gas, reflux, and belching
- Fatigue and difficulty with focus
- In severe cases: vitamin deficiencies and weight loss

It's also worth noting that SIBO has been associated with autoimmunity, fibromyalgia, and rosacea, so if one of those is an issue for you, you may want to investigate the bacterial connection with your doctor. The kind of bacteria overgrowing matters in terms of how you experience SIBO. For example, some metabolized bile salts could lead to fat malabsorption and foul-smelling diarrhea. Others may not lead to elimination issues but may cause severe bloating. Yet others may produce toxins like ammonia that cause inflammation and can cause gut barrier dysfunction or mimic other conditions.

Unlike with IBS, there is testing available for SIBO: the breath test and (less commonly) small intestinal culture. Recently, a consensus standard for testing has been proposed, but the diagnostic criteria are still a bit all over the place in practice. Breath testing usually measures both hydrogen and methane exhaled after consuming a test dose of either glucose or lactulose. These tests can produce false negatives but at this point, it's the best we've got—if you can access practitioners who do breath testing. Not all of us can.

I hope it goes without saying that something this serious should not be self-diagnosed or self-managed. Take the information in this book to your practitioner so you can customize an approach that is right for you.

Is It IBS or SIBO?

IBS and SIBO can look pretty similar, so there is a decent amount of research investigating the distinction between the two. These studies are conflicting: some show that SIBO and IBS are one and the same or that one causes the other. For example, SIBO can cause damage to the intestinal cells, reducing the activity of brush border enzymes that metabolize double sugars like lactose and fructose—two FODMAPs that can lead to diarrhea in those with IBS. The degree of SIBO in IBS has been estimated to be anywhere between 4 and 78 percent, with some believing that maybe a third of those with IBS have SIBO. Because IBS has strong diagnostic criteria, it is easier to diagnose; however, it could be wise to do SIBO testing to rule it out as a root cause of the IBS symptoms, especially if the usual approaches—low-FODMAP diet, stress management, probiotics—aren't working.

Severe SIBO can lead to inflammatory damage to the intestinal cell, making it difficult to distinguish from celiac disease—and it is suggested that those with unresponsive celiac disease may want to consider SIBO as a cause.

How to Get SIBO Moving

If you search the internet, you'll see a lot of very restrictive diets that are supposed to "starve out" SIBO. In reality, they are going to starve you and leave you so weak it will be hard to heal. I've seen it plenty of times.

Let me give it to you straight: diet alone is unlikely to improve SIBO, and dietary therapies for SIBO are poorly researched. If poor motility is thought to be a primary cause in overgrowth, we need to start there. For example, if motility is connected to low thyroid function, how is your iodine intake? Most of us tossed our iodized salt in the garbage when we discovered sea salt—but if you're on a plant-based diet, getting your daily iodine is critical to the healthy function of your thyroid. Everything in your body is connected—so be sure to explore all possible causes with your doctor.

In my practice, meal spacing and prokinetics are an important part of a good offensive. Whenever possible, I encourage my clients to go eleven to twelve hours overnight without food to allow for multiple MMC cycles. In addition, I encourage clients to eat filling and balanced meals so they can snack less; ideally waiting four to five hours between meals so that the third-phase MMC wave will activate in between meals. Now, in saying this, I do not want you to ignore your hunger signals. If you're hungry in between meals, have a light snack. I just want you to be mindful of the "always be eating" culture we're immersed in and consider whether it's making things better or worse.

When it comes to prokinetics, ginger, Iberogast, and melatonin are worth considering in consultation with your practitioner. Physicians also have pharmaceutical options available.

How to Feed Yourself without Overfeeding SIBO

In SIBO, it is expected that carbohydrates feed the bacteria that are overgrowing, particularly ones that are less quickly absorbed. Every time you eat, your small intestine is awash in nutrients coming from your stomach, making it difficult to avoid feeding the bacteria there.

Some believe in starving out the bacteria, while others believe that bacteria need to be fed and replicating to make them easier to kill with antimicrobials (talk to your doctor for more information). Some opt for a low-fibre, easily-digestible carbohydrate approach, such as eating white rice rather than beans. Others choose the specific carbohydrate approach. But what is more common amongst health professionals is the low-FODMAP elimination diet, even though there is very little evidence for its use in SIBO.

A low-FODMAP diet could help in a few ways, for example, reducing double sugars like lactose and fructose. If SIBO damages the brush border enzymes, malabsorption could occur that could lead to more fermentation and symptoms. It will decrease the poorly absorbed fermentable carbohydrates, which may help underfeed overgrowing bacteria without being totally low carb. In a couple of trials, a low-FODMAP diet has been shown to create small decreases in hydrogen on the breath test.

However, I would also encourage avoiding added sugars and low-FODMAP refined starches like rice cakes in favour of whole foods like intact grains, vegetables, and small portions of fruit if you can. The recipes marked Heal in this book are all low-FODMAP and most have minimal added sugars. A low-FODMAP diet is not meant to be long term, as it may alter the beneficial bacteria in the colon—and it's not a treatment for SIBO, just a support for antimicrobial protocols. We may find that while low-FODMAP lowers symptoms, it's not actually making the issue better. The idea here is to eat in a way that encourages motility and the growth of beneficial microorganisms so that once the antimicrobials do their work, your gut will be strong enough to prevent it from happening again. It's also strongly recommended to avoid alcohol, which can decrease motility and brush border enzyme activity and cause injury to the gut.

Should You Take a Probiotic?

The evidence is scarce for SIBO, but there are some *theoretical* reasons why probiotics might help:

- May increase transit time/motility
- May stimulate the MMC
- May help heal gut barrier dysfunction (leaky gut)
- May reduce hypersensitivity in the gut
- May fight off potentially harmful microbes

In the research, it is suggested that probiotics may be effective in helping decrease SIBO, but may also make it worse. Think about it: if our issue is bacterial overgrowth, putting more bacteria in there could potentially be a bad idea. Other trials have suggested that probiotics will work well as a complementary therapy to antimicrobial protocols—kill the bad guys while protecting the good.

While probiotics are not a first line of defence, I have recommended that some clients take them before bed. In theory, nighttime probiotics won't be "fed" at mealtimes or interfere with antimicrobials from your doctor, and they'll be exposed to a few cycles of MMC waves to reduce their ability to overgrow. You have to make this decision with your practitioner—and proceed with caution. If they appear to make symptoms worse in a way that doesn't subside over three to four days, discontinue use.

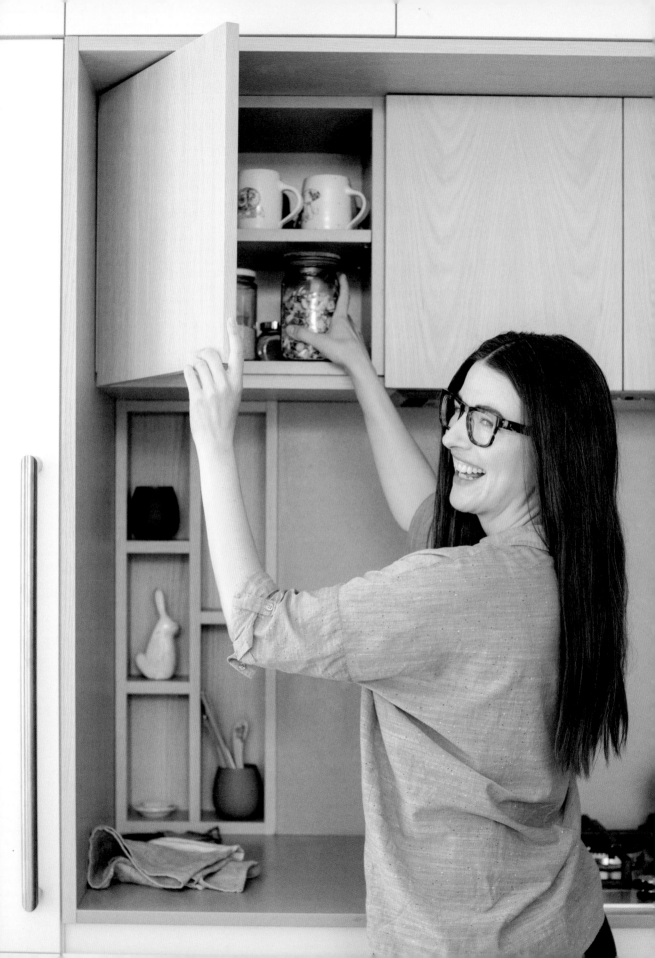

6

Gut-Healing Nutrition

You were built to heal. Everything you need to feel better is already within you; it just needs a little help. Your body has built-in repair functions that are kind of amazing, but they can get worn down by the daily assaults of modern living. So you eat some good food to nourish those healing pathways, with perhaps a little functional support if your gut is spasming or sluggish. You ease up on the factors—alcohol, added sugars, lack of fibre—that make it harder to heal. And you channel your inner yogi with a lot of stress release so that the nervous system can calm down.

Nutrition books will often jump into the "what to eat" conversation without helping you first understand your body or that nutrition isn't 100 percent of healing. I think that's a mistake, for a few reasons:

- Understanding your body is foundational for reducing your fears and anxiety about your condition. It will allow you to see that your symptoms are actually messages from your body and that, no, it is absolutely not betraying you. It's just trying to get your attention.
- Understanding your body on a deeper level is also critical to helping you assess how best to heal. I have sat across from numerous clients who've had surprisingly little information about their condition, besides what they had read on the internet, which left them adrift in a sea of advice, half-heartedly trying everything and feeling frustrated when it didn't work.

- Understanding your body also helps you find the motivation to make change. If you're not sure why FODMAPs matter, what's going to keep you going when you get tired of avoiding garlic in week two?

Understanding your body also strengthens your ability to observe and listen to the messages it is sending you. This far in, you've seen just how complex digestive health is—and only *you* are in your body. I can educate you about your body and share the tools that research suggests might help. But it is up to you to be a good observer, so you can advocate for yourself with your health-care practitioner and decide the path forward. The people on your health-care team are guides. You need to take our advice and view it through the lens of your own experience.

The focus of this chapter is the low-FODMAP diet along with supplements and lifestyle practices to support the gut-brain connection. If you have irritable bowel syndrome (IBS), there is a good chance that your doctor has suggested you try the low-FODMAP diet, and with good reason. In the research, a low-FODMAP approach has been found effective in as high as 80 percent of people who try it. So let's dive into what that actually looks like and how to make it happen.

FODMAPs

FODMAP is the acronym for fermentable oligosaccharides, disaccharides, monosaccharides, and polyols. FODMAPs are essentially carbohydrates that, due to their chemical structure—or your digestive tract function—are not completely digested and absorbed. Because they aren't absorbed, they remain in your gut where they can be fermented by the microbes living there.

For most of us, this is a good thing. You want to feed those microbes so they (and you) thrive. High-FODMAP foods are some of our healthiest, highest-fibre, most anti-inflammatory foods such as apples, garlic, and chickpeas.

- Oligosaccharides (multi-sugar chains): galacto-oligosaccharides and fructans
- Disaccharides (double sugars): lactose
- Monosaccharides (single sugars): fructose
- Polyols (sugar alcohols): sorbitol and xylitol

In IBS, it's thought that FODMAPs interact with your irritable gut in two main ways. The first is in your small intestine, where FODMAPs like fructose will draw more water into the gut, increasing the speed of your motility and loosening up stools. The second is in the large intestine, where trillions of hungry bugs start fermenting the FODMAPs, creating gas.

How these two things cause IBS symptoms is a little less certain than you'd expect. For example, in theory, your colon should be able to reabsorb all that extra water, but it doesn't. Yes, fermentation causes gas, but some studies show that people with IBS aren't making a huge amount of gas, despite eating FODMAPs. It's that their gut is hypersensitive to normal amounts of gas. In the research, a couple of new theories (unproven at this point) are also popping up. A low-FODMAP diet may help to normalize serotonin levels in the gut, improving motility, and may decrease levels of bacterial endotoxins called lipopolysaccharides, decreasing low-grade inflammation.

The Low-FODMAP Elimination

A low-FODMAP elimination means strictly eliminating all high-FODMAP foods for a defined period of time. Low-FODMAP eating doesn't actually eliminate FODMAPs from your diet; instead, it cuts FODMAPs down by about half—which is enough to drop FODMAP levels below your threshold for tolerating them. You want to keep in mind that FODMAP response is *dose-dependent*. Think of your FODMAP tolerance as a cup: if you overfill it, you get symptoms. The low-FODMAP elimination is going to drain that cup, and help you figure out how big your tolerance cup is when we slowly reintroduce FODMAPs to keep you symptom-free.

If you want the clearest response, you have to commit 100 percent: it doesn't really work to have one or two low-FODMAP meals a day, or to have six low-FODMAP days and one normal day a week. So I don't want you to try this unless this feels like a positive and empowering step in restoring your health. A few questions you want to ask yourself before you decide to begin:

1. **DO I HAVE A THOROUGH DIAGNOSIS?** Don't self-diagnose IBS. Reread Chapter 5 if you need to remind yourself why this can be a bad idea. Then, visit your doctor.

2. **IS THIS THE RIGHT TIME IN MY LIFE TO DO THIS?** If you're under a major deadline at work and working long hours or it's two weeks before winter holidays, maybe now is not the time. Make a plan to go low-FODMAP once the event has passed so it doesn't add stress, which can muddy your results.

3. **CAN I WORK WITH A DIETITIAN TO SUPPORT ME?** This will be 100 percent easier with a registered dietitian by your side to ensure that you aren't suffering from deficiencies or to answer all the questions that pop up. I totally understand that a dietitian isn't always available near you or affordable, which is why this book is in your hands.

In the research, low-FODMAP eliminations are typically between two and six weeks, but in practice, I find that four to eight weeks is an effective time frame. The reason for this slight difference is that I want you to be able to work on healing while you're free of high-FODMAP triggers. This looks like stress management and minding sugar and alcohol while eating a lot of healthy plant foods, getting rest, exercise, and (often) probiotics. All of these things need time to do their work to support a healthier microbiome and a calmer nervous system and inflammatory response.

Don't stay low-FODMAP long term, though. I've had plenty of clients who are nervous about reintroducing FODMAPs because they've seen such a massive improvement in their symptoms. But there are too many questions about how the low-FODMAP diet will affect your gut microbiome for me to be

I totally get that low-FODMAP might not feel right for you. Maybe all you need is to eat fewer hyper-processed foods and more plant-rich, anti-inflammatory meals like the ones in this book. Refer to Chapter 3 to see which nutrition strategies might work for you.

If you're not going low-FODMAP, you need to tap into your powers of observation and intuition. I highly recommend keeping a food and symptoms journal to see if any foods, such as fried foods, garlic, or caffeine, appear to cause immediate symptoms. Then, you can try avoiding them one at a time to see if your symptoms improve. Look for patterns that may exacerbate your symptoms, such as midweek stress, takeout food, weekend alcohol, and the "Sunday Scaries."

Be sure to make stress management a focus and consider a supplement or two. I also want to mention that there has been a FODMAP-lite approach suggested in the literature, where you avoid the following:

- Apples
- Cauliflower
- Dried fruit
- Leeks
- Legumes
- Milk
- Mushrooms
- Onions
- Pears
- Stone fruit, like peaches
- Watermelons
- Yogurt

The idea is that these foods have the biggest impact on symptoms for some. I'm not a huge fan of this approach yet, because there isn't a well-defined endgame or research base to support it. It's your call if you want to try this approach for a couple of weeks to see how it goes.

comfortable advising long-term use. I've also seen clients who have been low-FODMAP for a year or more come to me because they still don't feel great. I think that there are probably two main reasons for this: nutrient and fibre deficiencies plus the impact of long-term FODMAP avoidance on mind and body.

Rocking Low-FODMAP Life

There are a lot of healthy foods to choose from on the low-FODMAP diet, but navigating food choices means referring to your low-FODMAP food list until you know it by heart. It's a bit cumbersome, so I've tried to make it easier for you. If you're low-FODMAP, there are a lot of delicious recipes in this book—they are labelled Heal. I set aside my deep love of garlic and onions to create flavourful dishes for you to cook and feel better.

I recommend choosing a start date a week or so in advance so you have time to plan your meals and grocery shop. You can choose to freestyle your eating plan with the Heal recipes in this book plus the low-FODMAP food on pages 98 to 105 or you can try my seven-day meal plan (page 301) so you can set it and forget it. Whatever you do, do not try to wing it for the first few weeks. Low-FODMAP living means reading labels and making sure you have low-FODMAP food on hand. You need to know what you're going to eat ahead of time. Otherwise, you could find yourself starving at lunch and trying to do the mental math on which takeout option is going to be low-FODMAP and then feeling really frustrated. Takeout food is not a good option and unlikely to be low-FODMAP.

Give yourself the time and space you need to care for yourself during the elimination and challenge. What can you let go of? What can you get help with? Go for a walk instead of dusting. Say no to that extra project so you can say yes to cooking. It's worth it. You are worth it.

Plant-Based Eating and Low-FODMAP Can Work Together

Plant-based, low-FODMAP recipes are a bit hard to find, which is why I included so many low-FODMAP recipes in this book. Just in case someone has told you this, you do not have to give up your dietary preference for your therapeutic diet. If you are 100 percent plant based, you may be eating a little bit less protein than normal unless you really commit to that tofu-tempeh-hemp-heart life. Try to do your best to consume low-FODMAP portions of nuts, seeds, and beans as often as possible to bulk up your protein count, and remember it's just temporary. I've made sure that many of the Heal recipes contain protein because it's going to keep the hangries at bay.

There are a few nutrients that appear to be lower during FODMAP eliminations: fibre, calcium, and iron are most at risk *for all eaters*, not just plant-based ones. For plant-based eaters, reducing your intake of beans, nuts, and seeds is going to make it a bit harder to get your minerals. Therefore, a simple multivitamin and mineral supplement may help keep you topped up for the next couple of months. If you eat animal products, know that eggs, seafood, and meat don't have FODMAPs because they don't have carbohydrates, although dairy does. Low-lactose dairy is widely available, as are plant-based alternatives.

Other Dietary Approaches to Support Low-FODMAP Living

I want to give you a nudge about your intake of caffeine, alcohol, and added sugars before you embark on your low-FODMAP journey. The evidence doesn't clearly link any of these with symptoms; however, we also know that they aren't really gut friendly from a functional perspective. Caffeine can impact motility. If you drink only one small cup of coffee a day, I am less concerned—unless you know it has you running to the bathroom. And, of course, if you're constipated, it may be helping.

Alcohol, on the other hand, is worth avoiding while you're doing the elimination. Alcohol can cause irritation and temporary gut barrier leakiness that will make symptoms worse. It also can further inflammation, which is the exact opposite of what you're hoping to achieve right now. One or two glasses of wine a week won't really hurt, but you're putting so much work into healing, so do take care.

What about sugar? Table sugar is 100 percent okay on a low-FODMAP diet because the body metabolises the fructose in table sugar differently than free fructose in foods. However, eating a lot of added sugar isn't going to do you any favours. Remember, sugar isn't evil or toxic or dangerous, but a high-sugar dietary pattern is detrimental to the gut. So enjoy a bit of sugar to sweeten whole foods if you need to. Moderation is key, so don't consume too much sugar.

I also want you to consider two other helpers: probiotics and psyllium. Early evidence suggests that probiotics are supportive of symptom control in IBS and may help mitigate the effects of the low-FODMAP diet on your microbiome. If it's in the budget, give it a try for the full duration of your elimination and challenge.

When you reduce high-FODMAP grains and beans in your diet, it's easy to eat less fibre. Something that might help is taking 1 to 3 teaspoons (5 to 15 mL) of psyllium husk daily. Psyllium is a soluble fibre, so it shouldn't irritate the gut. It's also not very fermentable, meaning it won't lead to excess gas, but it will help regulate elimination, whether you have diarrhea or constipation. Just remember to drink plenty of water. See page 36 for more about psyllium.

How to Reintroduce FODMAPs

A low-FODMAP elimination is often called a short-term learning diet. This is where the learning part comes in. You eliminate the triggers, take time to heal, and then systematically reintroduce the FODMAPs to see just how sensitive you are. Typically, you will reintroduce very specific foods while you are still low-FODMAP. It can take six to eight weeks to do a classic reintroduction, which means you might be low-FODMAP for as long as four months.

If that seems okay to you, awesome. Go slow and steady; if you haven't been well for a long time, four months of effort to feel better is worth it. However, I also get that a bit of anxiety might have crept up just now and you're not sure if you can last that long. If so, revisit whether now is the right time for you and consider a bit of an accelerated path.

If you get a very clear signal that the low-FODMAP diet is working for you at the three-week mark, start your accelerated reintroductions at the four-week point. On the other hand, if you have no symptom improvement after four weeks, ditch the elimination. If it's not working, don't keep at it. Nothing works for 100 percent of people. I know it is disappointing, especially after you've made all the effort. As you think about your experience, it's worth checking if perhaps you were inadvertently eating FODMAPs during the trial or if stress was a big culprit. But sometimes FODMAPs aren't the thing and it's more about the nervous system.

But what if you're better, but not all the way? Or you were better at first then got a bit worse? That's when you might consider extending your elimination while you double down on stress management and explore supplementation options.

What to Eat During Your Reintroduction

You have four or five categories of food to reintroduce, depending on whether you eat dairy. You can do the reintroductions in any order you wish. If you're really missing beans, start with galacto-oligosaccharides (GOS). The only catch is that you have to eat the foods I recommend. We eat these foods specifically because they are high in only one type of FODMAP. Many foods have more than one type of FODMAP, so if you react to them, you can't be sure which FODMAP is the issue.

You'll take each category of foods through the accelerated four-day or conservative seven-day cycle below. If any symptoms come up, note which food introduction appeared to cause them. You'll avoid that food for now, wait until you are symptom-free (probably a couple of days), and continue with the next category of food.

Once you complete the trials and know which foods are causing issues, you have a couple of options. If the symptom was strong, you may choose to avoid that category as you restore the other FODMAPs to your diet—this is called the customization phase of the diet. Or you could choose to try the reintroduction again once you are feeling good to see if the symptom was a blip caused by stress or something else.

WEEK ONE: POLYOLS

Food One: **4 dried apricots**

Food Two: **½ cup (125 mL) mushrooms**

WEEK TWO: DAIRY (if you don't consume dairy, skip and go to Week Three)

Food One: **½ cup (125 mL) milk**

Food Two: **¾ cup (175 mL) plain yogurt**

WEEK THREE: FRUCTOSE

Food One: **1 teaspoon (5 mL) honey or 1 tablespoon (15 mL) agave syrup**

Food Two: **½ mango**

WEEK FOUR: FRUCTANS

Food One: **2 slices whole-grain bread**

Food Two: **1 garlic clove**

WEEK FIVE: GOS

Food One: **20 raw almonds**

Food Two: **½ cup (125 mL) cooked chickpeas**

I'm giving you two different options for reintroducing foods: an accelerated four-day cycle and a conservative seven-day cycle. Remember that you need to stay low-FODMAP during the reintroductions, so a four-day cycle will help you get through them faster. If you are nervous about symptom response or think that you're quite sensitive to FODMAPs, the seven-day cycle might improve your tolerance.

FOUR-DAY FOOD TRIAL CYCLE

Day One: serving of Food One

Day Two: serving of Food Two

Day Three: serving of Foods One and Two

Day Four: no trial food, see how you feel

SEVEN-DAY FOOD TRIAL CYCLE

Day One: serving of Food One

Day Two: no trial food

Day Three: serving of Food One

Day Four: no trial food

Day Five: serving of Food Two

Day Six: serving of Foods One and Two

Day Seven: no trial food, see how you feel

Once you've completed the reintroductions, I hope you'll have a clearer sense of which foods cause an issue. This experience is about putting you in the driver's seat and eliminating uncertainty and food anxiety. For example, perhaps you'll realize that you react to GOS, but know that sometimes you just want to eat chickpeas. You know that they may leave you feeling a little gassy or bloated, but you'll also know why. That's your call and kind of how I live my life.

You may find that you seem to tolerate all of the reintroductions. If so, what gives? Remember that it is all about dose. So a bit of FODMAP in a lower-FODMAP life is no big deal. But a giant bowl of garlicky cashew Alfredo might set you over the edge. If that's the case, continue to enjoy low-FODMAP meals and foods while you sprinkle in higher FODMAPs to find your happy medium.

Food Elimination Isn't Without Risk

Food elimination is just one tool in the toolkit for digestive health—one I am pretty cautious about using. Why? Because elimination makes it harder to get all of the nutrition your body needs to heal. It can mess with your head a bit too, making eating stressful and diminishing your enjoyment of food. In online wellness spaces, it's common to see people who eliminate food groups present themselves as being "in the know" or eating "healthier" than people who don't, but that's not knowledge. It is a disordered eating mindset. I highly recommend that if you have a history of disordered eating, you do not proceed with food elimination. Instead, work with a dietitian to determine a non-restrictive path forward.

Know that even if you and food have a solid relationship, it is not uncommon for food aversion to develop when you eliminate, especially if you feel so much better on a low-FODMAP diet. In fact, fear can create a bit of a placebo effect where you experience symptoms upon reintroduction because you expect them to occur. This gut-brain stuff is tricky. At this point, you should know that both cognitive behavioural therapy and hypnotherapy have been shown to be of benefit in IBS, so do not hesitate to seek counselling help if that option is available to you, especially if you also have depression or anxiety.

Don't Go Much? Let's Chat About Constipation-Predominant IBS

Because of all of this diarrhea talk, you might be wondering what the heck you are supposed to do if you have constipation-predominant IBS (IBS-C). How should you eat? What about supplements? Well, it depends. For example, while a low-FODMAP diet may work in IBS-C, it's not my first-line approach. In fact, my primary focus is always on the *constipation* part of the diagnosis. So be sure to review the recommendations on constipation in Chapter 2.

Why talk about constipation and not the brain-gut aspect? Because I've had a lot of clients who've come to me with diagnosed IBS, yet they were actually just super constipated. We fixed the constipation and the IBS went away. If you've been chronically constipated for years, you're going to be bloated, gassy, and in pain a lot of the time. So if you have a low-fibre diet, you don't drink a lot of water or eat a lot of vegetables, and you're not very active, I want you to start with the basics and see how you do.

When it comes to true IBS-C, it's a bit trickier. When I see that there is room for you to move toward a more gut-friendly, plant-forward life, that's where I start. But if you are already eating enough fibre, drinking plenty of water, and moving your body daily yet are still constipated, there are fewer tools in my toolkit for you. In practice, I will focus on motility with prokinetics and meal spacing (those MMC waves) as well as the microbe connection. If ginger or Iberogast doesn't work for you, your doctor will have other prescription promotility agents that may help.

Research also suggests that targeting the microbiome will help IBS-C. Remember how methane producers can slow down your motility? Dr. Mark Pimentel, a prominent gastroenterologist and researcher, has advocated for special antibiotic protocols that may help rebalance the gut flora in IBS-C, so that's a conversation to be had between you and your doctor.

I always want you to be fully informed and aware of how complex nutrition can be, but I don't want to give you the impression that elimination is always negative. If you've been unwell for a while, elimination can feel liberating—like you finally have some positive and effective action you can take to feel better. This is where that listening comes in: What is your body telling you? How do these choices feel? That's how you know the path forward.

Supplements to Support the Gut-Brain Connection

There are a lot of supplements marketed for gut health, from probiotics and prebiotics to enzymes and collagen. Despite the loud choruses of people singing collagen's praises, there is close to zero research on collagen for the gut.

You could easily spend hundreds of dollars on supplements, but I promise you, they won't have the impact that a solid diet and stress-reduction strategy will. Supplementing a gut-busting diet is like buying yourself a fancy new fridge when the foundation of your house is crumbling. There are, of course, a few supplements that can help boost your efforts when you're on the healing path. We've already talked about probiotics and prebiotics, the most evidence-based of the bunch, so I want to briefly discuss a few supplements we haven't fully explored yet, including peppermint oil, licorice, l-glutamine, and Iberogast.

PEPPERMINT OIL

Enteric-coated peppermint oil is perhaps one of my favourite supplements. It's inexpensive and one of the only evidence-based natural supplement options in IBS. It's an effective antispasmodic, meaning that it helps to reduce muscular spasms, thereby calming pain in the gut. It also has anti-inflammatory and pain-relieving effects. One recent review confirms that peppermint oil can improve abdominal pain and global symptoms of IBS; it's one I rely on a lot.

Enteric-coated peppermint oil can be taken on an as-needed basis or consistently to get symptoms under control. It is taken before each meal, typically in a 200 mg dose. Watch out because not all peppermint oil caps are vegan, so if you're vegan, be sure to check the label. Also, know that this isn't just peppermint essential oil. It's food grade and enteric-coated so it won't open in the stomach. Because peppermint oil soothes muscle contractions, it might make you a bit reflux-y. So it goes without saying that it might not be a good option if you have gastroesophageal reflux disease (GERD).

LICORICE

Most people either love or hate licorice, but if you have reflux, you just might learn to love it. Licorice is used in traditional Chinese medicine as a digestive tonic, and lab studies suggest that licorice—which is high in flavonoids—offers anti-inflammatory benefits. In traditional use, licorice is thought to be a demulcent, meaning that it helps soothe irritated and inflamed tissues.

Unfortunately, we don't have a lot of human clinical trials to guide us. However, early evidence suggests that licorice may increase mucus production, which could ease reflux, dyspepsia, and ulcer. Licorice is also a component of Iberogast, which you'll read more about below.

You will often see supplemental licorice sold as DGL, or deglycyrrhizinated licorice. Glycyrrhizin in licorice extracts can increase blood pressure, so it's removed. Avoid licorice supplements if you are pregnant, and always check with your doctor or pharmacist first if you are on any other medications or have a heart condition. Licorice can react with medications and cause dangerously low potassium levels.

L-GLUTAMINE

L-glutamine is an amino acid that is used as an energy source by gut cells—kind of like a healthy snack for your gut lining. Your gut actually uses about 30 percent of your body's total l-glutamine supply. While not an essential amino acid in everyday life (your body can make it), in times of trauma such as severe burns, it's thought that glutamine becomes "conditionally essential" because your stores of glutamine go down.

There is plenty of theoretical research to suggest that l-glutamine supports gut barrier integrity and lessens inflammation. You'll find that the internet is chockful of blogs telling you how l-glutamine will heal your gut. The problem is that we don't have a lot of human clinical research to support its use in digestive health. For example, in inflammatory bowel disease, you would expect that the degree of gut destruction would respond well to l-glutamine, but so far, no. In IBS, I found one small trial that suggests it works well to improve gut barrier integrity in post-infectious IBS but the study was also criticized for being of poor quality.

I typically don't recommend the use of l-glutamine, and certainly not as a first line of defence. It's expensive and I would rather you prioritize healthy food in your budget. Now, if you are really interested in taking it and it fits the budget, know that the best use seems to be in gut barrier dysfunction (leaky gut) and perhaps post-infectious IBS. If you're taking l-glutamine or plan to, know that a little sprinkle won't be enough. Avoid the capsules; look for powdered products and take 2.5 grams twice a day. It needs to be taken on an empty stomach. First thing in the morning and before bed is good. You can take as much as 5 grams twice a day, but you should talk to your naturopath about anything beyond this amount, which you may need for serious issues such as celiac disease.

IBEROGAST

Iberogast is an herbal blend of nine extracts that has been around since the 1950s. It contains bitter herbs, carminatives (such as peppermint), and even licorice. The research on Iberogast suggests that it has multiple effects, helping to reduce symptoms of IBS and functional dyspepsia (FD)—improving spasms, gas, and bloating. You can take it as needed or consistently before each meal. Talk with your doctor or pharmacist before taking Iberogast, as it may not play well with other medications. Do not take Iberogast if you have anything wrong with your liver.

I want to close this section by talking a little bit about supplements for stress. If stress is a major trigger for your gut issues, it might be worth considering spending your supplement budget on a balm for your frazzled nerves. I am a big fan of adaptogens and find ashwagandha has a compelling evidence base for stress relief. Be sure to talk to your pharmacist or naturopath about these options.

Creating a Space for Healing

Committing to healing means making space for it to happen. I get how hard that can seem, but if you're honest with yourself, you can probably make at least a bit of space. It means doing a bit less, perhaps having a bit less. Take a deep breath. Your health is your greatest gift. Taking a bit of time out of each day for healing will actually save you from being sidelined completely when you crash.

It's a lesson that took me too long to learn. But the better you take care of yourself, the more you have to give at work, to your family, and to achieving your goals. So let's start by talking about *how* you're eating. We covered this in Chapter 2, so let's refresh by reminding you that stress and eating are a recipe for a gut-brain disaster. If you're stressed out at mealtime, remember two things:

1. Always do your deep breathing before you eat.
2. Chew each bite thoroughly and don't rush. Eat what you have time to eat right now.

Ideally, you would eat meals at roughly the same time each day and try to go eleven to twelve hours overnight without food to give your gut plenty of time in the post-absorptive state, but don't get too rigid about it.

In an ideal world, we wouldn't be stressed and we would have plenty of downtime. As someone who runs her own business and had young children in the house for a decade, I know that might feel like a pipe dream in some stages of your life. So you'll have to be sneaky about it. For example, you could diffuse relaxing essential oils during the morning chaos to give yourself a little reminder to breathe deeply. You could fit in a few laps around the track while your kid plays soccer. Or, you could do five minutes of square breathing each day before lunch. Make it work for you.

Stress-Management Techniques

1. **BREATHWORK.** Breathwork can take many forms (like the square breathing technique on page 58), but at its heart, it is a purposeful breathing exercise. Deep breathing can activate the parasympathetic nervous system so that even if for just five minutes, your nervous system can be calm. You can find any number of breathwork teachers and exercises online. In one trial, 30 minutes of diaphragmatic breathing to relaxing music improved quality of life in four weeks.

2. **JOURNALLING.** Journalling can be a healing exercise for many, whether it is free-form writing or something more structured like a gratitude journal. It's great to do before bed, especially if your mind starts to run as soon as you close your eyes. Get it onto the page and out of your head.

3. **MEDITATION.** Meditation is one of the best tools around for calming the nervous system and building your capacity to tolerate what life throws at you. There are so many ways of meditating and plenty of free tools online to help you get started if the process seems intimidating.

4. **OUTSIDE TIME.** I always recommend fresh-air time to my clients, daily if possible. If you have access to a beautiful park, trail, or beach, fantastic. If not, just going for a walk in the neighbourhood, free of distractions, is critical for creating mental space for healing. If you live in a hectic city, try listening to calming music as you walk to drown out the noise.

5. **READING A FAVOURITE BOOK.** I'm a big fan of reading—art helps us connect to our emotions and I find it extremely calming (unless it's a wild thriller). While I like to be informed, reading the news or scrolling social media does not count as relaxation reading. When was the last time you read something just for fun?

6. **TAKING A BATH.** I have become extremely regimented about evening baths. When you're a parent, taking a bath after the kids go to bed is one of the only times of the day you have to yourself. Epsom salts—the inexpensive kind that contain magnesium—can really add to the de-stressing experience. You can read a book, listen to an uplifting podcast or music, or do nothing at all for fifteen minutes.

7. **MOVEMENT.** Exercise blasts stress and strengthens your body at the same time. If you can exercise outside, even better. It's better to commit to fifteen sweaty minutes every day than not exercising at all because you don't have time for a full hour.

8. **SOCIAL TIME.** Research has shown that social connections are critical to better health outcomes. Even if you can't see each other in person, make time for a distraction-free chat with friends and family at least a couple of times a week. Go for a walk, play a game, or have a video call.

9. **THERAPY.** I mentioned before that talk therapy and hypnotherapy may be effective in improving symptoms of IBS. If it's available to you, exploring your first brain might really help you chill out your second brain.

10. **SINGING.** Singing (even gargling and chanting) helps activate the vagus nerve and calm you down. So instead of listening to a podcast in the car, why not turn on some tunes and sing your way home?

11. **BAKING.** Getting dinner on the table might not always feel like a meditative task, but for a lot of us, baking does. So make banana bread or some cookies. Getting your hands dirty is always therapeutic.

12. **CREATING ART.** We spend a lot of time in task mode, and many of us don't make space to create. When I look at how much time my kids spend drawing and colouring and making things, it makes me realize that adults shouldn't abandon these pursuits. Knit, paint, take a pottery class, and get yourself in maker mode.

13. **PRACTISING TINY RITUALS.** Mindfulness can enhance almost everything you do. Perhaps an 11 a.m. tea is your thing. Drink it from your favourite mug. Do deep breathing while the kettle boils. Take a big inhalation of the tea and enjoy your first two sips with your eyes closed. Think of all the ways you can create these tiny rituals throughout your day. It will have a positive impact on your well-being.

Low-FODMAP Food List

This is your "yes" list of low-FODMAP servings of foods that you can use to craft a low-FODMAP eating plan. Portion matters when it comes to FODMAP, as reactions are dose-dependent; eat a double portion of a food and it may put you over the FODMAP limit. FODMAPs are found only in carbohydrate-containing foods. So you won't see any pure proteins or fats here, such as eggs or olive oil. This list was compiled using data from Monash University, the world leader in low-FODMAP research. You can download the Monash University FODMAP diet app for the complete list. There is a small fee, but it all goes into furthering research on low-FODMAP diets. A few notes on FODMAPs and food:

FLOURS AND GRAINS

When it comes to IBS, the trouble with grains isn't the gluten—it's the oligosaccharides, consisting of fructans and GOS. Whole grains offer a ton of fibre, vitamins, and minerals, so don't skip out on these great low-FODMAP options.

FRUIT

Fructose is a monosaccharide found in all fruit. Whether it causes an issue depends on the presence of glucose. If present, fructose is efficiently absorbed; however, if fructose is in excess of glucose, it's malabsorbed. This attracts water to the bowel, causing symptoms. It is recommended to limit fruit intake to one serving per meal when on a low-FODMAP diet.

VEGETABLES

The FODMAPs in vegetables can be all over the place, including oligosaccharides (fructans and GOS), monosaccharides (fructose), and polyols (mannitol and sorbitol). Try to include low-FODMAP vegetables at every meal if you can—their fibre, vitamins, minerals, and phytonutrients are important for long-term gut health and fighting inflammation.

PLANT-BASED DAIRY AND PROTEIN

Lactose in milk-based dairy is a disaccharide FODMAP. Lactose-free dairy is available. Plant-based dairy contains no lactose; however, it may contain other FODMAPs, so choose your alternative carefully. Note that the Monash University app lists UK oat milk as higher FODMAP than other oat milks.

Plant-based proteins (legumes and beans) are well known for causing gas because they've got FODMAPs aplenty, known as oligosaccharides (fructans and GOS). You can reduce their oligosaccharide content in a few ways, such as draining and rinsing the canned versions. Soaking the dry versions for twenty-four hours, rinsing well, and cooking in fresh water also helps.

CONDIMENTS, HERBS, AND SPICES

Most condiments, herbs, and spices are low-FODMAP.

BEVERAGES

Different beverages have varying amounts of FODMAPs. Alcohol and regular, non-decaffeinated coffee have low to no FODMAPs. With juice and tea, the FODMAP levels vary based on the brand and on the tea steeping time. Drink plenty of water, which is always a good idea.

SWEETS

Most sugars are low-FODMAP; however, some in greater amounts are considered high-FODMAP, due to the monosaccharide (fructose) and/or galacto-oligosaccharide (fructans) content.

Low FODMAP-Friendly Foods

FLOURS AND GRAINS

Almond flour (¼ cup/60 mL)

Barley, sprouted (½ cup/125 mL)

Buckwheat flakes, cooked
(½ cup/125 mL)

Buckwheat groats, cooked
(¾ cup/175 mL)

Chickpea pasta, cooked
(1 cup/250 mL)

Corn flakes (½ cup/125 mL)

Corn flakes, gluten-free
(1 cup/250 mL)

Flour, arrowroot, corn, green
banana, maize, millet, quinoa,
rice, sorghum, organic sieved
spelt, teff, or pounded yam
(⅔ cup/150 mL)

Flour, buckwheat, regular or
wholemeal (⅔ cup/150 mL)

Flour, gluten-free all-purpose
(⅔ cup/150 mL)

Hominy, canned (½ cup/125 mL)

Millet, hulled, cooked
(1 cup/250 mL)

Nutritional yeast flakes
(1 tablespoon/15 mL)

Oat bran (2 tablespoons/30 mL)

Oat groats (¼ cup/60 mL)

Oats, quick, uncooked
(¼ cup/60 mL)

Oats, rolled, dry (½ cup/125 mL)

Pasta, gluten-free, cooked
(1 cup/250 mL)

Polenta, cooked (1 cup/250 mL)

Quinoa, black, red, or white,
cooked (1 cup/250 mL)

Quinoa flakes, uncooked
(1 cup/250 mL)

Rice, basmati glutinous, red,
white, or brown, cooked
(1 cup/250 mL)

Rice, puffed/popped
(½ cup/125 mL)

Rice bran
(2 tablespoons/30 mL)

Rice flakes, dry (¼ cup/60 mL)

Rice noodles/sticks, cooked
(1 cup/250 mL)

Starch, corn, potato, or
tapioca (⅔ cup/150 mL)

Tortillas, corn (2 tortillas)

Wheat grain, sprouted
(¼ cup/60 mL)

FRUIT

Acai powder
(1 tablespoon/15 mL)

Ackee, canned in brine
(1 cup/250 mL)

Avocado (⅛ fruit)

Banana, unripe (1 medium)
or ripe (⅓ medium)

Banana chips, dried (15 chips)

Blueberries (¼ cup/60 mL)

Cantaloupe (¾ cup/175 mL)

Carambola/star fruit (1 medium)

Citrus peel, mixed fruit
(⅓ cup/75 mL)

Clementine (1 medium)

Coconut, fresh (⅔ cup/150 mL)

Coconut, shredded, dry
(½ cup/125 mL)

Cranberries, dried
(1 tablespoon/15 mL)

Currants (1 tablespoon/15 mL)

Dragon fruit (1 medium)

Grapefruit (¼ cup/60 mL)

Grapes (1 cup/250 mL)

Guava, ripe (2 medium)

Honeydew melon, peeled,
seeded (½ cup/125 mL)

Kiwifruit, gold or green (2 small)

Kumquats (4 fruit)

Lemon juice (½ cup/125 mL)

Lime juice (1 cup/250 mL)

Longan (2 fruit)

Lychee (3 fruit)

Mandarin, imperial (2 small)

Mangosteen (2 medium)

Orange, navel (1 medium)

Papaya/pawpaw
(1 cup/250 mL)

Passion fruit (2 fruit)

Pear, prickly (1 medium)

Persimmon (½ fruit)

Pineapple, chopped
(1 cup/250 mL)

Plantain (1 medium)

Pomegranate seeds
(¼ cup/60 mL)

Raisins (1 tablespoon/15 mL)

Rambutan (3 fruit)

Raspberries (30 berries)

Rhubarb, chopped
(1 cup/250 mL)

Strawberries
(10 medium berries)

Tamarind (4 fruit)

Low FODMAP-Friendly Foods

VEGETABLES

Alfalfa sprouts (2 cups/500 mL)

Artichoke hearts, canned (½ cup/125 mL)

Arugula (2 cups/500 mL)

Bamboo shoots, canned (⅓ cup/75 mL)

Bamboo shoots, fresh (½ cup/125 mL)

Beans, green (15 beans)

Bean sprouts (¾ cup/175 mL)

Beetroot, canned (½ cup/125 mL)

Bell pepper, sweet, green, chopped (½ cup/125 mL)

Bell pepper, sweet, red (FODMAP-free)

Bok choy (1 cup/250 mL)

Broccoli, heads only or whole (¾ cup/175 mL)

Broccoli, stalks only (⅓ cup/75 mL)

Broccolini, heads only or whole (½ cup/125 mL)

Broccolini, stalks only (1 cup/250 mL)

Butternut squash (⅓ cup/75 mL)

Cabbage, common or red (¾ cup/175 mL)

Cabbage, savoy (½ cup/125 mL)

Callaloo, canned in brine (¼ cup/60 mL)

Carrot (FODMAP-free)

Casava (½ cup/125 mL)

Celeriac/celery root (¼ root)

Chayote (½ cup/125 mL)

Chicory leaves (½ cup/125 mL)

Chili, green or red (1 chili)

Choy sum (FODMAP-free)

Chrysanthemum greens (1 cup/250 mL)

Collard greens (1 cup/250 mL)

Corn, sweet (½ cob)

Corn truffle (½ cup/125 mL)

Cucumber, common (FODMAP-free)

Daikon, white (½ cup/125 mL)

Dulse flakes (2 teaspoons/10 mL)

Eggplant/aubergine (1 cup/250 mL)

Endive (FODMAP-free)

Fennel, bulb (½ cup/125 mL)

Gai lan (1 cup/250 mL)

Galangal (1½-inch/4 cm piece)

Ginger root (FODMAP-free)

Heart of palm, canned (½ cup/125 mL)

Jalapeño pepper, pickled (1 tablespoon/15 mL)

Jicama (½ cup/125 mL)

Kabocha squash (⅔ cup/150 mL)

Kale (FODMAP-free)

Kohlrabi (½ cup/125 mL)

Leek, leaves only (⅔ cup/150 mL)

Lettuce, includes radicchio and rocket (2 cups/500 mL)

Lotus root, frozen (1 cup/250 mL)

Mushrooms, oyster (1 cup/250 mL)

Okra (7 pods)

Olives, black or green, pitted (½ cup/125 mL)

Onion, spring, scallion, or green, green tops only (1½ cups/375 mL)

Onion, large, pickled (2 onions)

Parsnip (FODMAP-free)

Peas, canned green (¼ cup/60 mL)

Potato, regular, unpeeled (FODMAP-free)

Pumpkin, canned (⅓ cup/75 mL)

Pumpkin, Japanese (⅔ cup/150 mL)

Radish (4 radishes)

Rutabaga/swede (1 cup/250 mL)

Seaweed/nori (FODMAP-free)

Snake bean (1 cup/250 mL)

Spaghetti squash, cooked (1 cup/250 mL)

Spinach, baby (1½ cups/375 mL)

Spinach, English (2 cups/500 mL)

Squash, pattypan (FODMAP-free)

Sun-dried tomatoes (3 pieces)

Sweet potato/yam (½ cup/125 mL)

Swiss chard/silverbeet (1½ cups/375 mL)

Taro, diced (½ cup/125 mL)

Tomatillos, canned or fresh, diced (1 cup/250 mL)

Tomatoes, canned (½ cup/125 mL)

Tomatoes, cherry (5 tomatoes)

Tomato, Roma or common (1 small)

Turnip (½ turnip)

Wakame flakes (1 teaspoon/5 mL)

Water chestnuts (½ cup/125 mL)

Witlof/Belgian endive (1½ stalks)

Yucca root (½ cup/125 mL)

Zucchini/courgette/baby marrow (⅓ cup/75 mL)

Low FODMAP-Friendly Foods

PLANT-BASED DAIRY

Cheese, soy (2 slices)

Milk, almond (1 cup/250 mL)

Milk, coconut, canned
(¼ cup/60 mL)

Milk, coconut, unsweetened,
UHT (½ cup/125 mL)

Milk, macadamia or
unsweetened quinoa
(1 cup/250 mL)

Milk, oat (½ cup/125 mL)

Milk, rice (¾ cup/175 mL)

Milk, soy protein, not whole
soy bean (1 cup/250 mL)

Milk powder, coconut
(1 tablespoon/15 mL)

Yogurt, coconut
(½ cup/125 mL)

PLANT-BASED PROTEIN

Almonds (10 nuts)

Almond butter
(1 tablespoon/15 mL)

Beans, adzuki, canned,
drained (¼ cup/60 mL)

Brazil nuts (10 nuts)

Brown rice protein,
sprouted powder, organic
(2 tablespoons/30 mL)

Cashews, activated (10 nuts)

Chana dal, boiled
(¼ cup/60 mL)

Chestnuts, boiled (20 nuts)

Chestnuts, roasted (10 nuts)

Chickpeas/garbanzo beans,
canned, rinsed (¼ cup/60 mL)

Edamame, shelled
(½ cup/125 mL)

Flaxseed (1 tablespoon/15 mL)

Hazelnuts (10 nuts)

Lentils, canned, rinsed
(½ cup/125 mL)

Lentils, boiled green, or red
(¼ cup/60 mL)

Lima beans, boiled
(¼ cup/60 mL)

Lotus seed, popped
(1 cup/250 mL)

Macadamia (20 nuts)

Mixed nuts (18 nuts)

Mung beans, boiled
(¼ cup/60 mL)

Peanut butter
(2 tablespoons/30 mL)

Peanuts (32 nuts)

Pecans (10 halves)

Pine nuts (1 tablespoon/15 mL)

Seeds, chia, hemp, poppy,
or pumpkin (2 tablespoons/
30 mL)

Sesame seeds
(1 tablespoon/15 mL)

Tempeh, plain (3½ oz/100 g)

Tigernuts (1 handful)

Tofu, firm, drained; not silken
(⅔ cup/150 mL)

Walnuts (10 halves)

CONDIMENTS, HERBS, AND SPICES

Adobo (1 teaspoon/5 mL)

Allspice (1 teaspoon/5 mL)

Asafoetida (¼ teaspoon/1 mL)

Asian (garlic) chives
(1 cup/250 mL)

Basil, fresh (1 cup/250 mL)

Bay leaves (1 leaf)

Cacao/cocoa powder
(2 teaspoons/10 mL)

Capers, in vinegar, salted
(1 tablespoon/15 mL)

Caraway seeds
(2 teaspoons/10 mL)

Cardamom (1 teaspoon/5 mL)

Chili powder (1 teaspoon/5 mL)

Chives (1 tablespoon/15 mL)

Chutney (1 tablespoon/15 mL)

Cilantro/coriander, fresh
(1 cup/250 mL)

Cinnamon (1 teaspoon/5 mL)

Cloves (1 teaspoon/5 mL)

Coconut cream (¼ cup/60 mL)

Coriander seeds
(1 teaspoon/5 mL)

Cumin (1 teaspoon/5 mL)

Curry leaves, fresh (1 cup/250 mL)

Curry powder (1 teaspoon/5 mL)

Dill, fresh (1 cup/250 mL)

Fennel seeds (1 teaspoon/5 mL)

Fenugreek leaves, dried
(1 cup/250 mL)

Fenugreek seeds
(2 tablespoons/30 mL)

Low FODMAP-Friendly Foods

CONDIMENTS, HERBS, AND SPICES (CONTINUED)

Five-spice powder
(1 teaspoon/5 mL)

Garam masala (1 teaspoon/5 mL)

Gotu kola (½ bundle)

Horseradish
(2 tablespoons/30 mL)

Kaffir lime leaves (3 leaves)

Lemongrass
(4-inch/10 cm stalk)

Mint, fresh (1 bunch)

Miso paste (2 tablespoons/30 mL)

Mustard, all types
(1 tablespoon/15 mL)

Mustard seeds (1 teaspoon/5 mL)

Nutmeg, fresh (2 whole)

Oregano, dried
(1 teaspoon/5 mL)

Pandan leaves
(1-inch/2.5 cm leaf)

Paprika (1 teaspoon/5 mL)

Parsley, fresh (1 cup/250 mL)

Pepper, black (1 teaspoon/5 mL)

Rosemary, fresh (1 cup/250 mL)

Saffron (0.04 oz/1 g)

Sage, fresh (1 bunch)

Soy sauce
(2 tablespoons/30 mL)

Sriracha hot chili sauce
(1 teaspoon/5 mL)

Star anise (2 cloves)

Sumac (1 teaspoon/5 mL)

Tahini (2 tablespoons/30 mL)

Tarragon, fresh (1 cup/250 mL)

Thai basil, fresh (1 cup/250 mL)

Thyme, fresh (1 cup/250 mL)

Tomato paste
(2 tablespoons/30 mL)

Turmeric (1 teaspoon/5 mL)

Vinegar, apple cider, malt,
red wine, or rice wine
(2 tablespoons/30 mL)

Vinegar, balsamic
(1 tablespoon/15 mL)

Wasabi paste
(2 tablespoons/30 mL)

Watercress, fresh (1 cup/250 mL)

BEVERAGES

Beer, 1 bottle/can (12 oz/355 mL)

Coconut water, fresh or
packaged (3.38 oz/100 mL)

Coffee, instant
(2 teaspoons/10 mL)

Cranberry juice (6.76 oz/200 mL)

Espresso, regular, black
(¼ cup/60 mL)

Kombucha, tea (½ cup/125 mL)

Orange juice, reconstituted,
fresh 99% blend (½ cup/125 mL)

Spirits, gin, vodka, or whisky
(1 oz/30 mL)

Tea, black, weak; chai, weak;
dandelion, weak; green,
strong; peppermint, strong;
white, strong (1 cup/250 mL)

Wine, red, sparkling, sweet,
or white (5 oz/150 mL)

SWEETS

Agar (1 stick)

Agave syrup, dark or light
(1 teaspoon/5 mL)

Chocolate, dark 85%
(2 squares; 0.7 oz/20 g)

Golden syrup (1 teaspoon/5 mL)

Honey (1 teaspoon/5 mL)

Maple syrup
(2 tablespoons/30 mL)

Molasses (1 teaspoon/5 mL)

Sorghum syrup
(2 teaspoons/10 mL)

Stevia, powdered, no sugar
alcohols (2 teaspoons/10 mL)

Sugar, brown (¼ cup/60 mL)

Sugar, coconut
(1 teaspoon/5 mL)

Sugar, icing
(1 tablespoon/15 mL)

Sugar, palm, raw or white
(1 tablespoon/15 mL)

Syrup, rice malt
(1 tablespoon/15 mL)

Vanilla beans (2 pods)

Vanilla extract
(1 tablespoon/15 mL)

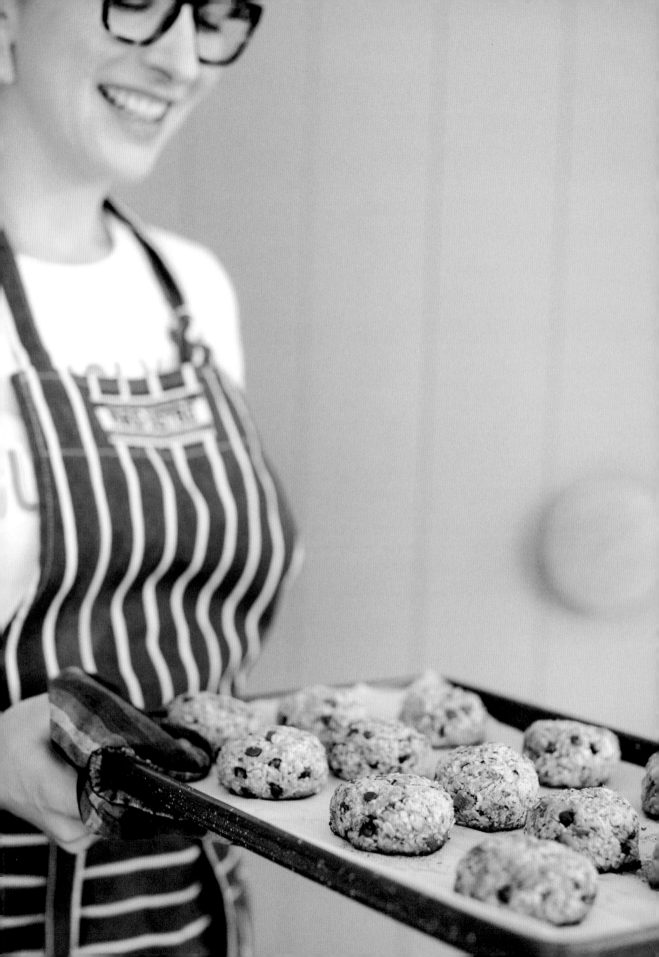

Mornings

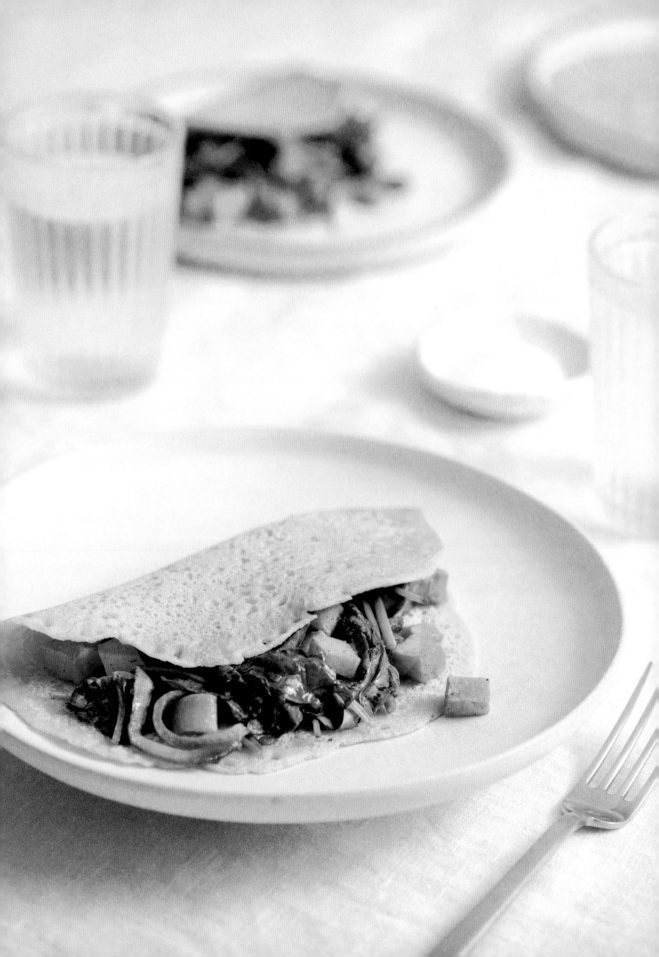

Chickpea Omelette with Curried Sweet Potato and Spinach Serves 4

When I was transitioning to a plant-based diet, dairy substitutes came easy to me, but I could not figure out how to recreate my favourite egg-based dishes. Then some genius figured out that chickpea flour—a staple in many South Asian kitchens—would work. Chickpea flour offers filling protein and plenty of minerals to make it a truly nutritious substitute. This omelette is one of my favourite breakfasts and it also transitions into a terrific dinner. Once you master it, you can stuff this omelette with any of your favourite fillings—from spinach and tofu feta cheese to roasted red peppers and onions.

DAIRY-FREE • GLUTEN-FREE • GRAIN-FREE • HIGH-FODMAP • NUT-FREE • VEGAN

ROASTED VEGETABLES

1 large sweet potato, scrubbed and chopped into ¾-inch (2 cm) cubes (about 3 cups/750 mL)

½ red onion, thinly sliced into half moons

1 tablespoon (15 mL) + 1 teaspoon (5 mL) avocado oil, divided, plus more for the pan

¾ teaspoon (3 mL) curry powder, divided

¼ teaspoon (1 mL) garam masala

¼ teaspoon (1 mL) salt, plus more for seasoning

4 cups (1 L) packed baby spinach

CHICKPEA OMELETTE

1 cup (250 mL) chickpea flour

¾ teaspoon (3 mL) salt

¼ teaspoon (1 mL) baking powder

¼ teaspoon (1 mL) ground turmeric

1¼ cups (300 mL) water

Tip You can make these omelettes ahead of time, which makes them great for meal prep. Keep the roasted vegetable mixture separately in an airtight container in the fridge. Store the omelettes, separated by parchment paper to avoid sticking, in a large airtight plastic bag in the fridge for up to 3 days. Reheat the omelettes in a nonstick skillet, covered, for a minute or so.

1. **Roast the vegetables:** Preheat the oven to 400°F (200°C). Line a baking sheet with parchment paper.

2. In a medium bowl, toss the sweet potato and red onion with 1 tablespoon (15 mL) of the avocado oil, ½ teaspoon (2 mL) of the curry powder, garam masala, and salt. Spread the vegetable mixture onto the prepared baking sheet, ensuring that the red onion is not close to the edges of the sheet to avoid burning. Roast until the sweet potato is fork-tender, 23 to 25 minutes.

3. Toss the spinach in the same bowl with the remaining 1 teaspoon (5 mL) avocado oil and ¼ teaspoon (1 mL) curry powder, and a pinch of salt. Place the spinach on top of the vegetable mixture and roast for 2 minutes more to wilt the spinach.

4. **Make the chickpea omelette:** In a medium bowl, whisk together the chickpea flour, salt, baking powder, and turmeric. Whisk in the water and let sit for 10 minutes to hydrate the flour.

5. Heat a medium nonstick skillet over medium heat and brush with a bit of avocado oil. When the oil is hot, pour ⅓ cup (75 mL) of the batter into the pan. (You should hear it sizzle. If the pan is not hot enough, it might be harder to flip the omelette.) Cook for about 1 minute. You'll see little bubbles on the surface, and it should look dry. Carefully run a spatula under the edges of the omelette, flip, and cook for 30 seconds. Transfer the omelette to a rack lined with parchment paper or keep warm in the oven. Cook the remaining 3 omelettes.

6. To serve, divide the roasted vegetables among the omelettes along one side and fold over.

Light As Air Waffles with Cardamom Sautéed Pears Makes twelve 4-inch waffles

Forget everything you know about whole grains being heavy! These waffles are crispy on the outside and light as air on the inside. Sunday morning waffles are a tradition in my house. Made with high-fibre pears and whole-grain flour, these waffles are the perfect brunch—as good for your body as they are for your soul. I like to make a double batch and then stash the rest in the freezer for midweek breakfasts.

DAIRY-FREE • HIGH-FODMAP • VEGAN

CARDAMON SAUTÉED PEARS

2 firm pears, cored and sliced (I use Bosc)

1 tablespoon (15 mL) freshly squeezed lemon juice

2 tablespoons (30 mL) water

1 tablespoon (15 mL) refined coconut oil or vegan butter

1 tablespoon (15 mL) pure maple syrup

½ teaspoon (2 mL) ground cardamom

Pinch of salt

WAFFLES

3 cups (750 mL) spelt or whole wheat flour

½ cup (125 mL) raw walnut pieces or chopped raw walnuts

3 tablespoons (45 mL) ground flaxseed

2 teaspoons (10 mL) baking powder

¾ teaspoon (3 mL) ground cardamom

½ teaspoon (2 mL) salt

⅓ cup (75 mL) avocado oil or refined coconut oil, melted, plus more for the pan

¼ cup (60 mL) pure maple syrup

1 tablespoon (15 mL) pure vanilla extract

1 tablespoon (15 mL) freshly squeezed lemon juice or apple cider vinegar

2 cups (500 mL) unsweetened non-dairy milk

FOR SERVING

Vegan butter

Nut butter

Pure maple syrup

1. **Prepare the pears:** In a small bowl, toss the pears with the lemon juice to prevent browning. Set aside while you prepare the waffles.

2. **Make the waffles:** Preheat a waffle iron. Line a baking sheet with parchment paper and place it in the oven. Preheat the oven to 200°F (100°C).

3. In a large bowl, whisk together the spelt flour, walnuts, flaxseed, baking powder, cardamom, and salt.

4. In a small bowl, whisk together the avocado oil, maple syrup, vanilla, and lemon juice. Add the wet ingredients to the dry ingredients, along with the non-dairy milk. Whisk until thoroughly mixed.

5. These waffles are light and can be difficult to remove from the waffle iron. If your waffle iron has a tendency to stick, brush it with avocado or coconut oil. Pour about ½ cup (125 mL) of the batter into the waffle iron and cook until fully browned and crispy, 4 to 5 minutes. Remove the waffle by gently loosening an edge with a heatproof rubber spatula or tongs, transfer to the prepared baking sheet, and keep warm in the oven. Repeat until all the batter is used.

6. **Sauté the pears:** Heat the water in a medium nonstick skillet over medium-high heat. Add the pears and cover with a lid. Cook for 1 minute to help soften the pears. Discard any remaining lemon juice. Remove the lid, reduce the heat to medium, and add the coconut oil, maple syrup, cardamom, and salt. Cook, stirring occasionally, until the liquid looks syrupy and the pears are soft and golden, 5 to 7 minutes.

7. Serve the waffles with vegan butter and/or your favourite nut butter, maple syrup, and sautéed pears.

FODMAP Note Spelt flour contains gluten and FODMAPs, so it is not suitable for those with celiac disease or following a low-FODMAP diet. For those who find traditional wheat flour irritating, spelt flour may be better tolerated.

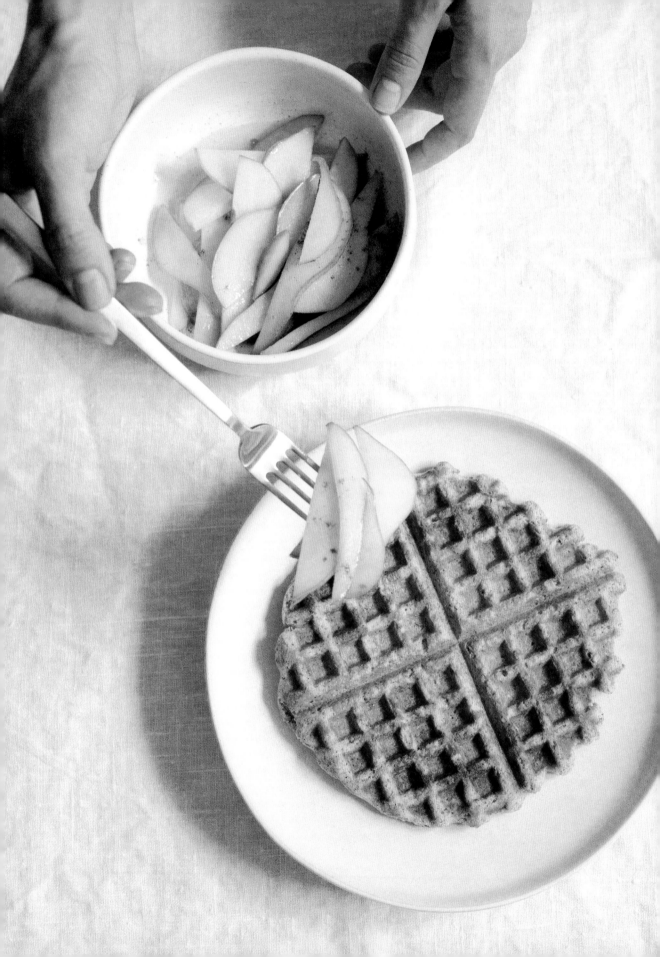

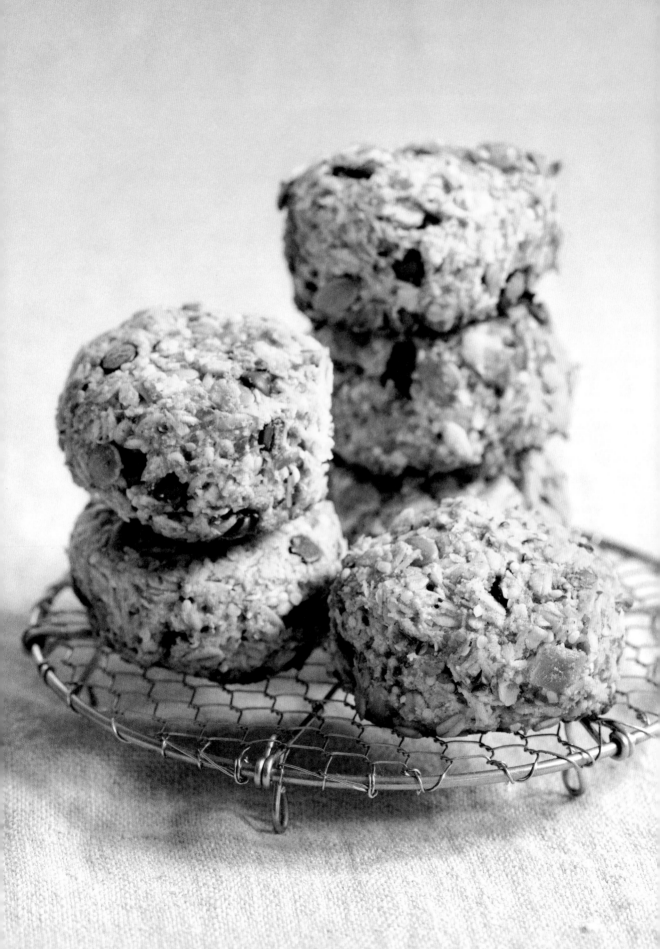

Breakfast Cookies Makes 16 cookies

Who doesn't want to eat cookies for breakfast? These cookies are truly a healthy start that will keep you energized. With almost no added sugars, and packed with nuts, seeds, and tummy-soothing ginger, they are the perfect grab-and-go breakfast with a piece of fruit. I have been making some variation of breakfast cookies for years and this variation is my favourite. Plenty of fibre, lots of minerals, and just a bit of chocolate. A single cookie is also low-FODMAP.

DAIRY-FREE • GLUTEN-FREE • LOW-FODMAP • VEGAN

1. Preheat the oven to 375°F (190°C). Line a large baking sheet with parchment paper.

2. In a large bowl, whisk together the rolled oats, coconut, almond flour, hemp hearts, pumpkin seeds, flaxseed, cinnamon, baking powder, and salt. Stir in the crystallized ginger and chocolate chips.

3. In a small bowl, mix together the banana, olive oil, and maple syrup until well blended. Add the banana mixture to the dry ingredients and stir to combine.

4. Working with wet hands so the batter does not stick too much, scoop ¼ cup (60 mL) of the batter and pat into 2-inch (5 cm) circles. Place evenly spaced on the prepared baking sheet. If the batter starts to stick to your hands, simply rinse them off and keep working with wet hands. The cookies will not spread, so you can easily fit them on one baking sheet. Bake until the cookies are golden on the bottom and starting to brown on top, 17 to 19 minutes. Cool on the baking sheet for 5 minutes, then transfer to a wire rack to fully cool. Store in an airtight container on the counter for up to 3 days or in the freezer for up to 1 month.

1 cup (250 mL) gluten-free old-fashioned rolled oats

1 cup (250 mL) unsweetened shredded coconut

¾ cup (175 mL) almond flour

½ cup (125 mL) hemp hearts

¼ cup (60 mL) raw pumpkin seeds

3 tablespoons (45 mL) ground flaxseed

1 teaspoon (5 mL) cinnamon

1 teaspoon (5 mL) baking powder

½ teaspoon (2 mL) salt

¼ cup (60 mL) crystallized ginger, finely diced

¼ cup (60 mL) dairy-free dark chocolate chips

1⅓ cups (325 mL) mashed bananas (about 3 medium)

¼ cup (60 mL) extra-virgin olive or avocado oil

2 tablespoons (30 mL) pure maple syrup

Raspberry and Chocolate Rye Muffins Makes 12 muffins

Rye is an underappreciated grain. It is flavourful and high in fibre, including fermentable fibres that feed the gut microbiota. With their tart raspberries and luscious chocolate, these muffins taste like a treat that happens to be packed with protein and omega-3 fatty acids from hemp and even a sneaky vegetable. They're nut-free and perfect for lunch boxes—children might not even realize they're health food.

DAIRY-FREE • HIGH-FODMAP • NUT-FREE • VEGAN

2 tablespoons (30 mL) ground flaxseed

¼ cup (60 mL) hot water

1 cup (250 mL) rye flour

½ cup (125 mL) spelt flour

½ cup (125 mL) hemp hearts

2 teaspoons (10 mL) baking powder

1 teaspoon (5 mL) baking soda

½ teaspoon (2 mL) salt

½ teaspoon (2 mL) ground cardamom

½ teaspoon (2 mL) cinnamon

1 cup (250 mL) grated zucchini, squeezed to drain water

1 cup (250 mL) mashed banana (2 to 3 medium)

½ cup (125 mL) extra-virgin olive oil

¼ cup (60 mL) pure maple syrup

2 teaspoons (10 mL) pure vanilla extract

1 cup (250 mL) fresh or frozen raspberries

⅓ cup (75 mL) dairy-free dark mini chocolate chips

1. Preheat the oven to 375°F (190°C). Line a 12-cup muffin tin with paper liners.

2. In a small bowl, stir the flaxseed with the hot water. Set aside.

3. In a large bowl, whisk together the rye flour, spelt flour, hemp hearts, baking powder, baking soda, salt, cardamom, and cinnamon.

4. In a medium bowl, mix together the zucchini, banana, olive oil, maple syrup, and vanilla. Add the flaxseed mixture and stir to combine.

5. Add the wet ingredients to the dry ingredients and stir until almost fully mixed. Add the raspberries and chocolate chips into the mixture. Stir to combine; be careful not to overmix.

6. Fill each muffin cup with about ⅓ cup (75 mL) of the batter. Bake until golden brown and a toothpick inserted in the centre of a muffin comes out clean, 18 to 22 minutes. Let the muffins cool in the pan for 15 minutes before turning them out onto a rack to cool completely. Store loosely covered on the counter for up to 3 days.

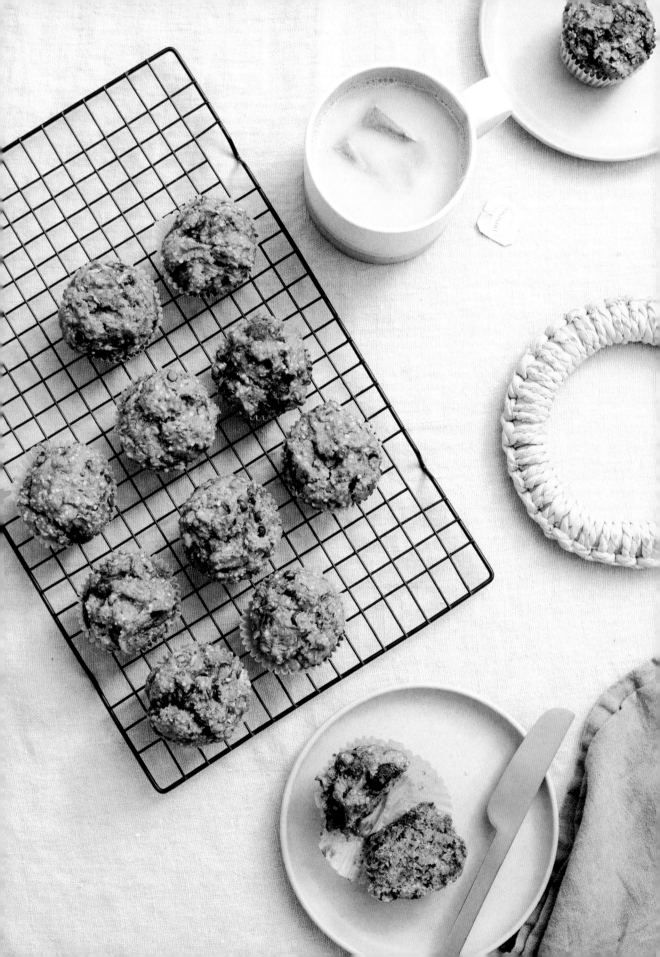

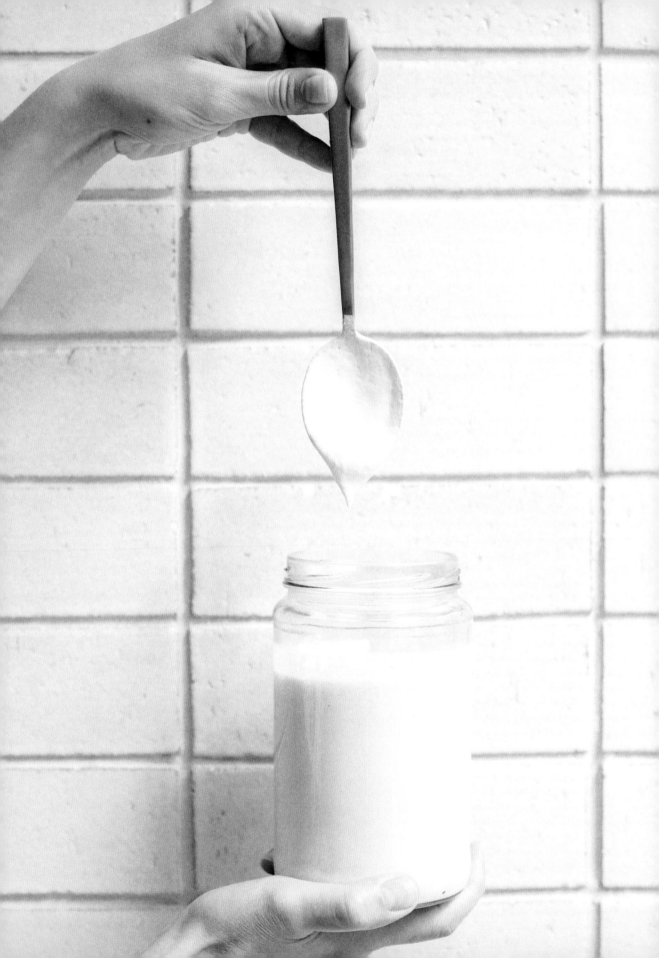

Fermented Cashew Yogurt Makes about 2½ cups (625 mL), serves 4 to 6

You are not going to believe how easy it is to make real, thick yogurt that is as good as any Greek yogurt I have ever tasted. This cashew yogurt is far more nutritious than coconut-based varieties. Cashew is high in prebiotic FODMAPs, making this recipe a true gut health all-star. Perfect with a little sprinkle of Crunchy Grain-Free Granola (page 128) and your favourite fruit.

DAIRY-FREE • GLUTEN-FREE • GRAIN-FREE • HIGH-FODMAP • VEGAN

1. Drain and rinse the cashews and transfer to a high-speed blender. Add the water, maple syrup, and salt. Blend until smooth. Carefully break open the probiotic capsules and pour the powder into the cashew cream. Pulse for a few seconds to blend. Discard the capsules. Pour the mixture into a clean 3-cup (750 mL) mason jar and cover with a double layer of cheesecloth, secured with an elastic band. Keep in a warm area wrapped in a clean kitchen towel. In cooler months, storing in the oven with the door closed and the oven light turned on provides great warmth. Ferment for 24 hours.

2. After 24 hours, stir in the lemon juice and a drizzle of maple syrup, if desired. (I prefer mine without the extra maple syrup.) Place the lid on tightly and store in the fridge for up to 2 weeks.

Tip When using a high-potency probiotic, the mixture continues to ferment a bit as it chills. After 3 or 4 days, it becomes tangier and a bit savoury and works well as a labneh or yogurt cheese. It would also make a great base for tzatziki.

2 cups (500 mL) raw cashews, soaked in warm water for 2 to 4 hours

1 cup (250 mL) water

1 tablespoon (15 mL) pure maple syrup, more as desired

Pinch of salt

Two 50 billion CFU probiotic capsules (I use Bio-K+; see Tip)

1 tablespoon (15 mL) freshly squeezed lemon juice

CCF Tea Makes about 1 quart (1 L)

CCF stands for cumin, coriander, and fennel—the trio of seeds that creates the base of this traditional Ayurvedic tea for digestion. A few modern studies suggest these phytochemical-rich seeds may be supportive in improving overall digestion and perhaps even beneficial for IBS, although not suitable while following a low-FODMAP diet. The cinnamon and ginger balance the savoury cumin for a mildly spicy tonic that is warming and comforting.

DAIRY-FREE • GLUTEN-FREE • GRAIN-FREE • HIGH-FODMAP • NUT-FREE • VEGAN

2 tablespoons (30 mL) coriander seeds

2 tablespoons (30 mL) fennel seeds

1 tablespoon (15 mL) cumin seeds

2 tablespoons (30 mL) grated fresh ginger

2 cinnamon sticks, broken into pieces

8 cups (2 L) water

1. Using a mortar and pestle or a rolling pin, gently crush the coriander seeds, fennel seeds, and cumin seeds.

2. In a medium saucepan, add the crushed seeds, ginger, cinnamon, and water. Bring to a boil over high heat. When the water is boiling, reduce the heat to maintain a gentle boil until the water is reduced by half, 25 to 30 minutes. Remove from the heat and let cool slightly. Strain into mugs. (Alternatively, you can let the tea cool completely then strain into a 1-quart/1 L mason jar, cover with a lid, and store in the fridge for up to 4 days. Warm before serving.)

Tip This tea contains a large amount of spices. If pregnant, please consult your doctor or midwife before consuming, as many herbal teas are not safe in pregnancy.

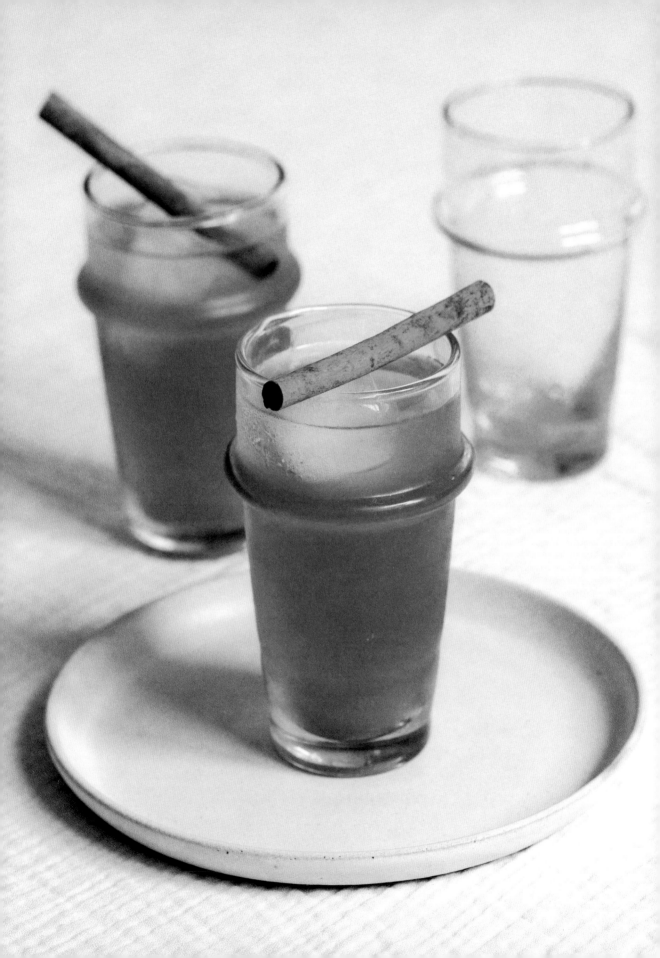

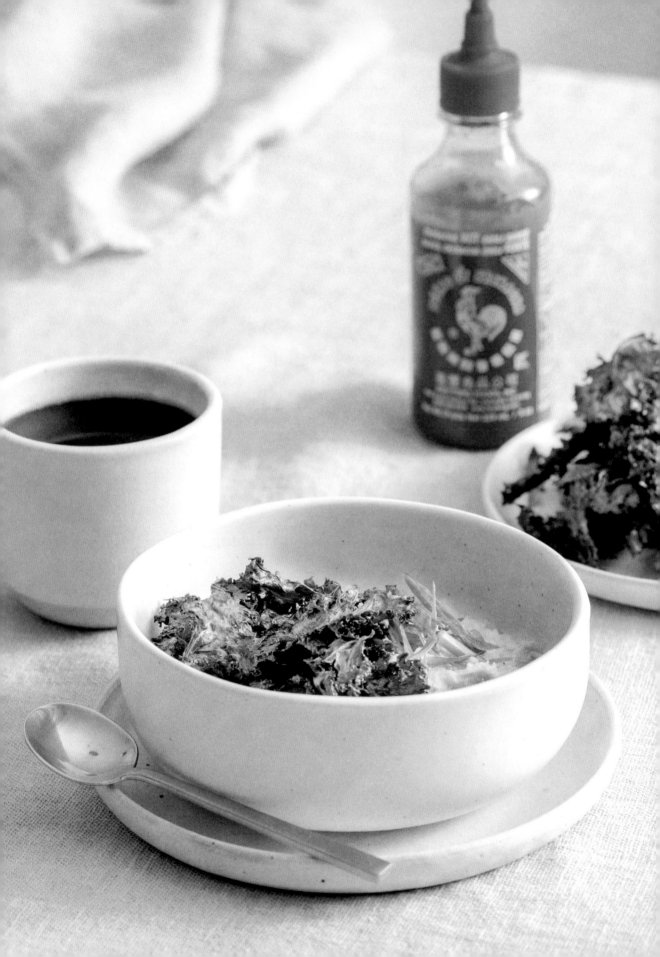

Savoury Miso Porridge with Crispy Kale Serves 2

Savoury porridges are common all over the world, which is especially exciting when you are not a huge sweet breakfast person like I am. You can also enjoy this porridge for dinner. Just think of it as a risotto made of oats. Oatmeal is hands down one of the greatest gut-health foods. It is easy on the irritated gut and filled with soluble beta-glucan fibre to help regulate digestion and feed beneficial bacteria in the gut. White (shiro) miso is mild in flavour but contains beneficial microbes. Always add miso at the end of cooking to preserve its benefits.

DAIRY-FREE • GLUTEN-FREE • LOW-FODMAP • NUT-FREE • VEGAN

1. **Make the crispy kale:** Preheat the oven to 400°F (200°C). Line 2 baking sheets with parchment paper.

2. In a large bowl, toss the kale with the avocado oil, salt, and chili flakes. Do not be tempted to add too much chili flakes or salt, as the seasonings will intensify as the kale cooks. Evenly spread the kale between the prepared baking sheets. Do not overcrowd the pans. Bake the kale for 5 minutes. Rotate the pans and bake until the kale is a bit crispy, but not completely dehydrated like kale chips, 3 to 6 minutes. Watch carefully so that the kale does not burn. (If you are using only one baking sheet, the kale cooks more quickly.) Set aside.

3. **Meanwhile, make the savoury miso porridge:** Bring the water to a boil in a small pot over high heat. Add the rolled oats and salt. Reduce the heat to medium and cook with the lid slightly ajar until desired consistency, 5 to 7 minutes. Remove from heat.

4. In a small bowl, mix the tahini with the miso until smooth and no clumps remain. Stir the mixture into the porridge until creamy. Add the chickpeas and stir again. Divide the porridge between bowls. Garnish with the green onions, crispy kale, and a drizzle of hot sauce, if using.

Tip If you use store-bought kale chips, this recipe comes together in about 15 minutes. Carefully read the label and watch for high-FODMAP ingredients such as garlic powder.

FODMAP Note Only canned chickpeas are low-FODMAP. If you are not following a low-FODMAP diet, you can use home-cooked chickpeas. It's also nice to add ½ clove grated garlic to the oats while cooking.

CRISPY KALE

1 large bunch kale, destemmed and torn into large pieces

1 tablespoon (15 mL) avocado oil

¼ teaspoon (1 mL) salt

Pinch of red chili flakes

SAVOURY MISO PORRIDGE

2 cups (500 mL) water

1 cup (250 mL) gluten-free old-fashioned rolled oats

⅛ teaspoon (0.5 mL) salt

2 tablespoons (30 mL) tahini

1 tablespoon (15 mL) white miso

½ cup (125 mL) canned chickpeas, rinsed and drained

GARNISHES

1 green onion, (green parts only), thinly sliced on the diagonal

Hot sauce (optional)

Pumpkin Oat Pancakes Makes 8 to 9 pancakes (3 low-FODMAP servings)

Pancakes are a weekend staple in my house, so I am always looking for ways to change up the flavours and make them even more nutritious. I love these pancakes because they are made with rolled oats that are rich in the soluble fibre beta-glucan to soothe and support an irritated gut. Pumpkin adds an abundance of anti-inflammatory nutrients, such as beta-carotene, and gives these treats a cozy, sweater weather vibe.

DAIRY-FREE • GLUTEN-FREE • LOW-FODMAP • NUT-FREE • VEGAN

1½ cups (375 mL) gluten-free old-fashioned rolled oats

1 tablespoon (15 mL) baking powder

½ teaspoon (2 mL) baking soda

½ teaspoon (2 mL) salt

½ teaspoon (2 mL) cinnamon

1 cup (250 mL) unsweetened pumpkin purée

½ cup (125 mL) unsweetened non-dairy milk (see Tip)

3 tablespoons (45 mL) organic cane sugar

3 tablespoons (45 mL) refined coconut oil, melted, or avocado oil, plus more for cooking

1 tablespoon (15 mL) freshly squeezed lemon juice or apple cider vinegar

2 teaspoons (10 mL) pure vanilla extract

TOPPINGS (OPTIONAL)

Finely chopped raw pecans

Finely chopped raw walnuts

2 tablespoons (30 mL) pure maple syrup

2 tablespoons (30 mL) natural peanut butter

1 tablespoon (15 mL) natural almond butter

1. In a high-speed blender, add the rolled oats, baking powder, baking soda, salt, and cinnamon. Pulse until it resembles panko crumbs. Add the pumpkin purée, non-dairy milk, cane sugar, coconut oil, lemon juice, and vanilla. Blend until combined. Let the batter sit for 5 minutes to thicken.

2. In a large nonstick skillet, heat 1 tablespoon of the coconut oil over medium heat. Cooking in batches, pour about ⅓ cup (75 mL) of batter per pancake into the pan and cook for 2 to 3 minutes. The pancakes will not bubble a lot like regular pancakes. The edges should look cooked and the bottom golden brown. Carefully flip the pancakes and cook for another 1 to 2 minutes. If the oil starts smoking or the pancakes brown too quickly, lower the temperature. Repeat to use the remaining batter, adding more coconut oil to the pan as needed. Serve with your favourite toppings, if using.

Tip I like to use almond milk to make these pancakes because of its light texture, but oat or rice milk will work if there is a nut allergy in your home. Oat and rice milk are also low-FODMAP in this serving size.

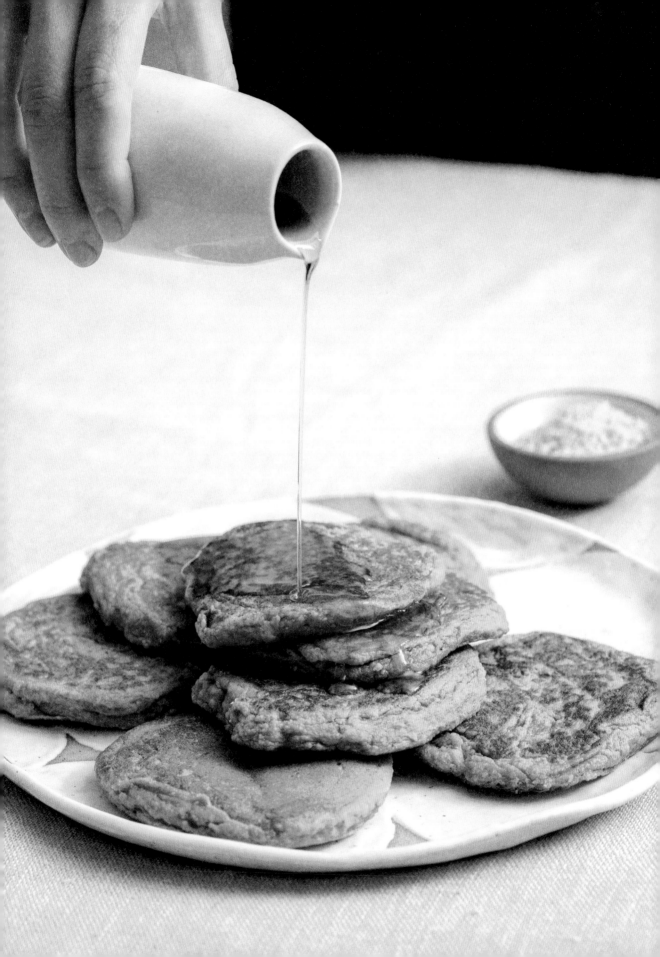

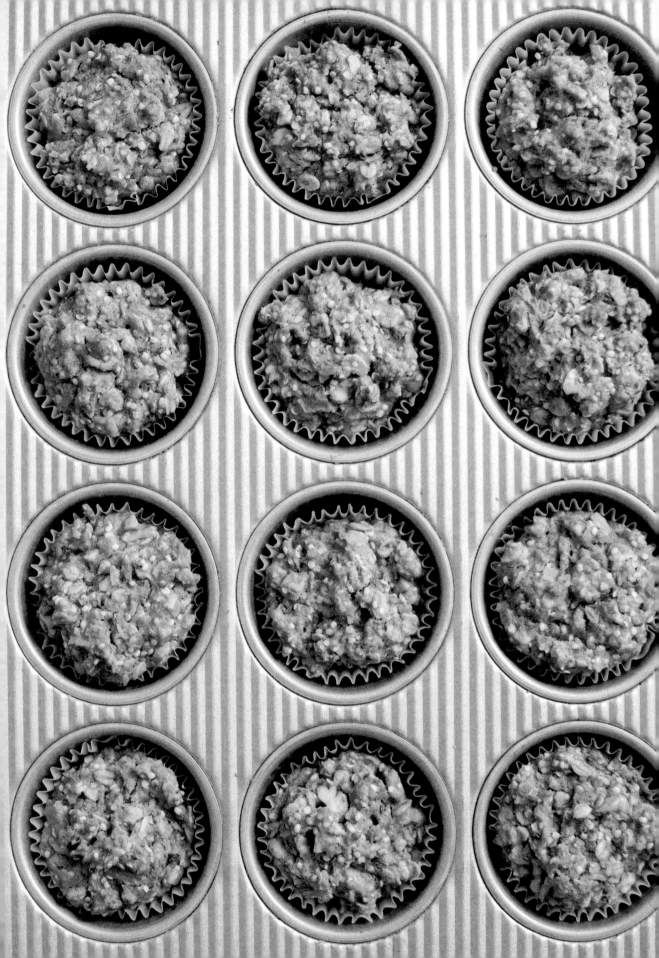

Carrot Cake Muffins Makes 12 muffins

Carrot cake is a favourite of my mine, which is probably no surprise given my affection for vegetables. I wanted to put everything I love about carrot cake into a nutrient-dense, low-FODMAP muffin. Low-FODMAP muffins tend to be mostly starch with very little nutritional value. Not these little gems! They are packed with soluble beta-glucan fibre from oats, and omega-3 fatty acids and plant-based protein thanks to hemp hearts and vitamin A–rich carrots.

DAIRY-FREE • GLUTEN-FREE • LOW-FODMAP • VEGAN

1. Preheat the oven to 350°F (180°C). Line a 12-cup muffin tin with paper liners.

2. In a medium bowl, whisk together the flour, rolled oats, hemp hearts, baking powder, cinnamon, baking soda, and salt.

3. In a small bowl, stir together the carrot, avocado oil, maple syrup, almond milk, apple cider vinegar, and vanilla. Stir the wet ingredients into the dry ingredients. Fold in the walnuts.

4. Fill each muffin cup with ¼ cup (60 mL) of batter. Bake until the top of the muffins are slightly crisp around the edges, 30 to 34 minutes. Let the muffins cool in the pan for 10 minutes, then turn out onto a rack to cool completely. (This is important for the best texture. The muffins will look a bit gummy when warm, but this disappears when cool.) Store loosely covered on the counter for up to 4 days or in an airtight container in the freezer for up to 1 month.

Tip Be sure to check that your 1:1 flour mix is low-FODMAP, for example, contains no chickpea flour. Also note that many 1:1 flour mixes contain xanthan gum as a stabilizer. If yours does not include xanthan gum, add 2 "flax eggs" to the wet ingredients. To prepare the flax eggs, stir 2 tablespoons (30 mL) ground flaxseed with ¼ cup (60 mL) warm water and let sit for 5 minutes before adding to the wet ingredients.

1 cup (250 mL) gluten-free 1:1 flour mix (I use Bob's Red Mill; see Tip)

1 cup (250 mL) gluten-free old-fashioned rolled oats

½ cup (125 mL) hemp hearts

2 teaspoons (10 mL) baking powder

2 teaspoons (10 mL) cinnamon

½ teaspoon (2 mL) baking soda

½ teaspoon (2 mL) salt

2 cups (500 mL) lightly packed, grated carrot (about 2 medium)

½ cup (125 mL) avocado oil

½ cup (125 mL) pure maple syrup

¼ cup (60 mL) unsweetened almond milk

1 tablespoon (15 mL) apple cider vinegar or freshly squeezed lemon juice

1 teaspoon (5 mL) pure vanilla extract

½ cup (125 mL) raw walnut pieces, finely chopped

Clarity Latte Serves 2

When life gets hectic, I will take as much clarity as I can get. I designed this adaptogenic latte to help calm frazzled nerves and bust the brain fog that can accompany digestive troubles. Matcha is a high-antioxidant powdered green tea that offers focused energy without the jitters, thanks to L-theanine, an amino acid that helps moderate the effects of caffeine. Coconut butter makes this latte extra creamy and offers energizing fats. Rhodiola is an adaptogenic herb that is uplifting and stress busting, while lion's mane supports cognitive function. Even without the adaptogens, this is a wonderful treat to help perk you up.

DAIRY-FREE • GLUTEN-FREE • GRAIN-FREE • LOW-FODMAP (SEE NOTE) • VEGAN

1¾ cups (425 mL) hot water

½ cup (125 mL) unsweetened almond or macadamia milk

2 tablespoons (30 mL) coconut butter (manna; see FODMAP Note)

1 tablespoon (15 mL) pure maple syrup

2 teaspoons (10 mL) good-quality matcha powder

1 teaspoon (5 mL) MCT oil (see Tip)

½ teaspoon (2 mL) rhodiola powder (optional; see Tip)

½ teaspoon (2 mL) lion's mane powder (optional; see Tip)

1. In a high-speed blender, add the hot water, almond milk, coconut butter, maple syrup, matcha, MCT oil, rhodiola powder (if using), and lion's main powder, if using. Cover the blender lid with a clean kitchen towel and blend until smooth. Pour into mugs.

Tips 1. Before you start taking adaptogens such as rhodiola or lion's mane, please check with your doctor to see if they will affect any medications you are on. Do not take them if you are pregnant or nursing.

2. MCT oil is a purified oil that consists of medium-chain triglycerides. It gives a little boost of energy, and some feel it may support feelings of mental clarity. You can find it in the supplement or natural food section of your supermarket. You can also omit it if you like.

FODMAP Note At the time of writing, coconut butter (manna) has not been tested for FODMAP. However, based on the fact that other forms of coconut are low-FODMAP in larger amounts, I am considering coconut butter (manna) low-FODMAP.

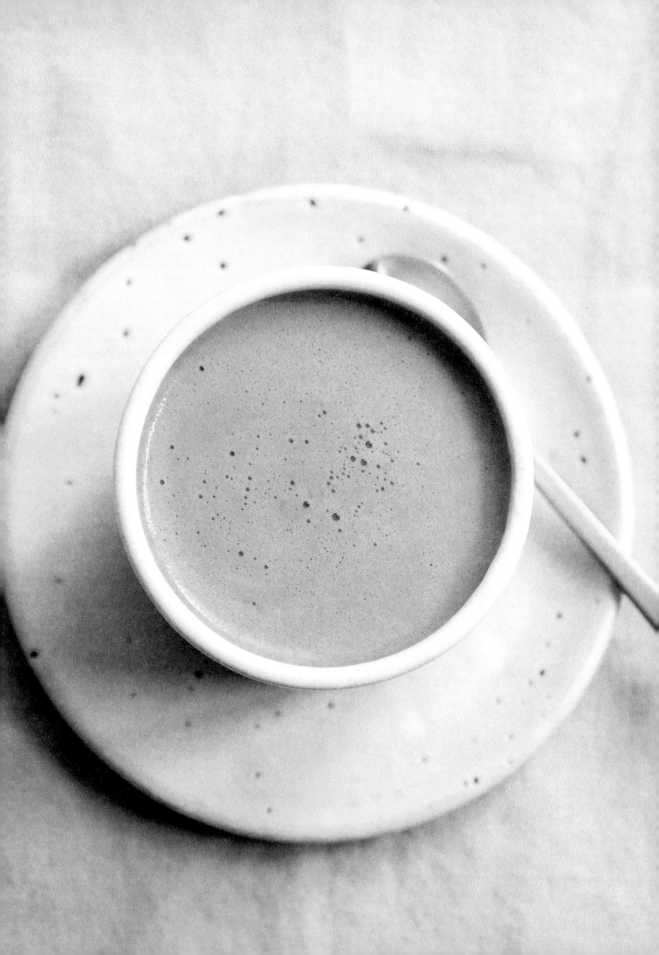

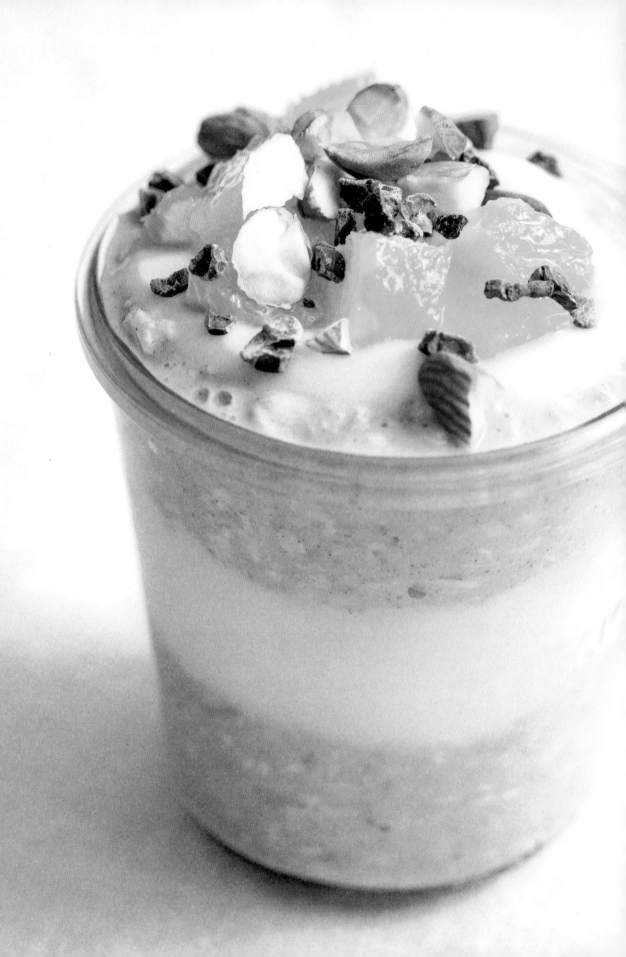

Cinnamon Orange Bircher Serves 2 to 3

It is so satisfying to wake up in the morning knowing that breakfast is ready to go. This sweetly scented Bircher has plenty of soothing soluble fibre from oats and oranges, alongside vitamin C to support the immune system. You can use any of your favourite toppings, but I love pairing cacao nibs with the orange. It is like the health food version of those chocolate oranges I loved as a kid. If you use low-FODMAP yogurt or dairy-free milk, this is a great breakfast treat for those with IBS. But, if you want a richer treat, pair it with my Fermented Cashew Yogurt (page 115).

DAIRY-FREE • GLUTEN-FREE • LOW-FODMAP • VEGAN

1. In a small bowl, stir together the rolled oats, almond milk, orange zest, orange juice, maple syrup, vanilla, cinnamon, ginger, and salt. Cover and store in the fridge overnight. Soaked oats will keep in the fridge for up to 4 days.

2. In the morning, stir in the yogurt to loosen it up, then divide the Bircher among bowls. Top with the chopped orange and your favourite toppings, if using.

1 cup (250 mL) gluten-free old-fashioned rolled oats

½ cup (125 mL) unsweetened almond milk

Zest and juice of 1 orange

1 tablespoon (15 mL) pure maple syrup

½ teaspoon (2 mL) pure vanilla extract

½ teaspoon (2 mL) cinnamon

¼ teaspoon (1 mL) ground ginger

Pinch of salt

FOR SERVING

½ cup (125 mL) coconut yogurt or unsweetened almond milk

1 orange, peeled, white pith removed, and chopped

Slivered almonds, hemp hearts, cacao nibs, or dairy-free dark chocolate chips (optional)

Crunchy Grain-Free Granola Makes about 5 cups (1.25 L), serves 10 to 12

Many store-bought granolas should be labelled as dessert, not breakfast. But not this delicious and healthy granola! Packed with filling fibre and protein, it is crunchy, flavourful, and just sweet enough. If I have an IBS flare, I find that a couple of grain-free weeks can help set me right again. This granola has plenty of anti-inflammatory omega-3 fatty acids as well as zinc to support healing. Enjoy this granola with Fermented Cashew Yogurt (page 115), with your favourite plant milk, or as a topping for a fruit salad.

DAIRY-FREE • GLUTEN-FREE • GRAIN-FREE • HIGH-FODMAP • VEGAN

1 banana

¼ cup (60 mL) extra-virgin olive oil

¼ cup (60 mL) pure maple syrup

1 teaspoon (5 mL) pure vanilla extract

1 teaspoon (5 mL) cinnamon

1 teaspoon (5 mL) ground turmeric

¼ teaspoon (1 mL) salt

1½ cups (375 mL) raw almonds, chopped

1 cup (250 mL) raw pumpkin seeds

1 cup (250 mL) uncooked millet

½ cup (125 mL) hemp hearts

½ cup (125 mL) dried cherries, apricots, or cranberries

1 tablespoon (15 mL) ground flaxseed

1. Preheat the oven to 325°F (160°C). Line a baking sheet with parchment paper.

2. In a large bowl, mash the banana. Whisk in the olive oil, maple syrup, vanilla, cinnamon, turmeric, and salt until well blended.

3. Add the almonds, pumpkin seeds, millet, hemp hearts, dried cherries, and flaxseed and stir to combine. Spread the mixture evenly onto the prepared baking sheet. Bake until the millet is super crunchy, 30 to 35 minutes. Stir every 10 minutes throughout baking. Let the granola cool completely on the baking sheet. The granola will continue to crisp as it cools. Store in an airtight container on the counter for up to 3 weeks.

Tip How can a grain-free granola contain millet? Millet is actually a seed and not a grain. If you are following a paleo plan that does not include millet, you can swap it for more nuts or another seed like pumpkin seed. However, the granola will not be as crunchy.

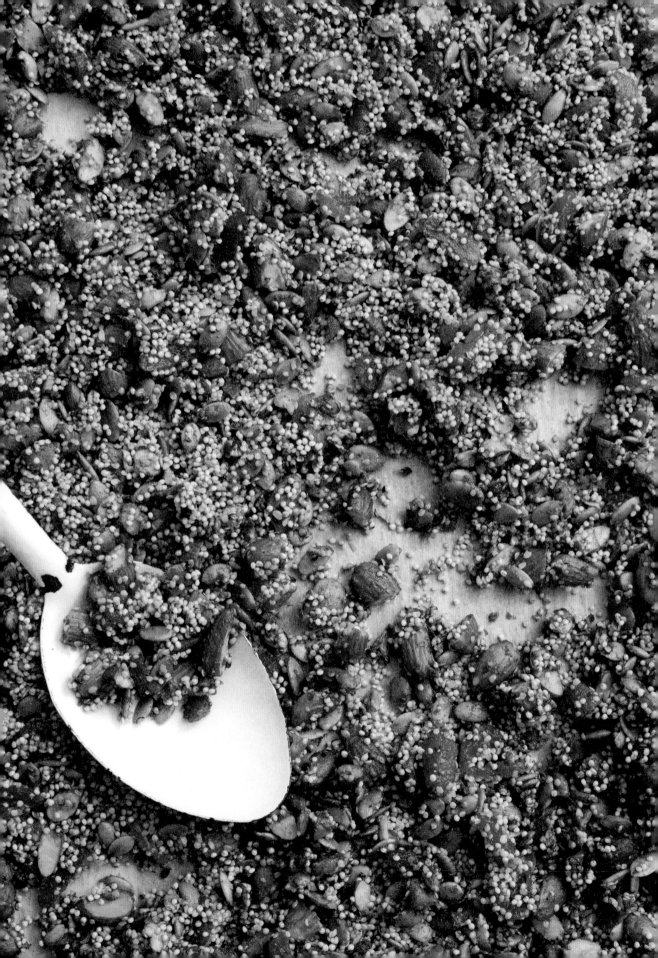

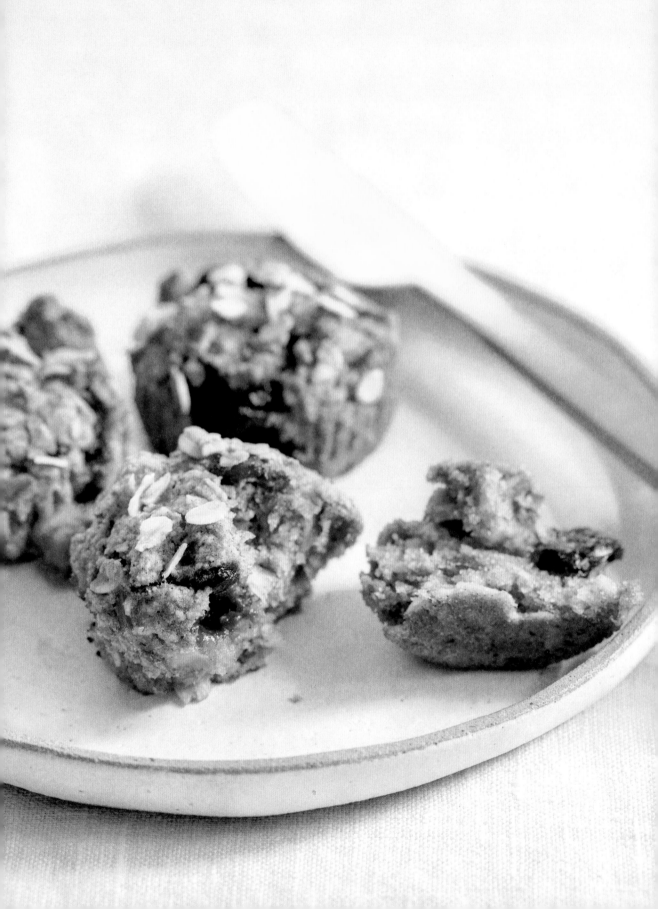

Cherry Almond Muffins Makes 12 muffins

My kids gobble up these muffins, which is saying a lot because they don't usually eat the muffins I bake. These gluten-free muffins have a soft crumb and look like a white flour muffin. They're so delicious, no one will ever know they're quite low in sugar and packed with healthy soluble fibre and plant-based protein. Cherries, almonds, and cardamom are a match made in heaven. Perfect for a light on-the-go breakfast or an afternoon pick-me-up.

DAIRY-FREE • GLUTEN-FREE • HIGH-FODMAP • VEGAN

1. Preheat the oven to 350°F (180°C). Line a 12-cup muffin tin with paper liners.

2. In a medium bowl, whisk together the rolled oats, almond flour, all-purpose flour, baking powder, cinnamon, baking soda, cardamom, and salt.

3. In a small bowl, stir together the applesauce, maple syrup, coconut oil, almond milk, lemon juice, and vanilla. Add the wet ingredients to the dry ingredients and stir to blend well. Fold in the cherries and almonds. Fill each muffin cup with ⅓ cup (75 mL) of batter. Bake until a toothpick inserted in the middle of a muffin comes out clean and the edges are golden, 27 to 28 minutes. Let the muffins cool in the pan for 10 minutes, then turn out onto a rack to cool completely. Store loosely covered on the counter for up to 4 days or in an airtight container in the freezer for up to 1 month.

1¼ cups (300 mL) gluten-free old-fashioned rolled oats

½ cup (125 mL) almond flour

½ cup (125 mL) gluten-free all-purpose flour

1 teaspoon (5 mL) baking powder

1 teaspoon (5 mL) cinnamon

½ teaspoon (2 mL) baking soda

½ teaspoon (2 mL) cardamom

¼ teaspoon (1 mL) salt

½ cup (125 mL) unsweetened applesauce

⅓ cup (75 mL) pure maple syrup

⅓ cup (75 mL) refined coconut oil, melted

2 tablespoons (30 mL) unsweetened almond milk

1 tablespoon (15 mL) freshly squeezed lemon juice

1 teaspoon (5 mL) pure vanilla extract

1 cup (250 mL) fresh or frozen pitted cherries, quartered

¼ cup (60 mL) raw almonds, chopped

Calming Rose Smoothie Serves 2

Do you want more calm in your life? Consider this smoothie your little oasis in a hectic morning. This delicately scented smoothie features rosewater to soothe frazzled nerves, along with easy-to-digest banana and ground psyllium to soothe and regulate an irritated gut. Hemp hearts are high in calming magnesium and give you your daily intake of omega-3 fatty acids. As delicate and easy-drinking as this smoothie is, it still provides anti-inflammatory phytochemicals and fibre from raspberries—a whopping 8 grams per cup.

DAIRY-FREE • GLUTEN-FREE • GRAIN-FREE • NUT-FREE • VEGAN

2½ cups (625 mL) water

1 frozen banana

2 cups (500 mL) frozen raspberries

¼ cup (60 mL) hemp hearts

2 tablespoons (30 mL) rosewater
(see Tip)

1 tablespoon (15 mL) pure maple syrup

2 teaspoons (10 mL) psyllium husk
(or 4 teaspoons/20 mL ground
flaxseed)

1. Place the water, banana, raspberries, hemp hearts, rosewater, maple syrup, and psyllium into a high-speed blender. Blend until smooth and pour into glasses.

Tip The strength of rosewater varies. I usually purchase Lebanese rosewater that has a water-like consistency and mild flavour. If you have a more concentrated variety, start with just 1 or 2 teaspoons (5 or 10 mL). You can also leave out the rosewater or replace it with 1 teaspoon (5 mL) pure vanilla extract.

Chocolate Cherry Rebuilder Smoothie Serves 1

This chocolate cherry delight is a delicious way to start your day—and it is designed with an irritated gut in mind. Anti-inflammatory polyphenols from cherries and cacao help lessen markers of inflammation. Zinc, from hemp hearts, chickpeas, and cacao, is a critical mineral for both your gut cells and immune system. Fermentable soluble fibres from cherries and chickpeas help boost your gut microbiota. I swear you will not taste the chickpeas!

DAIRY-FREE • GLUTEN-FREE • GRAIN-FREE • HIGH-FODMAP • NUT-FREE • VEGAN

1 cup (250 mL) water

1 to 2 pitted Medjool dates, depending
on desired sweetness (see Tip)

1 cup (250 mL) fresh or frozen pitted
cherries

⅓ cup (75 mL) cooked chickpeas

2 tablespoons (30 mL) hemp hearts

1 tablespoon (15 mL) raw cacao powder
or cocoa powder

1 teaspoon (5 mL) pure vanilla extract

2 to 3 ice cubes
(optional; to make it frostier)

1. Place the water, dates, cherries, chickpeas, hemp hearts, cacao powder, vanilla, and ice cubes (if using) into a high-speed blender. Blend until smooth and pour into a glass.

Tip Medjool dates are large, soft, caramel-like dates. If using another kind of date, like Deglet Noor, use 2 for each Medjool date. Soak in hot water for 10 minutes to soften and improve blending.

Green Smoothie Serves 2

This smoothie has it all: nutrient-dense greens, anti-inflammatory omega-3 fatty acids, and tummy-soothing and fermentable soluble fibre to boost beneficial bacteria in the gut. Oh, and it tastes good! This is an easy-to-drink smoothie that makes it easy to get more vegetables into your morning routine. If you need extra gut support, try adding 2 teaspoons (10 mL) of gut-regulating psyllium husk to the mix along with ¼ cup (60 mL) water.

DAIRY-FREE • GLUTEN-FREE • GRAIN-FREE • NUT-FREE • VEGAN

1. Place the water, banana, apple, zucchini, lemon, kale, cilantro, hemp hearts, and ice cubes into a high-speed blender. Blend until smooth and pour into glasses.

Tip To enjoy this smoothie as a meal, increase the protein by either doubling the hemp hearts (10 g protein per 3-tablespoon/45 mL serving) or adding a scoop of your favourite plant-based protein powder.

FODMAP Note For a low-FODMAP smoothie, swap 2 medium navel oranges, peeled, for the banana and apple. Serves 2.

1¼ cups (300 mL) water

1 small frozen banana

1 small apple, quartered and seeded

3-inch (8 cm) piece of zucchini

½-inch (1 cm) slice of lemon, skin-on

1 cup (250 mL) packed kale, inner tough rib and stem removed

½ cup (125 mL) lightly packed fresh cilantro

3 tablespoons (45 mL) hemp hearts

3 to 4 ice cubes

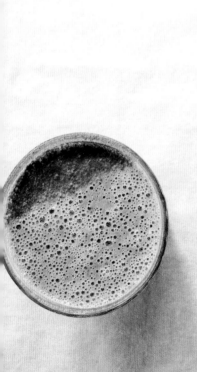
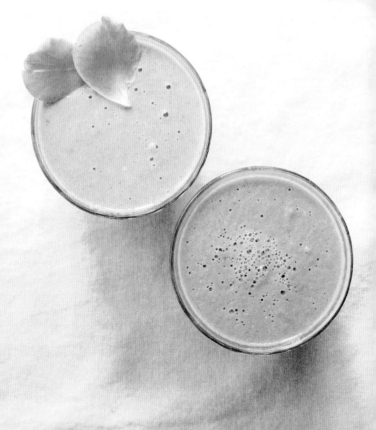

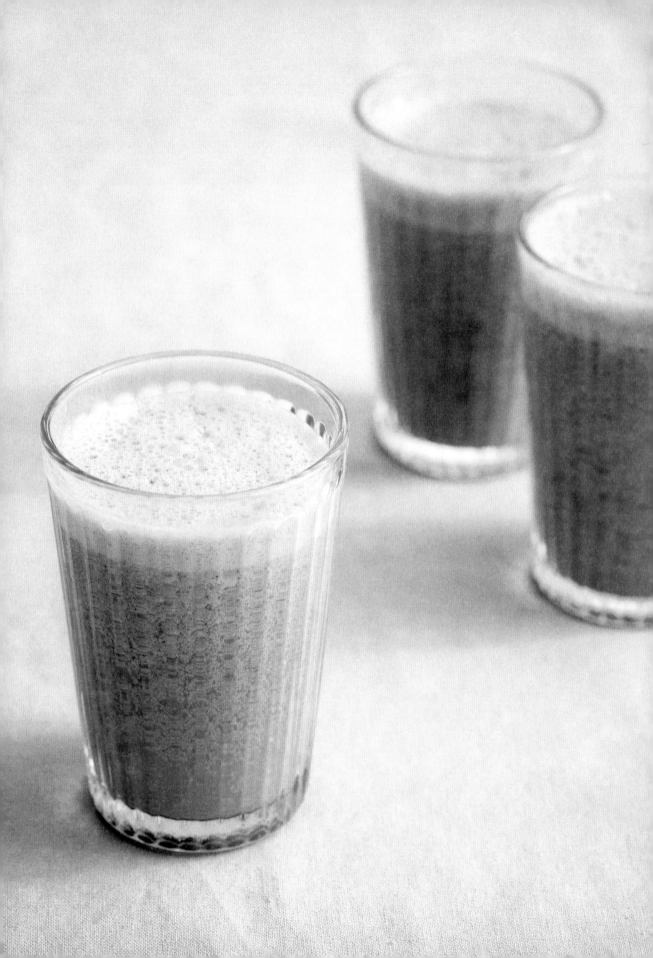

Blackberry Vanilla Hemp Milk Makes about 5 cups (1.25 L)

If you have been skeptical of making your own plant-based milk because you think it is too difficult, then this is the recipe to change your mind. No soaking or straining—just blend to enjoy a tasty milk rich in anti-inflammatory omega-3 fatty acids and more protein than most nut or seed milks. Blackberries are packed with fibre and phytochemicals, which along with the zinc in the hemp hearts make this a perfect beverage for boosting gut health.

DAIRY-FREE • GLUTEN-FREE • NUT-FREE • VEGAN

1. Place the water, blackberries, hemp hearts, maple syrup, vanilla, and salt into a high-speed blender. Blend until liquefied, 1 to 2 minutes. Taste and add more maple syrup if you like your milk a bit sweeter. Store in an airtight container in the fridge for up to 3 days.

Tip Blackberries are high in fibre, so this milk will have some seeds in it. If you prefer a perfectly smooth milk, you can strain it through a nut milk bag before refrigerating. Also, store-bought milk contains stabilizers, but homemade milk doesn't, so it will show signs of separation, which is normal. Shake it before enjoying.

4 cups (1 L) water

1½ cups (375 mL) fresh or thawed frozen blackberries (see Tip)

½ cup (125 mL) hemp hearts

2 tablespoons (30 mL) pure maple syrup, more as desired

1 tablespoon (15 mL) pure vanilla extract

Pinch of salt

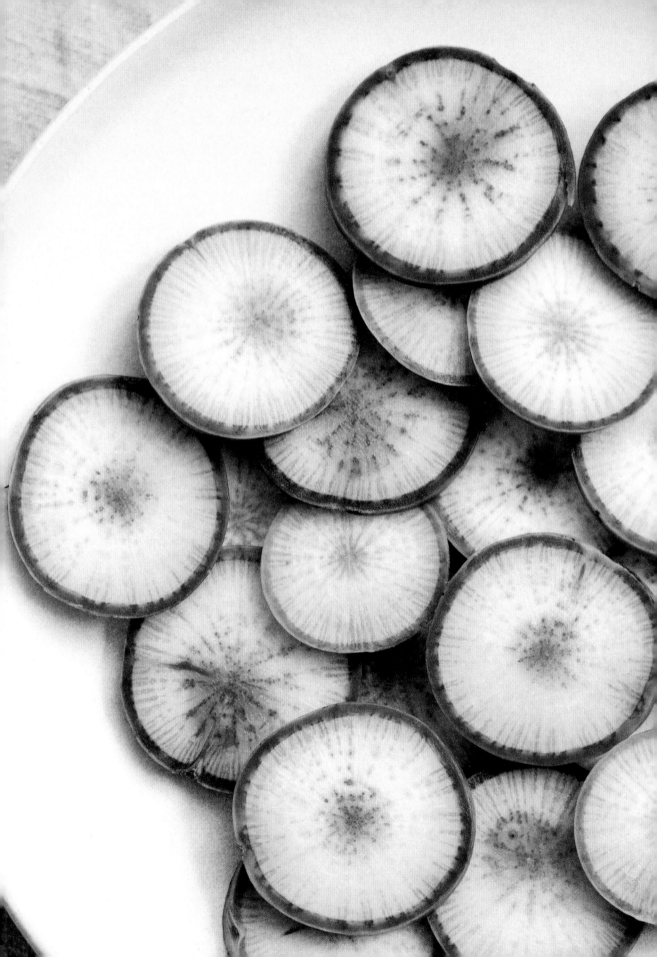

Quick and Simple Meals

Chickpea Shakshuka Serves 4

Everyone loves shakshuka. Hailing from North Africa and popular throughout the Middle East, shakshuka is a simple and flavourful meal of a rich tomato sauce with red peppers. It's often eaten with eggs as a breakfast, and the addition of chickpeas in this recipe makes it as filling as the original. This dish is loaded with spices—each with its own gut-calming benefits. I will happily eat this any time of day with a thick piece of sourdough toast.

DAIRY-FREE • GLUTEN-FREE OPTION • HIGH-FODMAP • NUT-FREE • VEGAN

2 tablespoons (30 mL) extra-virgin olive oil

1 large yellow onion, thinly sliced into half moons (I use a mandoline)

2 sweet red peppers, thinly sliced

4 cloves garlic, chopped

2 cans (14 ounces/398 mL each) chickpeas, drained and rinsed

1 tablespoon (15 mL) sweet paprika

1½ teaspoons (7 mL) ground cumin

1½ teaspoons (7 mL) dried oregano

1 teaspoon (5 mL) ground coriander

1 teaspoon (5 mL) salt

¼ teaspoon (1 mL) cardamom

Freshly cracked black pepper

Pinch of red chili flakes

1 can (28 ounces/796 mL) whole plum tomatoes

Freshly squeezed lemon juice, to taste

½ cup (125 mL) pitted Kalamata olives, chopped

½ cup (125 mL) fresh cilantro, chopped

FOR SERVING

Your favourite gluten-free or sourdough bread, toasted

1. In a large skillet or cast iron frying pan, heat the olive oil over medium-high heat. Add the onion and red peppers. Cook, stirring often, until the onion starts to soften, 5 to 7 minutes.

2. Reduce the heat to medium. Add the garlic and cook, stirring constantly, for 1 minute. Add the chickpeas, paprika, cumin, oregano, coriander, salt, cardamom, pepper, and chili flakes. Stir to combine. Crush the tomatoes with your hands into the skillet. Pour in any remaining juice from the can into the pan and simmer for 10 minutes to allow the flavours to combine. Taste and add lemon juice (I use 1 tablespoon/15 mL) to brighten the flavour. Stir in the olives. Ladle in bowls and top with the cilantro. Serve with your favourite toast.

Tip For gluten-free option, use gluten-free bread.

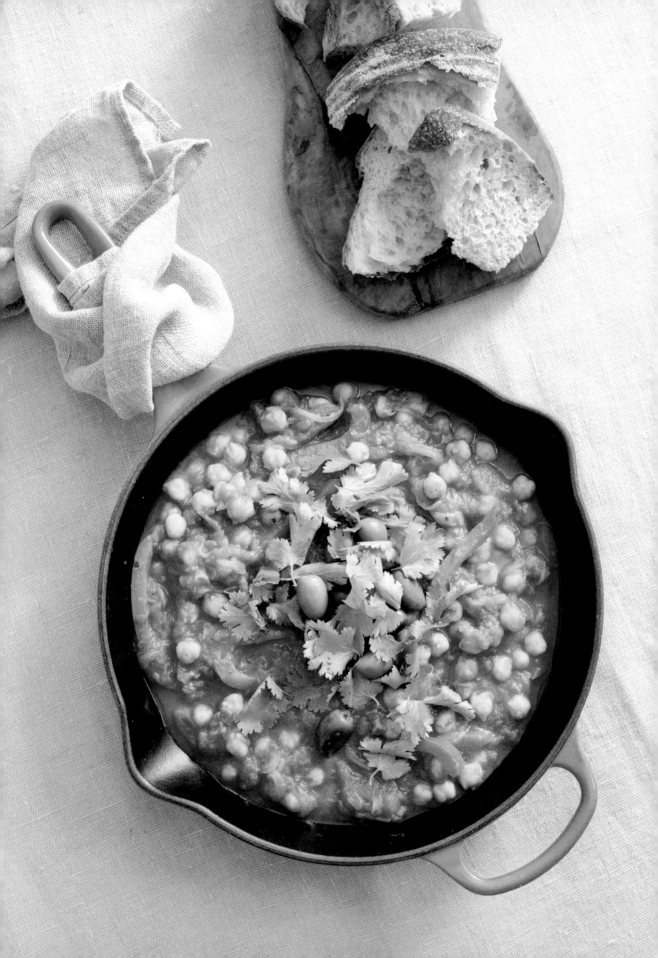

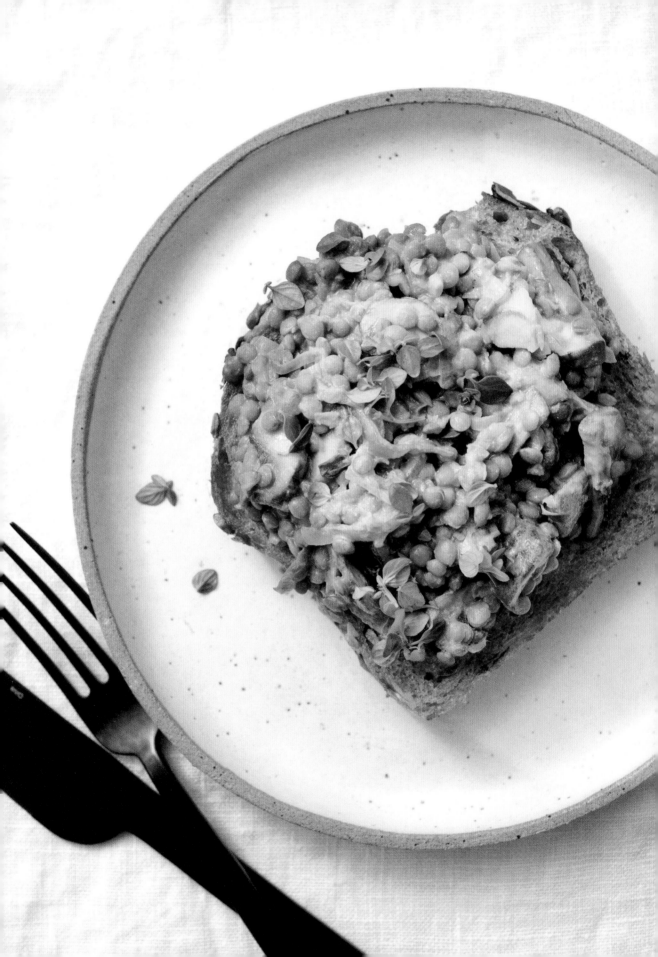

Creamy Mushroom Lentil Toast Makes 4 toasts

Stuff on toast is my life. Although all too often, what I'm piling on toast is leftovers! So I really enjoy dreaming up comforting meals that are custom-built for lavishing over a piece of toast. This is my version of a classic mushroom toast, bolstered by high-fibre lentils to boost plant-based protein and a host of minerals like zinc for gut health. It is creamy, savoury, and lemony. You could eat two pieces of toast for a filling, standalone meal or you could serve one toast with my Blistered Dijon Green Beans with Almonds (page 248) for an extra hit of green.

DAIRY-FREE • GLUTEN-FREE OPTION • HIGH-FODMAP • NUT-FREE • VEGAN

1. Preheat the oven to 200°F (100°C). Line a baking sheet with parchment paper.

2. Cut the garlic clove in half and gently rub each side of the bread with the garlic halves.

3. In a large skillet, heat 1 tablespoon (15 mL) of the olive oil over medium heat. Place the bread slices in the pan and fry until golden brown on the bottom, 1 to 2 minutes per side. You might need to fry the bread in batches. Sprinkle some flaky sea salt on the toast. Place the toast onto the prepared baking sheet and keep warm in the oven.

4. In the same skillet, heat the remaining 2 tablespoons (30 mL) olive oil over medium heat. Add the mushrooms and shallot. Cook, stirring occasionally, until water releases from the mushrooms and they start to brown, 7 to 9 minutes. Season with salt and pepper. Add the tamari and stir for 30 seconds, scraping up the brown bits from the bottom of the pan.

5. Reduce the heat to medium-low and add the lentils, soy milk, nutritional yeast, thyme, onion powder, and season with more salt, if needed. Cook until the lentils look creamy and most of the liquid is absorbed, 5 to 7 minutes. Remove from the heat, then stir in the lemon zest and vegan butter. Taste and adjust the salt and pepper, if needed. Top the slices of toast with the mushroom and lentil mixture. Store the mushroom and lentil mixture separately in an airtight container in the fridge for up to 4 days. Reheat with 1 tablespoon (15 mL) of water.

Tip For gluten-free option, use gluten-free bread.

1 clove garlic

4 slices of your favourite sprouted-grain, gluten-free, or whole-grain sourdough bread

3 tablespoons (45 mL) extra-virgin olive oil or avocado oil, divided

Flaky sea salt

½ pound (225 g) cremini mushrooms, sliced

1 medium shallot, halved and thinly sliced

½ teaspoon (2 mL) salt, plus more for seasoning

Freshly cracked black pepper

2 tablespoons (30 mL) gluten-free tamari

2 cups (500 mL) cooked brown or green lentils

½ cup (125 mL) unsweetened soy or oat milk

2 tablespoons (30 mL) nutritional yeast

1 tablespoon (15 mL) fresh thyme leaves

½ teaspoon (2 mL) onion powder

Zest of ½ lemon

1 tablespoon (15 mL) vegan butter

PROTECT

Chickpea Umami Burgers Makes 6 burgers

I turned to the power of umami to make what I think are my most delicious burgers yet. The word umami in Japanese roughly translates to "savoury deliciousness," which comes from a few amino acids naturally found in foods like sun-dried tomatoes, garlic, and soy sauce. Omega-3 fatty acids in walnuts and flaxseed help fight inflammation, while soluble fibre from beans and oats help regulate digestion and support beneficial bacteria in the gut. These soft, squishy, flavourful burgers are sure to be a hit with the family.

DAIRY-FREE • GLUTEN-FREE • HIGH-FODMAP • VEGAN

2 cups (500 mL) tightly packed
baby spinach

1 medium shallot, roughly chopped

½ cup (125 mL) raw walnuts

⅓ cup (75 mL) sun-dried tomatoes in oil,
drained and patted dry

2 cans (14 ounces/398 mL each) no-salt-
added chickpeas (or 3 cups/750 mL
cooked chickpeas)

½ cup (125 mL) gluten-free old-fashioned
rolled oats

2 tablespoons (30 mL) nutritional yeast

2 tablespoons (30 mL) ground flaxseed

1 teaspoon (5 mL) ground cumin

1 teaspoon (5 mL) garlic powder

¾ teaspoon (3 mL) salt

½ teaspoon (2 mL) onion powder

2 tablespoons (30 mL) water, more
if needed

3 tablespoons (45 mL) extra-virgin
olive oil, divided

1 tablespoon (15 mL) gluten-free tamari

Zest of ½ lemon

FOR SERVING (OPTIONAL)

Gluten-free buns

Spring salad mix

Vegan mayonnaise

Olive tapenade

1. Place the spinach in a colander over the sink. Slowly pour boiling water over the spinach to wilt it. Let sit to cool.

2. In a food processor, add the shallot, walnuts, and sun-dried tomatoes. Pulse until finely chopped. Add the chickpeas, rolled oats, nutritional yeast, flaxseed, cumin, garlic powder, salt, onion powder, water, 2 tablespoons (30 mL) of the olive oil, tamari, and lemon zest. Carefully squeeze all of the excess water from the spinach and add to the food processor. Pulse until about half the mixture looks like a paste, but you can still see plenty of distinct ingredients. You should be able to form a nice patty with ease. If the mixture is crumbly, pulse a bit more or add 1 to 2 tablespoons (15 to 30 mL) water, a bit at a time.

3. In a large nonstick skillet, heat the remaining 1 tablespoon (15 mL) olive oil over medium heat. Place the burgers in the pan and cook until a golden brown crust forms on the bottom, 3 to 4 minutes. Carefully flip and cook for another 3 to 4 minutes. The burgers will be soft and pleasantly squishy when warm, but they will firm up as they cool.

4. Serve the burgers with or without buns, layered with greens, a bit of vegan mayonnaise, and some olive tapenade, if using.

Tip If you want a more traditional, firmer burger texture, add ⅓ cup (75 mL) gluten-free bread crumbs. These burgers can be made ahead and refrigerated for up to 24 hours before cooking.

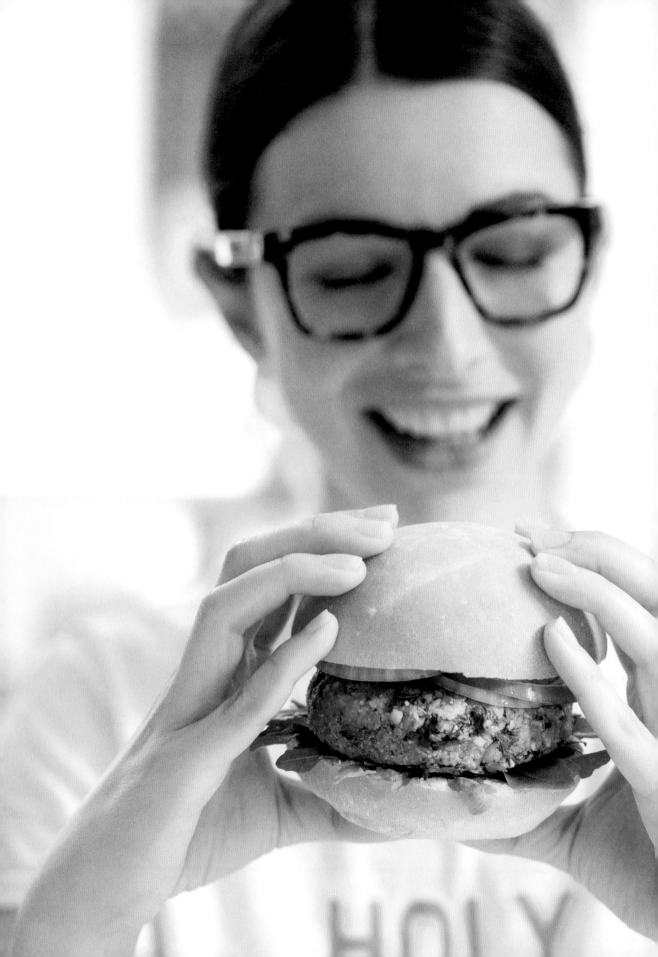

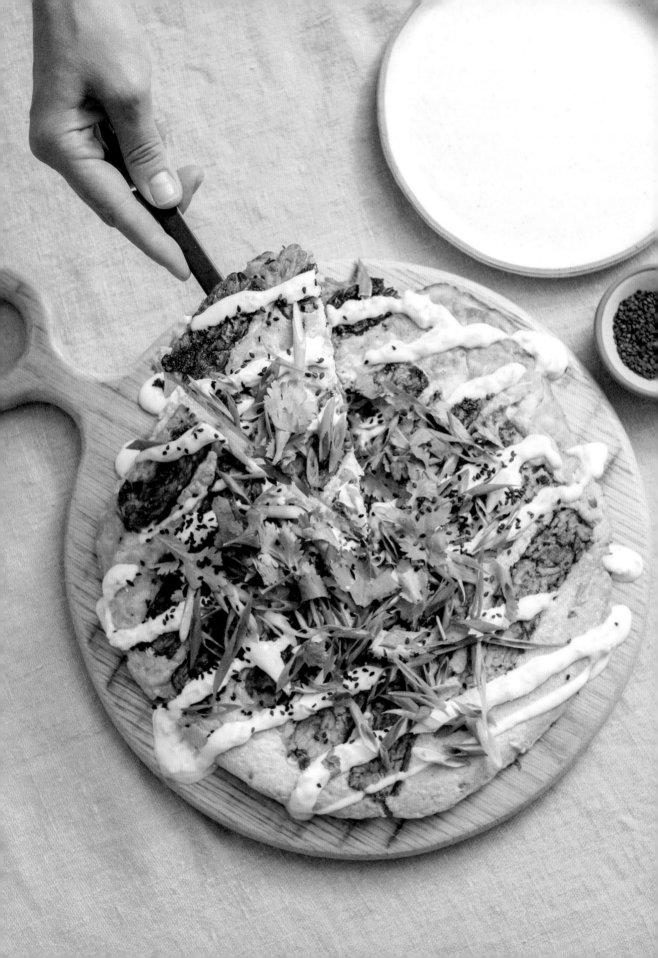

Tofu Okonomiyaki Serves 4

Okonomiyaki (pronounced oak-oh-no-mi-yaki) is a type of veggie- and protein-filled savoury pancake—the name literally means "whatever you want, grilled." I ate okonomiyaki for the first time in Osaka, Japan, at a restaurant where you can order your favourite fillings off the menu and grill it yourself at your table. This, of course, is a non-traditional version made with chickpea flour instead of eggs and topped with smoked tofu, inspired by a recipe from *Chatelaine* magazine I have made dozens of times over the years. It has so many gut-friendly foods on deck: fermented miso, glutamine-rich cabbage, and pickled ginger. It is a simple and satisfying main dish and is perfect served as a side salad.

DAIRY-FREE • GLUTEN-FREE • GRAIN-FREE • HIGH-FODMAP • NUT-FREE • VEGAN

1. **Make the ginger mayonnaise:** In a small bowl, mix together the vegan mayonnaise, pickled ginger, and pickled ginger juice. Set aside.

2. **Make the tofu okonomiyaki:** In a medium bowl, whisk together the chickpea flour, water, and salt. Stir in the cabbage and green onions. Let sit.

3. Cut the tofu into ¼-inch (5 mm) slices. In a small bowl, mix together the sesame oil and miso. Rub both sides of the tofu with the miso mixture.

4. In a medium nonstick skillet or cast iron frying pan, heat the avocado oil over medium heat. Place the tofu slices in the pan and cook until browned, about 3 minutes. Flip the tofu, then pour the chickpea mixture overtop. Cook for 3 minutes more to brown the tofu. Reduce the heat to medium-low, cover with a lid, and steam the okonomiyaki until set on the bottom, 3 to 4 minutes. Place a plate over the pan and flip the okonomiyaki onto a large plate. Carefully slide the okonomiyaki back into the pan, increase the heat to medium, and cook until golden brown on the bottom, 4 to 5 minutes. Cut into quarters and serve with a dollop of ginger mayonnaise overtop.

GINGER MAYONNAISE

⅓ cup (75 mL) vegan mayonnaise

¼ cup (60 mL) pickled ginger, minced

1 tablespoon (15 mL) pickled ginger juice

TOFU OKONOMIYAKI

1½ cups (375 mL) chickpea flour

1¼ cups (300 mL) water

1 teaspoon (5 mL) salt

2 cups (500 mL) finely shredded cabbage or coleslaw mix

3 green onions, thinly sliced

1 package (8 ounces/225 g) smoked tofu or tempeh

1 tablespoon (15 mL) sesame oil

1 tablespoon (15 mL) white miso

1 tablespoon (15 mL) avocado oil

Zucchini Cacio e Pepe Pasta with Pan-Fried Oyster Mushrooms Serves 3 to 4

This dish is inspired by Chef Matthew Kenney's delicious Kelp Noodle Cacio e Pepe. Cacio e Pepe is a classic Italian sauce traditionally made with Parmesan cheese and pepper that Chef Kenney recreates with cashews. I've substituted zucchini and pine nuts to make an unbelievably delicious low-FODMAP cream sauce that tastes garlicky, cheesy, and utterly craveable. Topped with beta glucan–rich, crispy, fried oyster mushrooms, it is a meal that will make you want to invite people over to share.

DAIRY-FREE • GLUTEN-FREE • LOW-FODMAP • VEGAN

1 package (12 ounces/340 g) gluten-free pasta (see Tip)

¼ cup (60 mL) pine nuts

5 tablespoons (75 mL) avocado oil, divided (see Tip)

1⅓ cups (325 mL) peeled and chopped zucchini (about 1 medium zucchini)

¾ teaspoon (3 mL) salt, divided, plus more for seasoning

½ teaspoon (2 mL) freshly cracked black pepper, plus more for seasoning

2 teaspoons (10 mL) nutritional yeast

1 pound (450 g) oyster mushrooms, trimmed and separated

1 tablespoon (15 mL) fresh thyme leaves

Tips 1. If you are not following a low-FODMAP diet, I highly recommend making this dish with chickpea pasta to provide extra fibre and enough protein to make it a more complete meal.

2. You cannot substitute olive oil in this recipe. The sauce has such a delicate flavour that any bitter notes in olive oil will throw it off.

FODMAP Note Most mushrooms are high-FODMAP, but oyster mushrooms are the exception. If oyster mushrooms are not available and you are following a low-FODMAP diet, do not substitute regular mushrooms. Instead, sauté some kale or another low-FODMAP vegetable to accompany the dish.

1. Bring a large pot of water to a boil. Cook the pasta according to package directions. Drain in a colander, reserving at least ¼ cup (60 mL) of the cooking liquid. Rinse the pasta under cool running water. Return the pasta to the pot off the heat.

2. Heat a medium skillet over medium heat. When hot, reduce the heat to medium-low and add the pine nuts. Toast, stirring often, until the pine nuts are fragrant and golden, 2 to 3 minutes. Transfer the pine nuts to a small food processor (or bullet blender).

3. In the same skillet, heat 1 tablespoon (15 mL) of the avocado oil over medium heat. Add the zucchini and cook, stirring occasionally, until softened, 6 to 7 minutes. If the zucchini is browning too quickly, reduce the heat to medium-low. You want the zucchini soft and golden, not crispy and brown. Season with ¼ teaspoon (1 mL) of the salt and some pepper. Transfer the zucchini into the food processor with the pine nuts. Wipe the pan clean.

4. To the food processor, add 2 tablespoons (30 mL) of the avocado oil, nutritional yeast, the remaining ½ teaspoon (2 mL) salt, and the pepper. Blend until smooth. It will be very thick at this point. Set aside.

5. In the same skillet, heat the remaining 2 tablespoons (30 mL) avocado oil over medium-high heat. Add the mushrooms and fry, shaking the pan occasionally so they don't stick, until golden brown and almost crisp on one side, about 4 minutes. Turn the mushrooms over and fry for 2 minutes more until golden brown. Sprinkle with a generous pinch of salt, more pepper, and the thyme.

6. Add 2 tablespoons (30 mL) of the reserved pasta cooking liquid to the sauce. Mix together to loosen up the sauce. (I like to blend with an immersion blender.) Toss the sauce with the pasta. If the sauce looks too thick, add more pasta cooking liquid, 1 tablespoon (15 mL) at a time, tossing after each addition, until the sauce coats the pasta well but is not runny. To serve, divide the pasta among shallow bowls and top with the mushrooms.

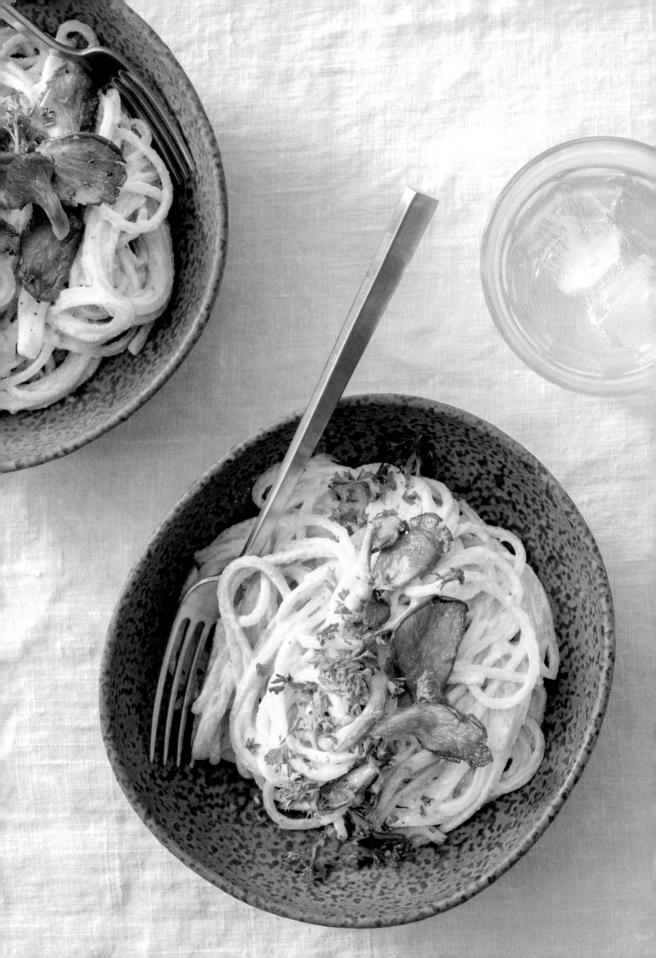

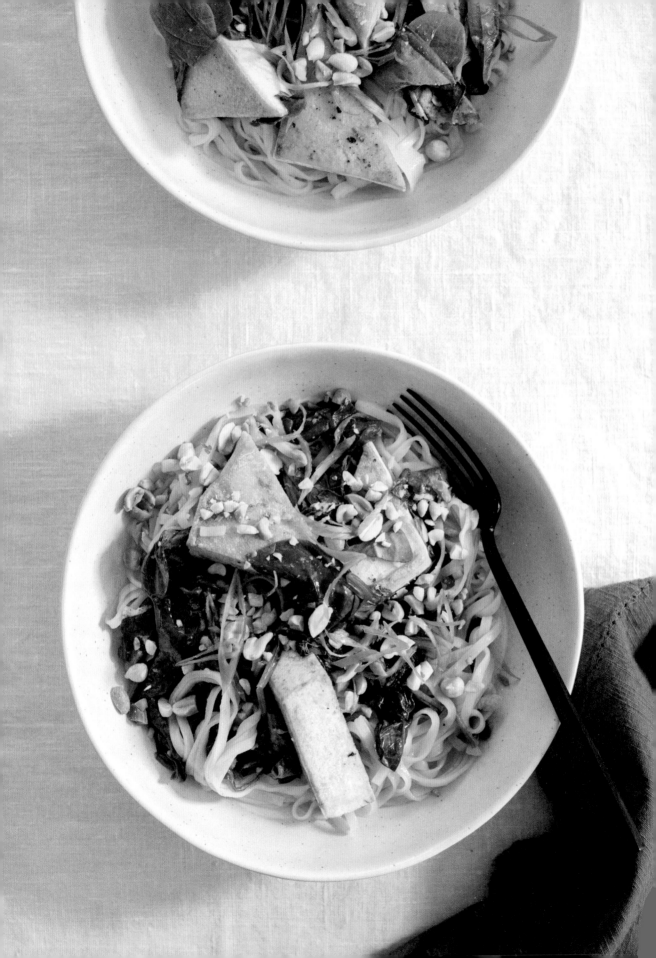

Turmeric-Fried Tofu with Spinach and Rice Noodles Serves 2 to 3

This dish is inspired by a Vietnamese dish called Cha Ca La Vong, which is fish fried in turmeric and served with greens, peanuts, and rice noodles. It really celebrates the earthy, rich flavour of turmeric—no hiding behind a curry powder or coconut milk here! It is a light and easily digestible dinner for irritable tummies, with plenty of immune-supporting protein and anti-inflammatory power from the turmeric and ginger.

DAIRY-FREE • GLUTEN-FREE • LOW-FODMAP • NUT-FREE OPTION • VEGAN

1. In a small shallow bowl, mix together the ginger, avocado oil, lime juice, and turmeric. Season well with salt and pepper.

2. Heat a dry nonstick skillet over medium heat. Dip both sides of the tofu slices in the marinade and place in the pan. Pour the remaining marinade over the tofu. Fry until golden brown on the bottom, 3 to 4 minutes. Turn the tofu over and cook until golden brown, 2 to 3 minutes. Remove from the heat.

3. Meanwhile, in a large pot, cook the rice noodles according to package directions. Drain in a colander and rinse quickly under cool running water.

4. In a small bowl, mix together the tamari, sesame oil, rice vinegar, and Sriracha.

5. Add the cooked rice noodles back to the pot, along with the spinach and tamari-sesame oil mixture. Toss to coat. The heat of the noodles and the pot will wilt the spinach.

6. To serve, divide the noodle mixture among bowls. Top with the tofu and garnish with the green onions and peanuts.

Tip For nut-free option, omit the peanuts or substitute with ¼ cup (60 mL) pumpkin seeds.

1 tablespoon (15 mL) peeled, diced fresh ginger

1 tablespoon (15 mL) avocado or refined coconut oil

1 tablespoon (15 mL) freshly squeezed lime juice

1 teaspoon (5 mL) ground turmeric

Salt and freshly cracked black pepper

1 package (12 ounces/340 g) extra-firm tofu, cut into 12 slices

½ pound (225 g) medium-width dried rice noodles

2 tablespoons (30 mL) gluten-free tamari

2 tablespoons (30 mL) sesame oil

1 tablespoon (15 mL) rice vinegar

1 tablespoon (15 mL) Sriracha sauce

1 package (5 ounces/140 g) baby spinach (about 8 packed cups/2 L)

GARNISHES

2 green onions (green parts only), thinly sliced

½ cup (125 mL) chopped salted peanuts (see Tip)

Kitchari Serves 4

You would not expect a lentil recipe to be low-FODMAP, but rinsed canned lentils are low-FODMAP in a ½-cup (125 mL) serving. I love keeping legumes in a low-FODMAP diet to support long-term gut health. Kitchari is a traditional Ayurvedic porridge of legumes, rice, and vegetables with as many variations as there are cooks. The ingredients list is long only because I have added a lot of anti-inflammatory and digestion-soothing spices here for a flavourful and comforting meal that is perfect when your tummy needs a little calming down. If you do not have all these spices, just use what you have, but make sure it is low-FODMAP.

DAIRY-FREE • GLUTEN-FREE • LOW-FODMAP • NUT-FREE • VEGAN

2 tablespoons (30 mL) avocado or refined coconut oil

1 cup (250 mL) diced carrots

1 cup (250 mL) diced parsnips

1-inch (2.5 cm) piece of fresh ginger, peeled and diced

1 teaspoon (5 mL) coriander seeds

1 teaspoon (5 mL) mustard seeds

1 teaspoon (5 mL) cumin seeds

½ teaspoon (2 mL) fennel seeds

½ teaspoon (2 mL) fenugreek seeds

1 teaspoon (5 mL) ground turmeric

½ teaspoon (2 mL) ground cumin

½ cup (125 mL) uncooked brown basmati rice

3 cups (750 mL) water

1 teaspoon (5 mL) salt

2 cups (500 mL) canned lentils, drained and rinsed

FOR SERVING

Lime

1 cup (250 mL) fresh cilantro leaves, minced

1. In a medium saucepan, heat the avocado oil over medium heat. Add the carrots, parsnips, and ginger. Cook, stirring often, until the vegetables begin to soften, about 3 minutes. Add the coriander seeds, mustard seeds, cumin seeds, fennel seeds, fenugreek seeds, turmeric, and cumin and cook, stirring constantly, for 30 seconds.

2. Add the rice, water, and salt. Bring to a boil, then reduce the heat to medium-low and simmer, covered, for 15 minutes.

3. Add the lentils. Stir, cover with the lid slightly ajar, and cook until the mixture reaches porridge consistency, 15 to 20 minutes. Add a big squeeze of lime; taste and adjust the salt, if needed. Divide among bowls and top with the cilantro. Store any leftovers in an airtight container in the fridge for up to 4 days.

Tip This recipe comes together quickly, so have all your ingredients ready before you start cooking. Measure out the seeds and spices into a small bowl before you begin.

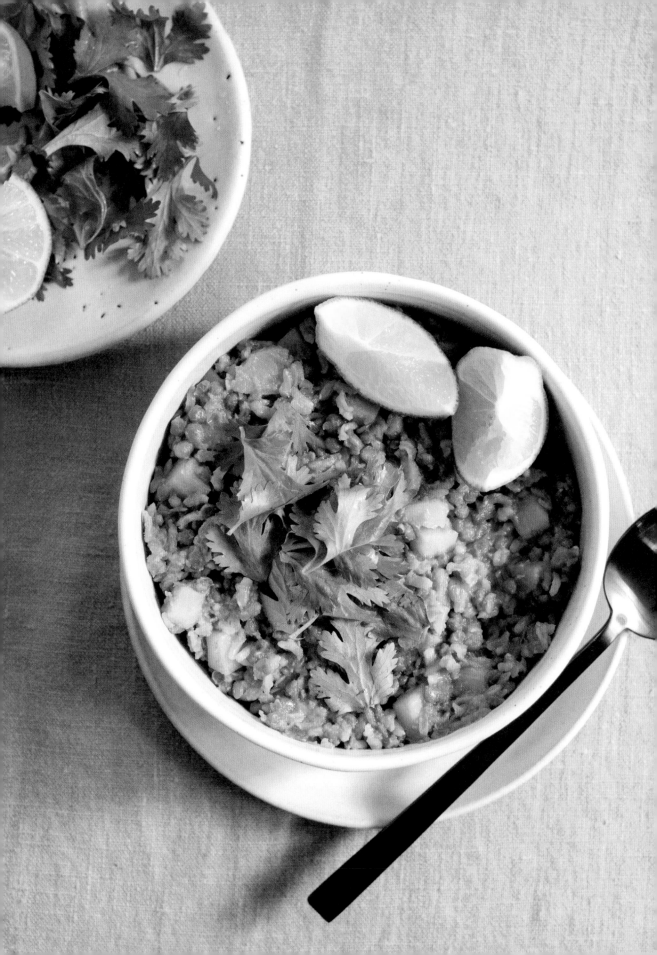

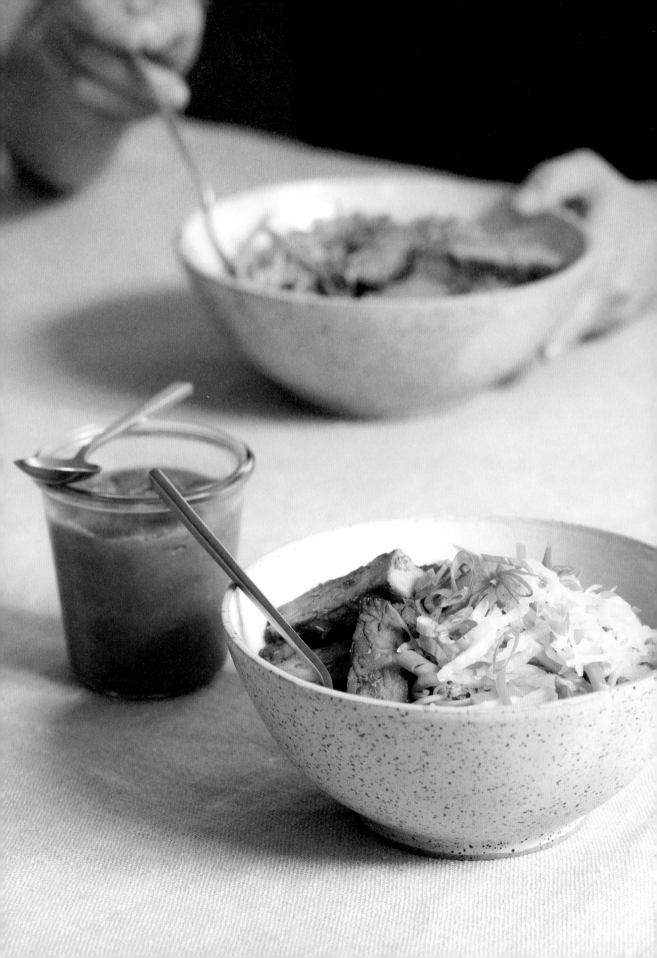

Soba with Napa Cabbage and Peanutty Tempeh Serves 4

Sometimes caring for an irritated gut and feeding the family means making separate meals. But this low-FODMAP dinner is easy on irritated tummies and family-friendly. Napa cabbage is one of those veggies that is easy to get into kids because it wilts down into a noodle dish perfectly. This is a quick weeknight meal that has it all—protein-packed tempeh, filling healthy fats from the peanut butter, and all the veggies. Building flavour into meals without garlic is possible.

DAIRY-FREE • GLUTEN-FREE • LOW-FODMAP • VEGAN

1. Bring a large pot of water to a boil. Cook the soba noodles according to package directions. Drain in a colander and rinse under cool running water. Set aside.

2. In a small bowl, mix together the peanut butter, ¼ cup (60 mL) of the water, rice vinegar, tamari, maple syrup, sesame oil, and hot sauce. Do not worry if it doesn't look mixed, it will come together in the pan.

3. In a large nonstick skillet, heat the coconut oil over medium heat. Place the tempeh in the pan and fry until browned, 3 to 4 minutes per side. Transfer the tempeh to a large plate.

4. In the same skillet over medium heat, add the cabbage, carrots, and remaining ¼ cup (60 mL) water. Cook, stirring frequently, until the cabbage wilts and the carrots are soft, 4 to 5 minutes. Transfer the vegetables to the plate with the tempeh.

5. Add the peanut sauce to the warm pan (off the heat) and gently whisk until the peanut butter melts into the sauce, about 2 minutes. Add the soba noodles, vegetables, and tempeh. Toss with the sauce. Divide among bowls and top with the green onions.

1 package (8 ounces/225 g) pure buckwheat soba noodles or gluten-free spaghetti

½ cup (125 mL) natural peanut butter

½ cup (125 mL) water, divided

¼ cup (60 mL) rice vinegar

3 tablespoons (45 mL) gluten-free tamari

2 tablespoons (30 mL) pure maple syrup

1 tablespoon (15 mL) sesame oil

1 tablespoon (15 mL) hot sauce

1 tablespoon (15 mL) coconut or avocado oil

1 package (8 ounces/225 g) smoked tempeh, cut in half and sliced

1 pound (450 g) Napa cabbage, chopped

2 medium carrots or parsnips, peeled and grated or cut into matchsticks

4 green onions (dark green parts only), thinly sliced

FODMAP Note If you are not following a low-FODMAP diet, feel free to use standard wheat-containing buckwheat soba noodles if you wish, and try adding ½ clove grated garlic to the sauce.

Roasted Eggplant and Tempeh Tacos with Cumin Lime Mayonnaise Serves 4

Time to shake up your Taco Tuesday. This 30-minute meal has it all—silky, spiced eggplant and earthy, protein-rich tempeh alongside a supporting cast of my favourites. Cilantro packs a surprising amount of good-for-you phytochemicals as well as trace amounts of immune-supportive beta-carotene and balancing potassium. These tacos make a nice, light meal on their own or are delicious served with Kale Salad with Spiced Corn and Jicama (page 208).

DAIRY-FREE • GLUTEN-FREE • LOW-FODMAP • NUT-FREE • VEGAN

ROASTED EGGPLANT AND TEMPEH FILLING

1 medium eggplant, cut into ½-inch (1 cm) cubes

1 teaspoon (5 mL) coarse salt

1 package (8 ounces/225 g) smoked tempeh, cut into ½-inch (1 cm) cubes

2 tablespoons (30 mL) avocado oil

1 teaspoon (5 mL) ground cumin

½ teaspoon (2 mL) ground coriander

¼ teaspoon (1 mL) red chili flakes

¼ teaspoon (1 mL) salt

Freshly cracked black pepper

CUMIN LIME MAYONNAISE

½ cup (125 mL) vegan mayonnaise

2 tablespoons (30 mL) freshly squeezed lime juice

½ teaspoon (2 mL) cumin

⅛ teaspoon (0.5 mL) salt

FOR SERVING

8 small corn tortillas

1 cup (250 mL) lightly packed fresh cilantro

Sliced pickled jalapeño peppers or hot sauce

1 lime, cut into 4 wedges

1. **Make the roasted eggplant and tempeh filling:** Preheat the oven to 375°F (190°C). Line a baking sheet with parchment paper.

2. In a fine-mesh strainer, toss the eggplant with the coarse salt. Set the strainer over a large bowl and let sit for 10 minutes to remove extra moisture. Rinse the eggplant and pat dry with paper towel.

3. In a medium bowl, toss the eggplant and tempeh with the avocado oil, cumin, coriander, chili flakes, salt, and pepper. Evenly spread the mixture on the prepared baking sheet. Be sure not to overcrowd the pan so the eggplant and tempeh roast, not steam. Roast until the eggplant is soft and a bit translucent (it will not brown much), about 25 minutes.

4. **Meanwhile, make the cumin lime mayonnaise:** In a small bowl, mix together the vegan mayonnaise, lime juice, cumin, and salt.

5. In a small skillet over medium-high heat, toast the tortillas, 1 to 2 minutes per side. Alternatively, you can skip warming the tortillas.

6. To serve, spread some cumin lime mayonnaise on each tortilla and top with the eggplant and tempeh mixture, cilantro, and jalapeño peppers. Serve with a lime wedge on the side.

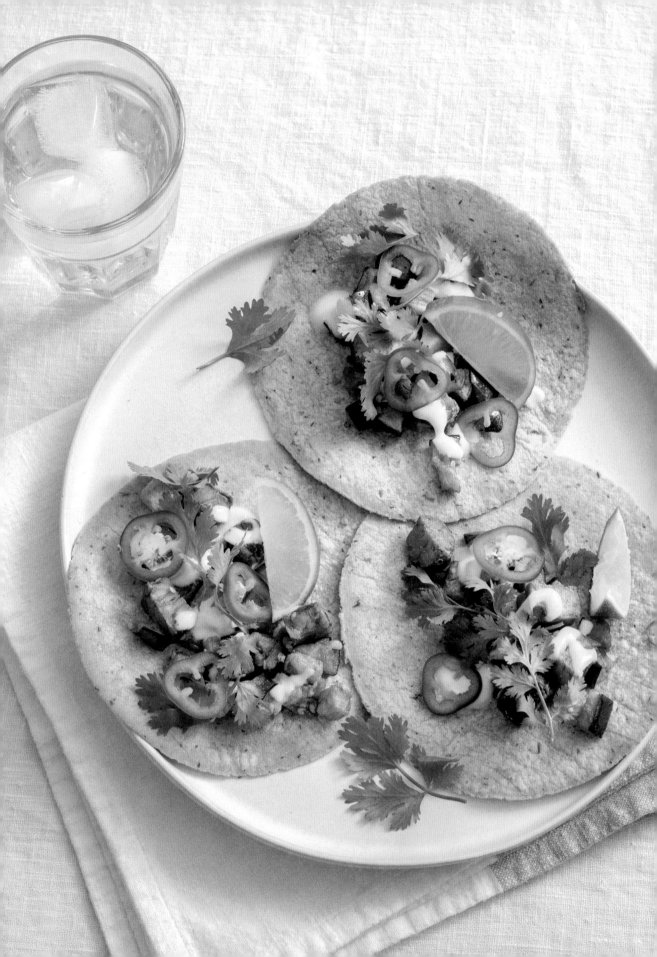

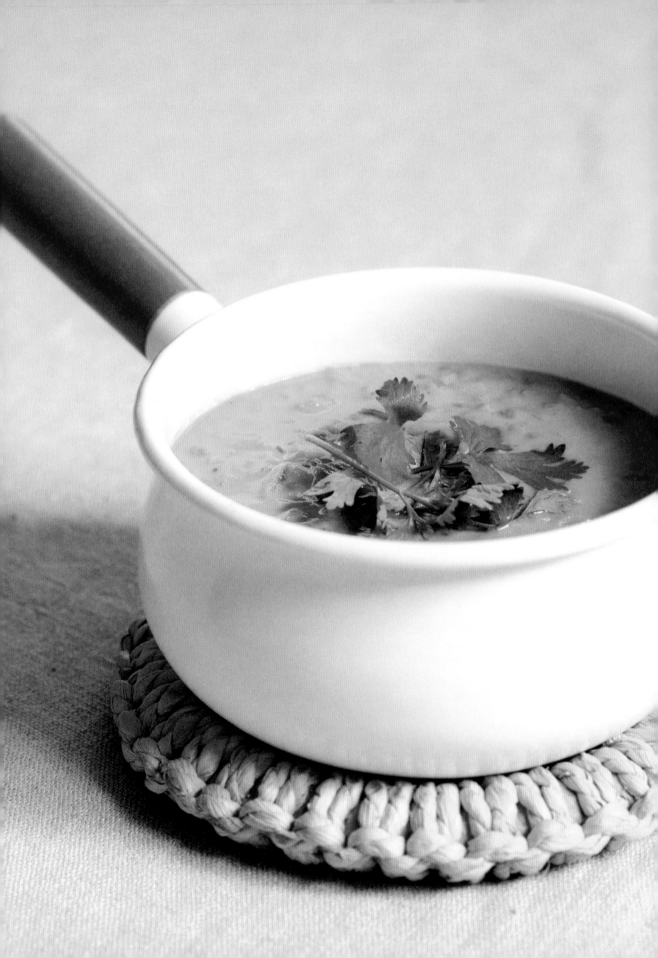

Tomato Coconut and Lentil Curry with Spinach Serves 4 to 6

I am always in the mood for a good curry, and this one is a treat. Richly spiced but not too spicy, the combination of tomatoes, coconut, and lime is umami-packed and sure to please. This flavourful curry is a gentler way to enjoy FODMAP-rich plants to help rebuild your gut. If need be, you can also purée the curry to make it even easier to digest. Served with your favourite grain, this curry is a hearty meal the whole family will enjoy.

DAIRY-FREE • GLUTEN-FREE • LOW-FODMAP OPTION • HIGH-FODMAP • NUT-FREE • VEGAN

1. In a medium pot, heat the coconut oil over medium heat. Add the onion and cook, stirring occasionally, until soft and glossy, 5 to 7 minutes. Add the garlic, curry powder, cumin seeds, coriander seeds, mustard seeds, turmeric, and garam masala. Cook, stirring constantly, until fragrant, 1 minute.

2. Add the lentils, tomatoes, coconut milk, lime peel, and salt. Bring to a boil over high heat. When the mixture is boiling, reduce the heat to medium-low and simmer, uncovered, for 10 minutes to allow the flavours to develop. Stir in the spinach to wilt and add the lime juice. Taste and adjust the salt and lime juice, if desired. Remove the lime peel, and serve with your favourite grain.

FODMAP Note To make this dish low-FODMAP, replace half the coconut milk with water and omit the onion and garlic. Add a pinch of asafetida, if desired.

2 tablespoons (30 mL) refined coconut oil

1 small yellow onion, diced

3 cloves garlic, diced

1 tablespoon (15 mL) curry powder

2 teaspoons (10 mL) cumin seeds

1 teaspoon (5 mL) coriander seeds

1 teaspoon (5 mL) mustard seeds

½ teaspoon (2 mL) ground turmeric

¼ teaspoon (1 mL) garam masala

2 cans (14 ounces/398 mL each) lentils, drained and rinsed

1 can (28 ounces/796 mL) diced tomatoes

2 cups (500 mL) canned full-fat coconut milk

2-inch (5 cm) piece of lime peel, white pith removed

1¼ teaspoons (6 mL) salt

5 ounces (140 g) baby spinach (about 8 packed cups/2 L)

1 to 2 tablespoons (15 to 30 mL) freshly squeezed lime juice

FOR SERVING

Cooked quinoa, millet, or brown rice

Raw Beet Ravioli with Macadamia Pesto Cheese Serves 2

I do not think I am cut out for a fully raw food life, but I do love a beet ravioli. Marinated beets are flavourful and make a bright contrast to the luscious, rich macadamia pesto cheese that is packed with plant power. Herbs are often overlooked as sources of anti-inflammatory phytochemicals—we really need to eat more. This is a very quick and satisfying light meal or appetizer.

DAIRY-FREE • GLUTEN-FREE • GRAIN-FREE • HIGH-FODMAP • VEGAN

MARINATED BEETS

2 large red beets, peeled and very thinly sliced with a mandoline

1 tablespoon (15 mL) avocado oil

1 tablespoon (15 mL) freshly squeezed lemon juice

⅛ teaspoon (0.5 mL) salt

MACADAMIA PESTO CHEESE

½ cup (125 mL) macadamia nuts

¼ cup (60 mL) water

½ cup (125 mL) lightly packed fresh basil

½ cup (125 mL) lightly packed fresh curly parsley, leaves and tender stems

2 tablespoons (30 mL) hemp hearts

1 tablespoon (15 mL) nutritional yeast

1 clove garlic, grated

¼ + ⅛ teaspoon (1.5 mL) salt

2 tablespoons (30 mL) avocado oil

1 tablespoon (15 mL) freshly squeezed lemon juice

1. **Marinate the beets:** Place the sliced beets in a medium bowl. Cover the beets with the avocado oil, lemon juice, and salt. Let marinate while you make the cheese.

2. **Make the macadamia pesto cheese:** In a small food processor, add the macadamia nuts and water. Blitz until the nuts are finely chopped. Add the basil, parsley, hemp hearts, nutritional yeast, garlic, and salt. Pulse until well minced. With the processor running, drizzle in the avocado oil and lemon juice. Taste and adjust the lemon juice and salt, if needed.

3. Depending on the size of the beets, you can either fold 1 tablespoon (15 mL) of the macadamia pesto cheese inside each beet slice or you can make little ravioli sandwiches with 1 tablespoon (15 mL) of cheese between 2 beet slices.

4. Leftover beet and pesto cheese can be stored separately in airtight containers in the fridge for up to 3 days. They are delicious tucked into a sandwich or added to a salad.

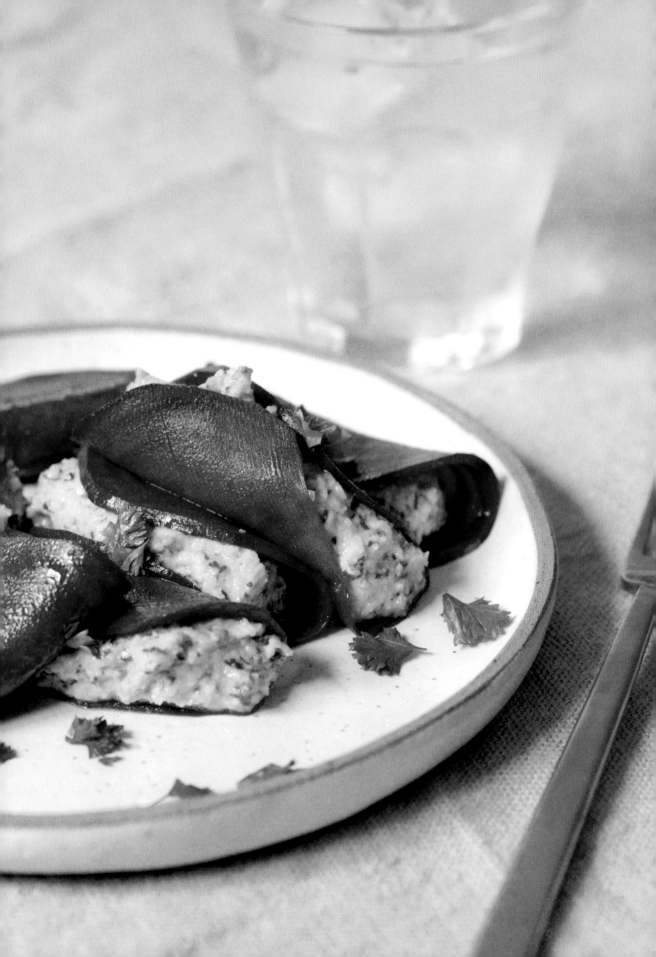

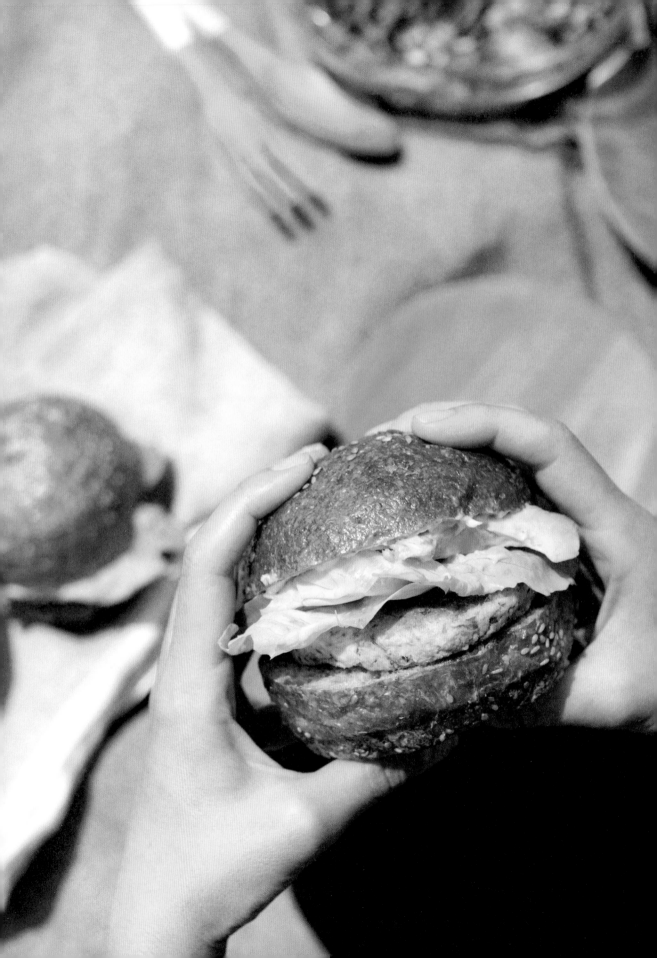

Mediterranean Artichoke Burgers Makes 4 burgers

Nothing beats a delicious plant-based burger that takes less than 20 minutes to make. These Mediterranean artichoke burgers are light, yet satisfying. I could have just as easily called these prebiotic patties for all of the prebiotic FODMAPs in the chickpea flour, artichokes, and garlic, but that does not sound as delicious! They have a vaguely fish burger vibe (without the fish) and are delicious in a bun with roasted potatoes and my Cabbage and Fennel Slaw with Jalapeño Grapefruit Dressing (page 216) or served on top of a salad, like the Kohlrabi Chopped Salad (page 219).

DAIRY-FREE • GLUTEN-FREE OPTION • HIGH-FODMAP • NUT-FREE • VEGAN

1. Squeeze the artichokes to drain excess liquid and place them in a food processor. Add the chickpea flour, parsley, green onions, mustard, lemon zest, garlic, salt, and oregano. Pulse until it looks flaky in texture but starting to come together. Divide the mixture into 4 portions and, using your hands, form into 1-inch (2.5 cm) thick patties.

2. In a large nonstick skillet, add a drizzle of avocado oil and heat over medium heat. Place the patties in the pan and cook until a golden brown crust forms on the bottom, 3 to 4 minutes. Carefully flip (they are soft) and cook for 3 to 4 minutes more. Serve on hamburger buns and with your favourite toppings.

Tip For gluten-free option, use gluten-free hamburger buns.

2 cups (500 mL) canned artichokes, drained and rinsed (about two 14-ounce/398 mL cans)

⅔ cup (150 mL) chickpea flour

½ cup (125 mL) lightly packed fresh curly parsley

2 green onions, chopped

1 tablespoon (15 mL) Dijon mustard

Zest of ½ lemon

1 clove garlic, grated

¾ teaspoon (3 mL) salt

½ teaspoon (2 mL) dried oregano

Avocado oil, for cooking

FOR SERVING

4 gluten-free or whole-grain hamburger buns

Vegan mayonnaise

Dijon mustard

Roasted red peppers

Arugula

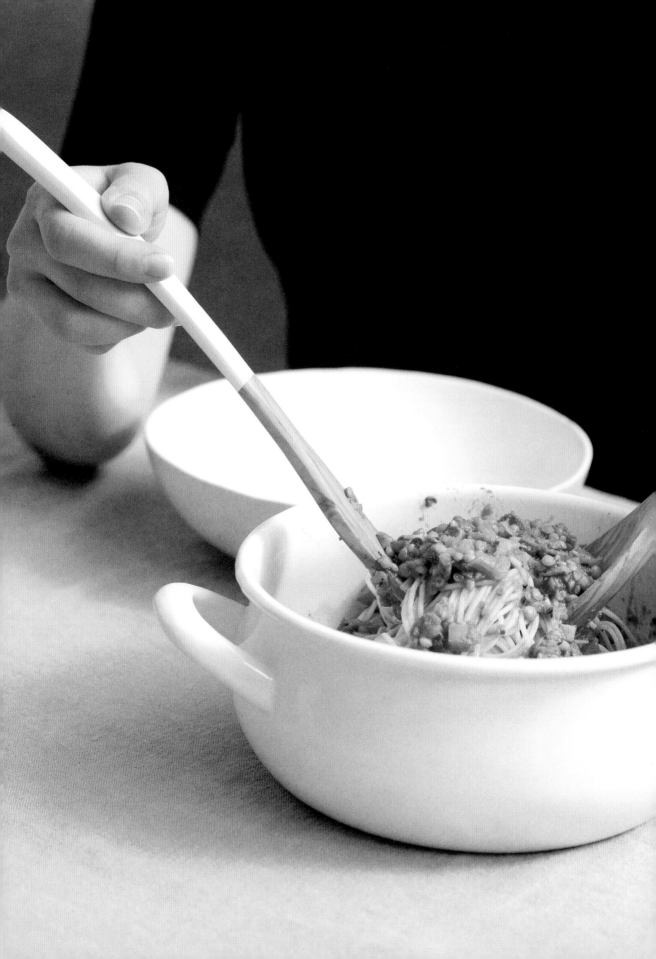

Heartier Meals

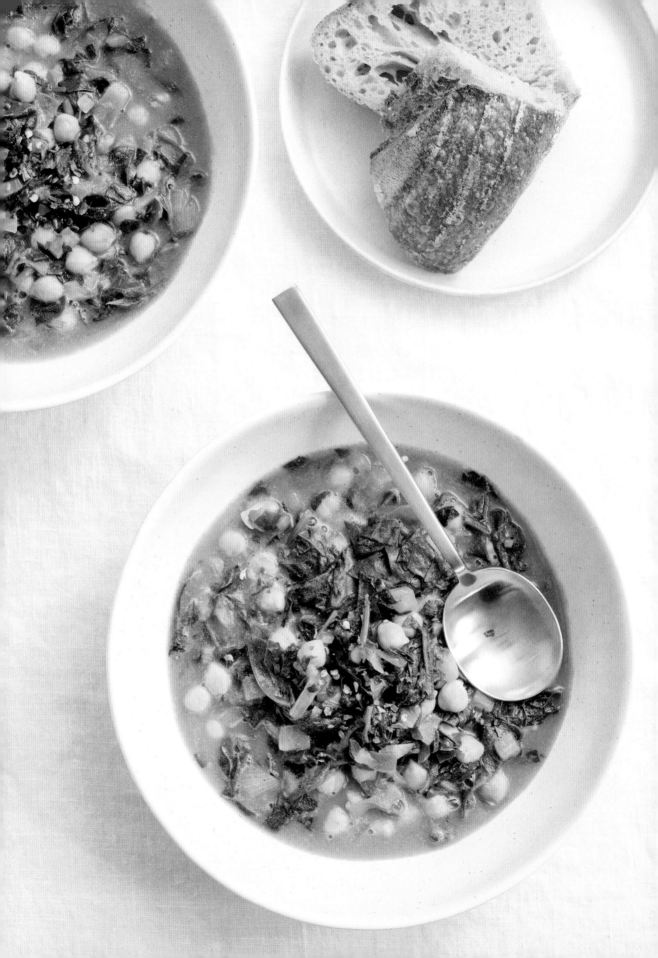

Spanish Chickpea and Spinach Stew Serves 4

This is a variation on a vegetable-forward dish that I came to rely on during a trip to Seville, Spain. It's a delicious stew found in almost every Spanish restaurant, packed with plant-based protein and microbiome-boosting fibre from chickpeas. Typically thickened with picada de pan, a slurry made from fried bread, this stew uses chickpeas and arrowroot powder to create a thick and creamy texture without the gluten. The dish is simple, yet deeply satisfying, and the combination of greens and beans is one of my favourites for keeping my gut happy and inflammation at bay.

DAIRY-FREE • GLUTEN-FREE • GRAIN-FREE • HIGH-FODMAP • NUT-FREE • VEGAN

1. In a large skillet, heat 2 tablespoons (30 mL) of the olive oil over medium heat. Add the whole garlic cloves and cook, stirring often, until fragrant, 2 to 3 minutes. Add ½ cup (125 mL) of the chickpeas, paprika, and cumin and cook, stirring constantly, until fragrant, 1 minute. Remove from the heat.

2. In a small food processor, carefully add the spiced chickpea mixture along with the reserved ½ cup (125 mL) chickpea liquid, arrowroot powder, and ¼ teaspoon (1 mL) of the salt. Purée until smooth. Set aside.

3. In the same skillet, wiped clean, heat the remaining 2 tablespoons (30 mL) olive oil over medium heat. Add the onion and cook, stirring occasionally, until soft and starting to brown, 3 to 4 minutes. Add the remaining chickpeas and tomato. Cook until the tomato juices thicken, about 5 minutes.

4. Add the spinach in 2 batches, stirring until wilted. Season with salt and pepper. Add the vegetable stock, chickpea slurry, and remaining ¾ teaspoon (3 mL) salt. Bring to a boil over high heat. When the mixture reaches a boil, reduce to a simmer over medium-low heat to allow the flavours to blend. Stir in the sherry vinegar and adjust seasoning, if needed.

5. Serve in bowls with bread or your favourite cooked grain, if desired. Store any leftovers in an airtight container in the fridge for up to 4 days.

¼ cup (60 mL) extra-virgin olive oil, divided

4 cloves garlic

2 cans (14 ounces/398 mL each) chickpeas, drained and divided, reserving ½ cup (125 mL) chickpea liquid

1 tablespoon (15 mL) sweet paprika, preferably Spanish

2 teaspoons (10 mL) ground cumin

1 tablespoon (15 mL) arrowroot powder

1 teaspoon (5 mL) salt, divided, plus more for seasoning

1 small yellow onion, diced

1 medium tomato, diced

½ pound (225 g) spinach, roughly chopped (about 8 packed cups/2 L)

Freshly cracked black pepper

2 cups (500 mL) low-sodium vegetable stock

1 tablespoon (15 mL) sherry vinegar, red wine vinegar, or freshly squeezed lemon juice

FOR SERVING (OPTIONAL)

Gluten-free bread

Cooked millet, brown basmati rice, or quinoa

Sunchoke Kale White Bean Gratin Serves 4

This is one of my favourite things to eat: earthy kale with a comforting mix of sunchokes and white beans, lavished with an addictively creamy and flavourful sauce that makes me insanely happy. With a trio of pre-biotic foods—cashews, beans, and sunchokes—this is gut-boosting comfort food at its finest. If you are new to high-FODMAP living, be aware that sunchokes are very high in prebiotic inulin and might make you a bit gassy. You can always substitute kohlrabi for sunchokes if you need a lower-fibre option or if sunchokes are unavailable.

DAIRY-FREE • GLUTEN-FREE OPTION • HIGH-FODMAP • VEGAN

1¾ cups (425 mL) water

1½ cups (375 mL) raw cashews

Zest of 1 lemon, divided

3 cloves garlic, minced, divided

1 sprig fresh rosemary, leaves only, chopped

1 tablespoon (15 mL) freshly squeezed lemon juice

1¼ teaspoons (6 mL) salt, plus more for seasoning

1¼ teaspoons (6 mL) onion powder

½ teaspoon (2 mL) garlic powder

½ teaspoon (2 mL) freshly cracked black pepper, plus more for seasoning

¼ teaspoon (1 mL) red chili flakes

½ cup (125 mL) regular or gluten-free panko bread crumbs (see Tip)

1 teaspoon (5 mL) extra-virgin olive oil

2 large bunches curly or Tuscan kale, inner rib and stems removed, torn into large pieces

2 cans (14 ounces/398 mL each) white beans (or 3 cups/750 mL cooked navy, cannellini, or butter beans)

½ pound (225 g) sunchokes, peeled and finely sliced

5 slices vegan cheese, torn into large pieces (I use Violife Provolone or Daiya Swiss Style)

1. Preheat the oven to 350°F (180°C).

2. In a high-speed blender, add the water, cashews, half of the lemon zest, 1 minced garlic clove, rosemary, lemon juice, salt, onion powder, garlic powder, pepper, and chili flakes. Blend until smooth. The cashew cream should taste a bit salty and tangy, but it will be toned down by the unseasoned kale. If not salty/tangy enough, add more salt and/or lemon juice. Set aside.

3. In a small bowl, mix together the remaining 2 minced garlic cloves, remaining lemon zest, panko, olive oil, and a small pinch each of salt and pepper.

4. Heat a large oven-proof skillet over medium heat. Add the kale and cover with a lid for 1 minute to start the wilting process. You do not want the kale fully wilted. Remove from the heat. Toss the white beans and sunchokes into the pan. Pour the cashew cream over the vegetables and stir to combine. Top with the torn cheese and then sprinkle with the panko mixture. Bake until the cashew cream is bubbling, the cheese is melted, and the topping is golden brown, 50 to 55 minutes. Remove from the oven and let cool slightly before serving.

Tips 1. If you don't have a high-speed blender, soak the cashews in hot water for 30 to 60 minutes prior to blending for a smoother consistency.

2. The cashew sauce also makes a delicious sauce for pasta or grain bowls.

3. For gluten-free option, use gluten-free panko bread crumbs.

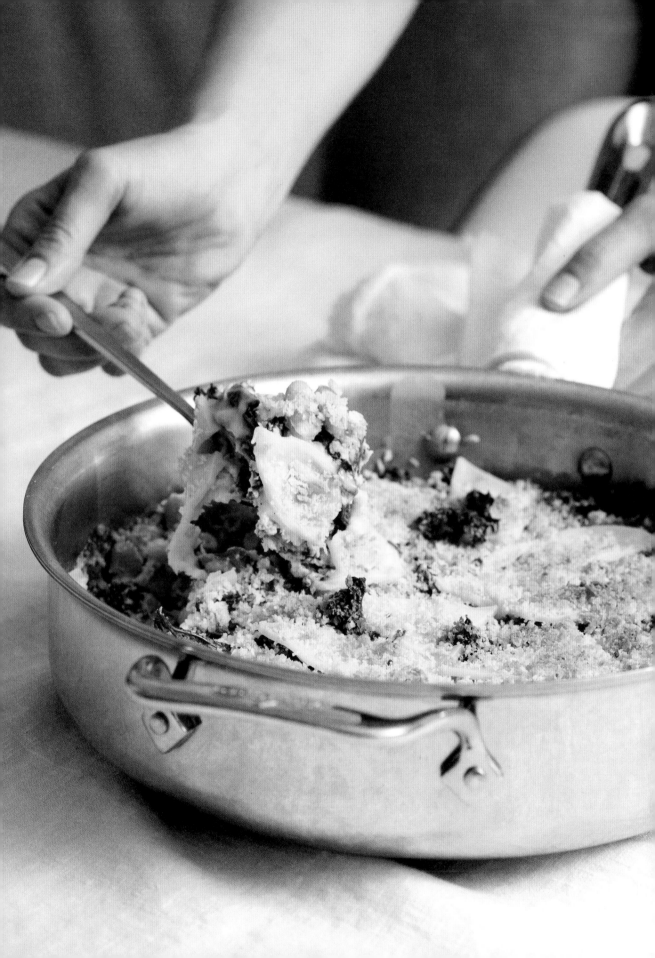

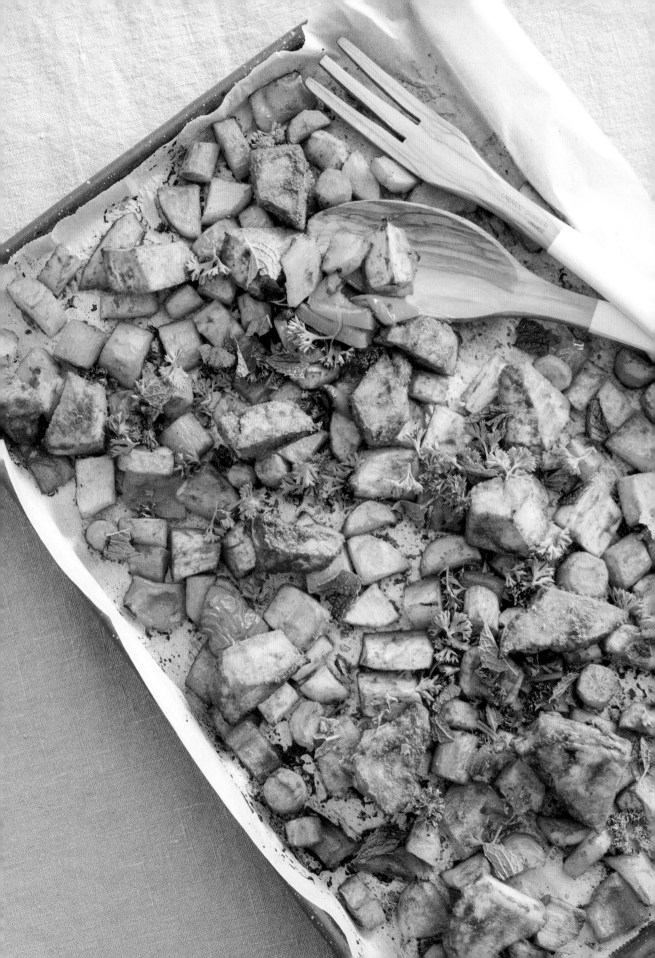

Sheet Pan Harissa Tofu and Veggies Serves 4

Whenever I am stuck for dinner ideas, roasting is in order. On its own, this is a flavourful and protein-rich light meal. Served with a whole grain like wheat berries or millet, it is hearty enough to satisfy even big appetites. The flavour and heat intensity of harissa really varies and can make or break the meal. Be sure to taste your harissa before it goes into the marinade! If it lacks heat, add some red chili flakes or hot sauce. Not enough flavour? Bump up the cumin and onion powder until your marinade has some serious zing.

DAIRY-FREE • GLUTEN-FREE • HIGH-FODMAP • NUT-FREE • VEGAN

1. Preheat the oven to 400°F (200°C). Line 2 baking sheets with parchment paper.

2. In a medium bowl, whisk together the avocado oil, harissa paste, lemon juice, cumin, salt, cane sugar, onion powder, and pepper. Toss the tofu in the sauce. Transfer the tofu to one of the prepared baking sheets, leaving the remaining sauce in the bowl. Toss the squash, carrots, parsnips, red pepper, and red onion into the sauce. Transfer the vegetables to the second baking sheet. Roast both sheets until the tofu is crispy around the edges and the vegetables are fork-tender, about 40 minutes. Rotate the sheets halfway through cooking. To serve, divide the cooked grain, tofu, and vegetables among bowls and sprinkle with the herbs.

Tip Cooking the tofu and vegetables on separate baking sheets ensures the torn edges of the tofu get crispy and the vegetables roast rather than steam.

¼ cup (60 mL) avocado oil

3 tablespoons (45 mL) spicy harissa paste

2 tablespoons (30 mL) freshly squeezed lemon juice

1 teaspoon (5 mL) ground cumin

1 teaspoon (5 mL) salt

1 teaspoon (5 mL) organic cane sugar or pure maple syrup

½ teaspoon (2 mL) onion powder

Freshly cracked black pepper

1 package (12 ounces/340 g) extra-firm tofu, sliced in half horizontally and torn into pieces

1 pound (450 g) butternut squash, peeled, chopped into ¾-inch (2 cm) cubes

4 medium carrots, scrubbed and chopped into ¾-inch (2 cm) cubes

2 medium parsnips, scrubbed and chopped into ¾-inch (2 cm) cubes

1 sweet red pepper, seeded and chopped into ¾-inch (2 cm) cubes

1 small red onion, peeled and chopped into ¾-inch (2 cm) cubes

FOR SERVING

Your favourite cooked grain, such as millet, brown rice, or quinoa

½ cup (125 mL) mixed fresh herbs (I like thinly sliced mint and curly parsley)

Skillet Flatbread with Tempeh and Cauliflower "Chorizo Verde" Serves 4

I love creating plant-based meals that mimic the depth of flavour that you might expect from a meat-containing meal. This flatbread dish does not disappoint! This fun and flavourful meal is a great way to introduce yourself to tempeh—a fermented soybean cake that has a rich, earthy flavour. It can feel intimidating to cook with at first, but crumbling a pre-marinated block of tempeh into a chorizo-spiced sauté will win over any tempeh skeptics. This recipe is fantastic for a weekend dinner with friends, served with a light salad such as Snap Pea Salad with Hazelnuts and Barley (page 203) or Shaved Fennel, Apple, and Celery Salad (page 200).

DAIRY-FREE • HIGH-FODMAP • NUT-FREE • VEGAN

TEMPEH AND CAULIFLOWER "CHORIZO VERDE"

1¼ cups (300 mL) water, divided

½ cup (125 mL) lightly packed fresh curly parsley, chopped

½ cup (125 mL) lightly packed fresh basil, chopped

3 tablespoons (45 mL) avocado oil, divided

3 cloves garlic, peeled and diced

1 jalapeño pepper, halved

1 teaspoon (5 mL) salt, divided

2 cups (500 mL) finely chopped cauliflower (about ½ medium head)

1 package (8 ounces/225 g) smoked tempeh, crumbled

1 tablespoon (15 mL) dried oregano

1½ teaspoons (7 mL) ground cumin

1 teaspoon (5 mL) onion powder

½ teaspoon (2 mL) garlic powder

½ teaspoon (2 mL) sweet paprika

1 to 2 tablespoons (15 to 30 mL) freshly squeezed lemon juice

FLATBREAD

2 cups (500 mL) whole wheat or spelt flour, plus more for dusting

2 teaspoons (10 mL) baking powder

½ teaspoon (2 mL) salt

⅔ cup (150 mL) water

Avocado oil, for cooking

TOPPINGS (OPTIONAL)

1 ripe avocado, pitted, peeled, and mashed

Hummus

Pizza sauce

1. **Make the tempeh and cauliflower "chorizo verde":** In a small food processor, add ¼ cup (60 mL) of the water, parsley, basil, 2 tablespoons (30 mL) of the avocado oil, garlic, jalapeño, and ½ teaspoon (2 mL) of the salt. Pulse until it resembles a loose pesto.

2. In a large skillet, heat the remaining 1 tablespoon (15 mL) avocado oil over medium heat. Add the cauliflower and crumbled tempeh and cook until the cauliflower starts to soften, stirring occasionally, 5 to 7 minutes. Add the oregano, cumin, onion powder, garlic powder, paprika, and remaining ½ teaspoon (2 mL) salt. Stir the mixture for 1 minute.

3. Add the herb mixture and the remaining 1 cup (250 mL) water to the skillet. Simmer over medium-low heat until most of the liquid has absorbed, about 10 minutes. Add 1 tablespoon (15 mL) of the lemon juice. Taste and adjust the lemon juice and/or salt, if needed. Set aside.

4. **Make the flatbread:** In a medium bowl, whisk together the whole wheat flour, baking powder, and salt. Add the water and, using your hands, mix together and form the dough into a ball. Cover with a clean kitchen towel and let the dough rest for 10 minutes.

5. Lightly dust a work surface with flour. Divide the dough into 4 portions. Flatten each with the palm of your hand or roll with a floured rolling pin into a 7-inch (18 cm) round flatbread, ¼ inch (5 mm) thick. This is a rustic whole-grain dough, so don't worry if it cracks.

6. Heat a large nonstick skillet slightly below medium-high heat. Brush the pan with a bit of avocado oil. Cook the flatbread, one at a time, until bubbles form on the surface and there are some char marks on the bottom, 1 to 2 minutes. Flip and cook for another 1 to 2 minutes. Reduce the heat if the oil is smoking.

7. To serve, spread preferred toppings (if using) on the flatbread and top with the tempeh and cauliflower "chorizo verde."

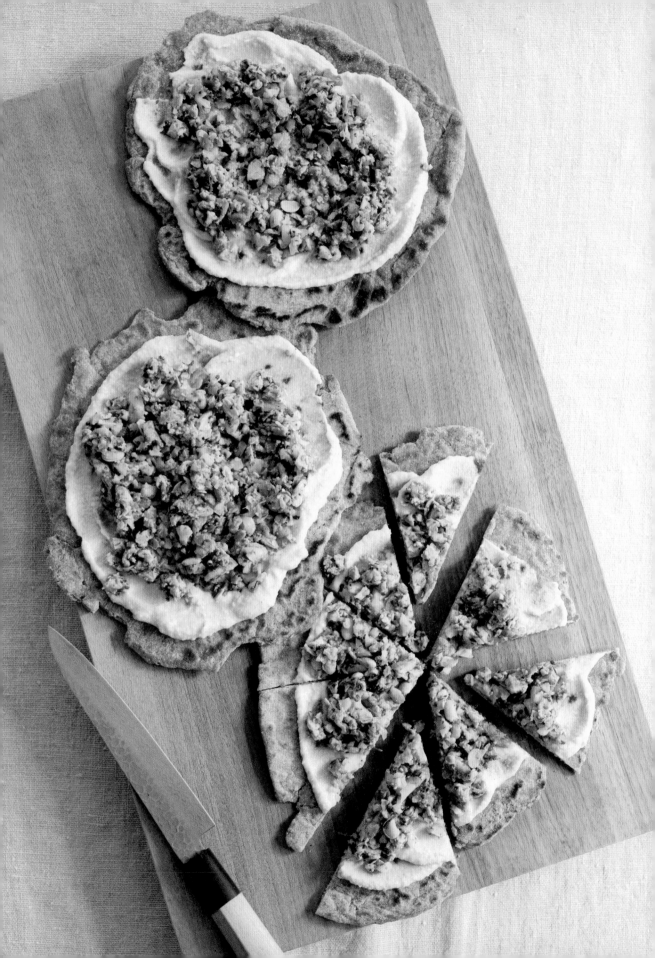

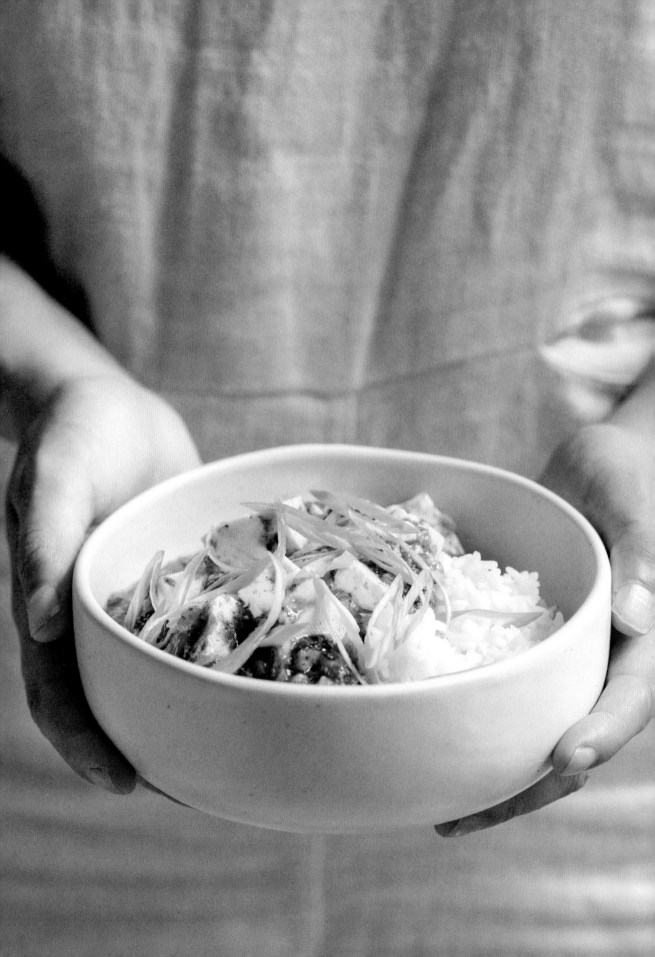

Mapo Tofu Serves 6

Mapo tofu is a signature dish from Chengdu in China's Sichuan province—also known for its fiery Sichuan peppercorns. Sichuan peppercorns have a numbing heat that is unlike the chili peppers you might be used to. I had the good fortune of eating a vegan Mapo Tofu that used spelt to mimic the chewiness of pork at the restaurant Planta Queen in Toronto while celebrating the launch of my book *Eat More Plants*. It was kind of genius—and I vowed to create my own version. I wanted to honour this recipe by using as many of the traditional ingredients as possible. I have created it with a level of spiciness that should work for most, but if you're up for it, bring the heat!

DAIRY-FREE • HIGH-FODMAP • NUT-FREE • VEGAN

1. Place the shiitake mushrooms in a small bowl. Cover the mushrooms with the boiling water and let sit for 10 minutes.

2. Drain the mushrooms, reserving 1 cup (250 mL) of the soaking water. In a food processor, add the shiitake and cremini mushrooms, shallot, ginger, and garlic. Pulse until finely chopped.

3. In a large skillet, heat the avocado oil over medium heat. Add the Sichuan peppercorns and Thai red chili. Let it sizzle, stirring occasionally, until fragrant, 3 to 4 minutes. Using a slotted spoon, carefully remove the peppercorns and red chili. Transfer to a small plate lined with paper towel and reserve for garnish, if desired. Add the mushroom mixture to the pan and cook, stirring often, until moisture is released, 3 to 4 minutes. Stir in the chili bean paste, Shaohsing cooking wine, black bean sauce, soy sauce, and five-spice powder. Mix well.

4. In a small bowl or measuring cup, mix the arrowroot powder with the reserved 1 cup (250 mL) mushroom soaking water, then stir into the skillet. Add the tofu and spelt. Reduce the heat to medium-low and cook until thickened and gravy-like, about 5 minutes. Try not to stir too much, as it will break up the tofu.

5. To serve, divide the rice, greens, and mapo tofu among bowls. Garnish with the green onions and the cooked Sichuan peppercorns and Thai red chili, if desired.

Tips 1. To pump up the heat, add another 1 tablespoon (15 mL) of Sichuan peppercorns and/or chili bean paste.

2. High in salt, this recipe is not suitable for a low-sodium diet.

1 ounce (28 g) dried shiitake mushrooms

1½ cups (375 mL) boiling water

½ pound (225 g) cremini mushrooms, cleaned and halved

1 shallot, peeled and quartered

2-inch (5 cm) piece of fresh ginger, peeled and roughly chopped

3 cloves garlic, peeled

¼ cup (60 mL) avocado oil or refined coconut oil

1 tablespoon (15 mL) Sichuan peppercorns

1 fresh Thai red chili, sliced

2 tablespoons (30 mL) chili bean paste (Toban Djan)

2 tablespoons (30 mL) Shaohsing cooking wine

1 tablespoon (15 mL) black bean sauce

1 tablespoon (15 mL) soy sauce

¼ teaspoon (1 mL) five-spice powder

1 tablespoon (15 mL) arrowroot powder

1 pound (450 g) medium-firm tofu, cut into 1-inch (2.5 cm) cubes

1 cup (250 mL) cooked spelt or wheat berries

FOR SERVING

Cooked brown rice

Steamed or roasted greens such as broccoli or bok choy

3 green onions, thinly sliced on the diagonal

Lentil Bolognaise Serves 6

Few dishes are more comforting than a hearty bolognaise. Slowly cooked with rich lentils and plenty of sneaky veggies, this sauce is high in fibre as well as filling protein. The mushroom, garlic, and shallot provide plenty of fermentable FODMAPs to boost your microbiome, and tummy-soothing fennel seeds give it just a hint of an Italian sausage vibe. This familiar favourite is a complete and satisfying meal that will appeal to even the plant-based skeptics at your table.

DAIRY-FREE • GLUTEN-FREE • HIGH-FODMAP • NUT-FREE • VEGAN

2 tablespoons (30 mL) extra-virgin olive oil

2 sweet red peppers, finely chopped

½ pound (225 g) cremini mushrooms, finely chopped

1 large shallot, diced

4 cloves garlic, chopped

Freshly cracked black pepper

2 tablespoons (30 mL) nutritional yeast

2 tablespoons (30 mL) balsamic vinegar

2 teaspoons (10 mL) dried basil

1 teaspoon (5 mL) dried oregano

½ teaspoon (2 mL) fennel seeds, lightly crushed

½ teaspoon (2 mL) organic cane sugar

Pinch of red chili flakes

1 can (28 ounces/796 mL) crushed tomatoes

2 cups (500 mL) cooked brown lentils

1 teaspoon (5 mL) sea salt, plus more for seasoning

1 pound (450 g) of your favourite dried gluten-free pasta (I like spaghetti)

Freshly squeezed lemon juice, to taste

1. In a large skillet, heat the olive oil over medium heat. Add the red peppers, mushrooms, shallot, and garlic and cook, stirring often, until the vegetables have softened and the water from the mushrooms has evaporated, 9 to 10 minutes. Season generously with salt and pepper.

2. Add the nutritional yeast, balsamic vinegar, basil, oregano, fennel seeds, cane sugar, and chili flakes. Stir for 30 seconds so the mixture becomes fragrant. Add the tomatoes, lentils, and salt. Simmer over medium-low heat until the sauce thickens, 20 to 25 minutes.

3. While the sauce simmers, cook the pasta according to package directions. Drain in a colander and rinse under cool running water.

4. When the bolognaise is thickened, taste and adjust seasoning as needed (lemon juice for acidity, a bit more cane sugar to mellow out flavours, or extra salt).

5. Serve the lentil bolognaise over pasta. Leftovers can be stored separately in airtight containers in the fridge for up to 3 days.

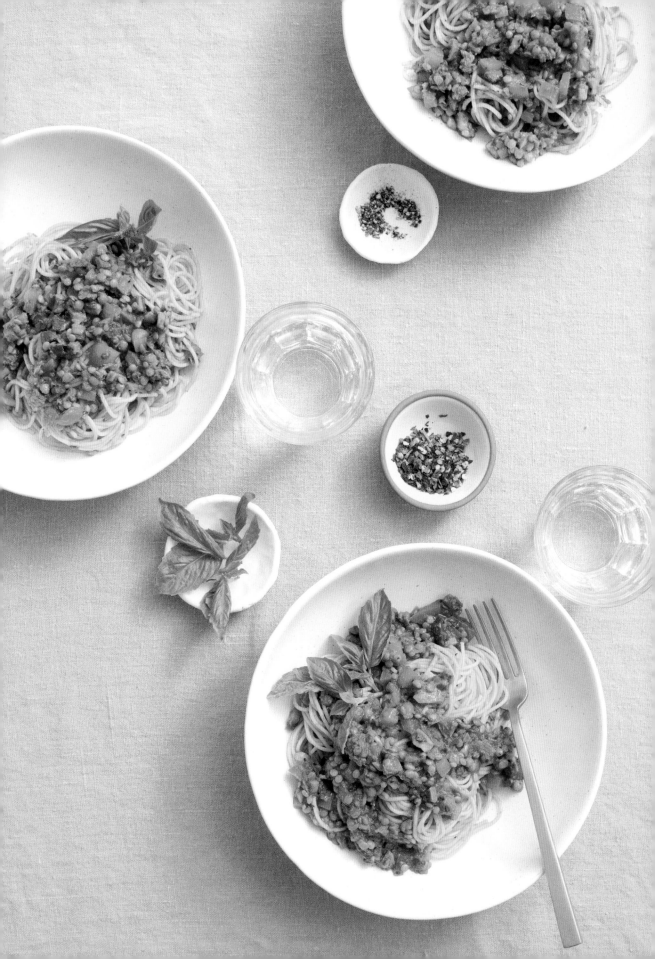

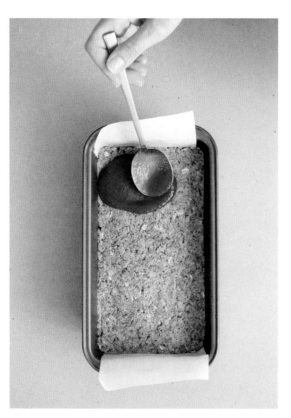

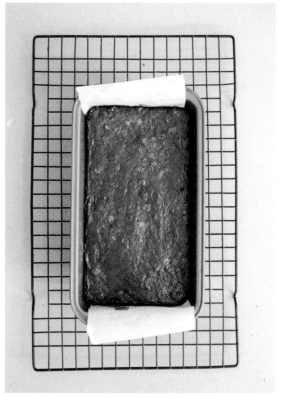

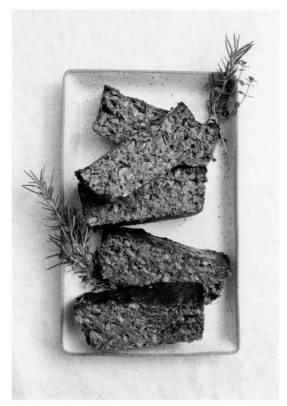

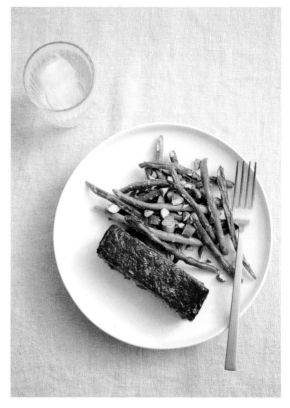

Lentil Walnut Loaf Serves 6 to 8

There is something so comforting about a lentil loaf. This loaf is inspired by Angela Liddon's Ultimate Lentil Walnut Loaf with a ketchup-based glaze. Angela is an author and the founder of Oh She Glows, and she completely changed my mind about lentil loaves! It's a hearty and incredibly nutrient-dense main packed with veggies. There is protein and healthy fats from walnuts, flaxseed, and lentils; omega-3 fatty acids; and even vitamin B12 from the nutritional yeast. This loaf makes a wonderful addition to a Sunday supper or holiday dinner. It also freezes really well, so make a double batch for quick weeknight meals.

DAIRY-FREE • GLUTEN-FREE • HIGH-FODMAP • VEGAN

1. **Make the lentil walnut loaf:** Preheat the oven to 350°F (180°C). Grease a 9 × 5-inch (2 L) loaf pan with olive oil and line with parchment paper.

2. Whisk the flaxseed with the hot water in a small bowl. Set aside.

3. In a medium skillet, toast the walnuts over medium heat until fragrant, 3 to 4 minutes. Toss the walnuts into a food processor.

4. In the same skillet, heat 1 tablespoon (15 mL) of the olive oil over medium heat. Add the onion and mushrooms and cook, stirring occasionally, until the mushrooms release their water and the onions start to soften and brown, 5 to 7 minutes. Add the celery, carrots, and garlic and cook, stirring often, until the carrots are soft, 5 to 7 minutes. Deglaze the pan with the tamari and balsamic vinegar, stirring, for 30 seconds. Season the vegetables generously with salt and pepper. Remove from the heat and let cool for a few minutes, then transfer the mixture to the food processor with the walnuts. Add the parsley and pulse until very finely chopped and the mixture starts to come together. Scrape the vegetable mixture into a large bowl. Add the lentils, bread crumbs, nutritional yeast, flaxseed mixture, rolled oats, remaining 1 tablespoon (15 mL) olive oil, maple syrup, thyme, oregano, onion powder, garlic powder, salt, and pepper. Using your hands, mix until well blended. Taste and add more salt, if needed. Scrape the mixture into the prepared loaf pan. Press down firmly to pack it together and smooth the top. Bake, uncovered, for 30 minutes.

5. **Meanwhile, make the glaze:** In a small bowl, whisk together the ketchup and tamari.

6. Spread the glaze evenly over the loaf and continue cooking until the edges of the loaf are lightly browned, about 15 minutes more. Cool the loaf in the pan for 10 minutes, then carefully transfer to a rack to cool for 5 minutes more before slicing.

Tip The loaf contains a lot of moisture and firms up as it cools. I recommend slicing it with a serrated knife.

LENTIL WALNUT LOAF

¼ cup (60 mL) ground flaxseed

½ cup (125 mL) hot water

1 cup (250 mL) raw walnuts

2 tablespoons (30 mL) extra-virgin olive oil, divided

1 medium sweet onion, diced

¼ pound (115 g) cremini mushrooms, chopped

2 ribs celery, finely diced

2 carrots, finely diced

4 cloves garlic, minced

2 tablespoons (30 mL) gluten-free tamari

1 tablespoon (15 mL) balsamic vinegar

Freshly cracked black pepper

½ cup (125 mL) packed chopped curly parsley

2 cups (500 mL) cooked brown lentils

½ cup (125 mL) gluten-free bread crumbs

¼ cup (60 mL) nutritional yeast

¼ cup (60 mL) gluten-free old-fashioned rolled oats

1 tablespoon (15 mL) pure maple syrup

1 tablespoon (15 mL) fresh thyme leaves (or 1 teaspoon/5 mL dried thyme)

1 teaspoon (5 mL) dried oregano

1 teaspoon (5 mL) onion powder

½ teaspoon (2 mL) garlic powder

½ teaspoon (2 mL) salt, plus more for seasoning

GLAZE

⅓ cup (75 mL) ketchup

1 tablespoon (15 mL) gluten-free tamari

Oat Milk Polenta with Burst Tomatoes, Crispy Tofu, and Arugula Serves 4

Polenta is simple comfort food at its finest—the creamy oat milk and nutritional yeast in this version give it a cozy, cheesy vibe that is irresistible. Calcium-rich oat milk and tofu make it a great bone-boosting meal. Oat milk is considered low-FODMAP in a ½-cup (125 mL) serving, except for some UK varieties. If uncertain, macadamia milk is another low-FODMAP alternative that could work here as well. Easy on the gut, this is a light, yet satisfying, meal.

DAIRY-FREE • GLUTEN-FREE • LOW-FODMAP • NUT-FREE • VEGAN

BURST TOMATOES, CRISPY TOFU, AND ARUGULA

1 package (12 ounces/340 g) extra-firm tofu

3 tablespoons (45 mL) avocado oil, divided

Freshly cracked black pepper

20 cherry tomatoes

1 teaspoon (5 mL) dried oregano

¼ teaspoon (1 mL) salt, plus more for seasoning

¼ cup (60 mL) drained capers, patted dry

4 large handfuls of arugula (or 2 cups/ 500 mL finely shredded spinach)

OAT MILK POLENTA

2 cups (500 mL) water

2 cups (500 mL) unsweetened oat milk

2 teaspoons (10 mL) low-FODMAP vegetable-based bouillon (see FODMAP Note)

½ teaspoon (2 mL) salt

1 cup (250 mL) polenta

¼ cup (60 mL) nutritional yeast

1. **Make the burst tomatoes and crispy tofu:** Slice the tofu in half, then in half again horizontally to create four thinner squares. Slice each thin piece of tofu diagonally. You should have 8 triangles. (This is my favourite way to prepare the tofu, but often I go with cubed tofu as shown in the photo. Either way works well.)

2. In a large nonstick skillet, heat 1 tablespoon (15 mL) of the avocado oil over medium heat. Place the tofu in the pan and cook until crisp and golden brown, 3 to 4 minutes per side. Transfer to a large plate and season with salt and pepper on both sides.

3. In the same skillet, add the remaining 2 tablespoons (30 mL) avocado oil and the tomatoes. Sprinkle the oregano and salt over the tomatoes and cook, stirring occasionally, until they start to burst, 7 to 9 minutes. Add the capers and cook, stirring often, for 1 minute more. Remove from the heat, add the cooked tofu, and cover with the lid slightly ajar to keep warm.

4. **Make the oat milk polenta:** In a medium pot, add the water, oat milk, bouillon, and salt. Bring to a boil over medium-high heat. Reduce the heat to medium-low, then add the polenta and nutritional yeast. Cook, whisking constantly, until the polenta is creamy and looks translucent, 10 to 12 minutes.

5. To serve, divide the polenta among bowls. Toss the arugula with the tofu and tomato mixture, then divide over the polenta.

Tips 1. If you are not following a low-FODMAP diet, I recommend using 1 pint (500 mL) of cherry tomatoes (or more) and adding 2 cloves of minced garlic in the last minute of cooking with the capers.

2. You can also substitute 2 teaspoons of Better Than Bouillon Seasoned Vegetable Base and omit the ½ teaspoon (2 mL) of salt in the polenta.

FODMAP Note Low-FODMAP bouillon can be found in some specialty and health food stores or online. I use Fody Vegetable Soup Base powder. Alternately, you can use another 1 teaspoon (5 mL) salt instead of the bouillon.

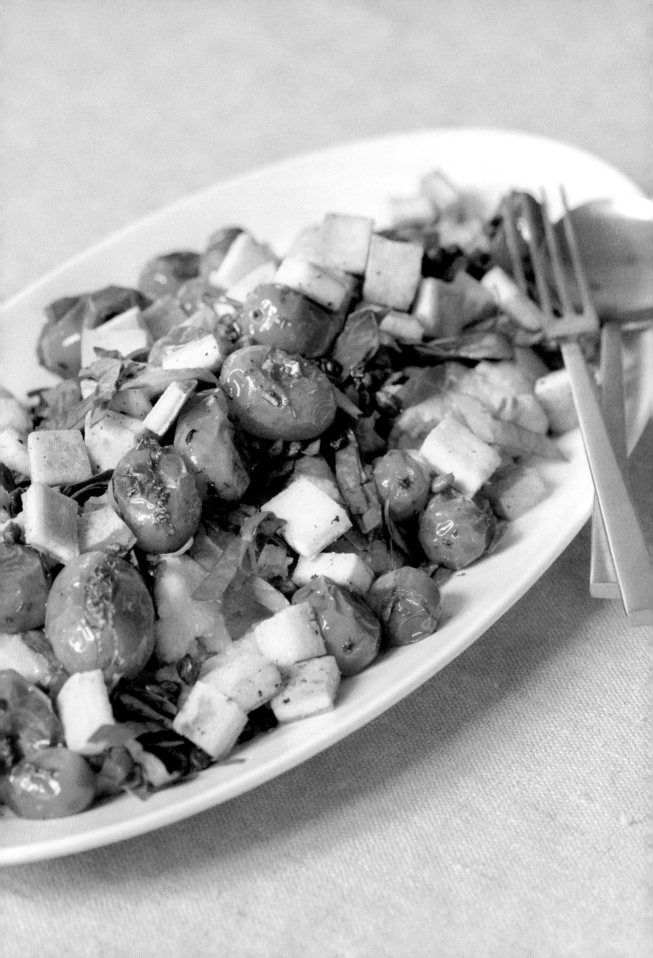

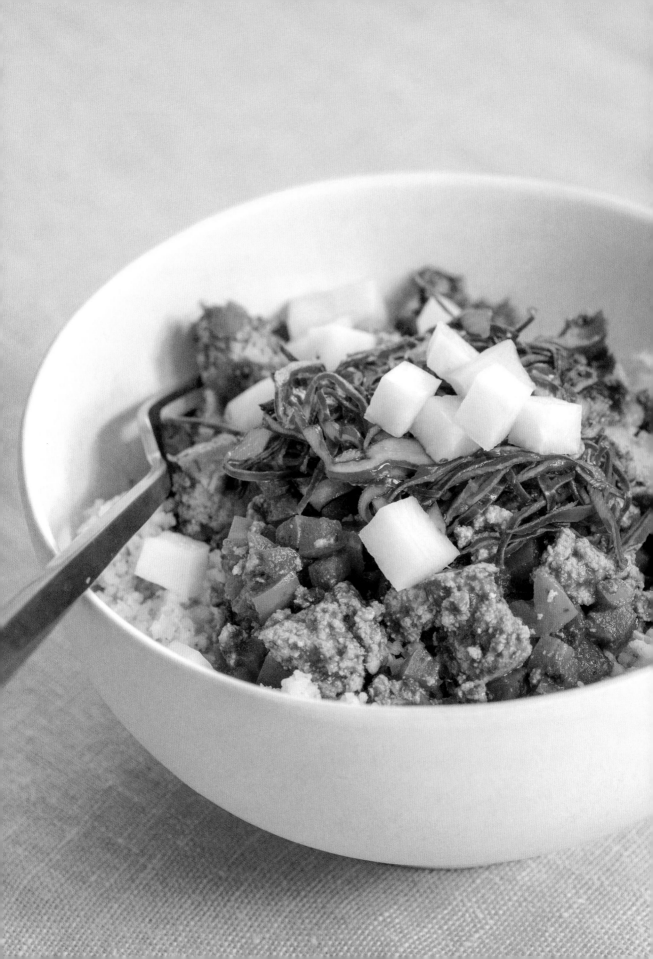

Tofu Sofrito Bowls Serves 4

Give me flavour and make it filling! Inspired by one of my favourite takeout dishes, this tofu sofrito bowl makes the most of those spices sitting in your pantry. Tofu is also a great way to get more protein, which is critical for supporting the immune system and rebuilding gut cells when following a low-FODMAP diet. The sofrito is great on its own but I have added even more flavour and texture with an easy marinated cabbage and diced kohlrabi. These bowls have everything you need to fight inflammation and boost gut health—plenty of veggies, plenty of fibre, and anti-inflammatory nutrients to support healing. This will keep well in the fridge for up to five days, so it is perfect for meal prep.

DAIRY-FREE • GLUTEN-FREE • LOW-FODMAP • NUT-FREE • VEGAN

1. In a medium bowl, add the cabbage, ½ teaspoon (2 mL) of the salt, cane sugar, and half the lime juice. Gently massage the cabbage for 1 minute to soften. Set aside.

2. In a small bowl, toss the kohlrabi with the remaining lime juice. Set aside.

3. Slice the tofu in half, then in half again horizontally to create four squares. In a large nonstick skillet, heat 1 tablespoon (15 mL) of the olive oil over medium-high heat. Place the tofu in the pan and cook until golden on the bottom, 3 to 4 minutes. Flip and cook until golden on the other side, 2 to 3 minutes. Transfer the tofu to a plate.

4. Reduce the heat to medium and add the remaining 1 tablespoon (15 mL) olive oil to the skillet. Add the red peppers and cook, stirring occasionally, until softened and starting to brown, 5 to 7 minutes. Reduce the heat to medium-low, then add the water, tomato paste, apple cider vinegar, molasses, oregano, cumin, chili powder, the remaining 1 teaspoon (5 mL) salt, chili flakes, and cinnamon. Stir until well combined. Simmer for 5 minutes.

5. Tear and crumble the cooked tofu into the sauce, stirring to coat, and let simmer for 5 minutes more to heat through and let the flavours blend.

6. To serve, divide the rice and tofu mixture among bowls. Top with the cabbage and kohlrabi.

¼ medium red cabbage, finely shredded with a mandoline

1½ teaspoons (7 mL) salt, divided

¼ teaspoon (1 mL) organic cane sugar

Juice of 1 lime, divided

2 cups (500 mL) peeled and diced kohlrabi

1 block (12 ounces/340 g) extra-firm tofu

2 tablespoons (30 mL) extra-virgin olive or avocado oil, divided

2 sweet red peppers, finely diced

½ cup (125 mL) water

¼ cup (60 mL) tomato paste

¼ cup (60 mL) apple cider vinegar

1 tablespoon (15 mL) blackstrap molasses (see FODMAP Note)

1 tablespoon (15 mL) dried oregano

2 teaspoons (10 mL) dried cumin

1 teaspoon (5 mL) chili powder

½ teaspoon (2 mL) red chili flakes

¼ teaspoon (1 mL) cinnamon

3 cups (750 mL) cooked brown rice, millet, or quinoa, for serving

FODMAP Notes 1. **Blackstrap molasses is a potentially high-FODMAP food. However, the ¼ tablespoon (4 mL) per portion serving size is low-FODMAP.**

2. **If you are not following a low-FODMAP diet, layer on some avocado too.**

Baked Potatoes Stuffed with Spiced Lentils and Kale Serves 4

I love baked potatoes. Luckily they are low-FODMAP and the perfect base for a hearty sauté of lentils, rich with spices and lashings of coconut milk. Instead of baking in foil, these potatoes get a little rubdown with avocado oil so their fibre-rich skin crisps up and adds another layer of texture to this filling and comforting meal.

If you are not following a low-FODMAP diet, the spiced lentils and kale are also delicious overtop of sweet potatoes.

DAIRY-FREE • GLUTEN-FREE • GRAIN-FREE • LOW-FODMAP • NUT-FREE • VEGAN

BAKED POTATOES

4 medium russet potatoes, scrubbed

Avocado oil or melted vegan butter

Salt and pepper, for seasoning

SPICED LENTILS AND KALE

1 tablespoon (15 mL) extra-virgin olive oil or avocado oil

1 large bunch curly kale, stems diced and leaves torn into bite-size pieces

Freshly cracked black pepper

2 cups (500 mL) canned lentils, drained and rinsed

¾ cup (175 mL) canned light coconut milk

1 teaspoon (5 mL) ground cumin

½ teaspoon (2 mL) cinnamon

½ teaspoon (2 mL) ground coriander

½ teaspoon (2 mL) ground turmeric

½ teaspoon (2 mL) salt, plus more for seasoning

¼ teaspoon (1 mL) garam masala

Pinch of red chili flakes

1 tablespoon (15 mL) pure maple syrup

1 tablespoon (15 mL) freshly squeezed lime juice

Vegan butter

1. **Bake the potatoes:** Preheat the oven to 425°F (220°C). Line a baking sheet with parchment paper or place a wire rack on top.

2. Prick the potatoes all over with a fork and then rub them with avocado oil. Season the potatoes with salt and pepper and place them onto the prepared baking sheet. Bake until fork-tender, 50 to 60 minutes.

3. **Meanwhile, make the spiced lentils and kale:** In a medium skillet, heat the olive oil over medium heat. Add the kale and cook, stirring occasionally, until bright green and starting to wilt, 3 to 4 minutes. Season with salt and pepper.

4. Add the lentils, coconut milk, cumin, cinnamon, coriander, turmeric, salt, garam masala, and chili flakes. Simmer over medium-low heat until creamy, but not overly liquidy, 5 to 6 minutes. Stir in the maple syrup and lime juice. Taste and adjust the salt, if needed.

5. Carefully cut along the top and about three-quarters of the way through the baked potatoes and pull back the skin. Split the potatoes a bit to make room for the filling. Add a bit of vegan butter to each potato. Divide the lentil mixture overtop of the potatoes and serve.

Tip For a faster version, use 1½ pounds (675 g) of halved baby potatoes instead of whole potatoes and roast for 20 to 25 minutes. Spoon the lentils and kale over the roasted potatoes.

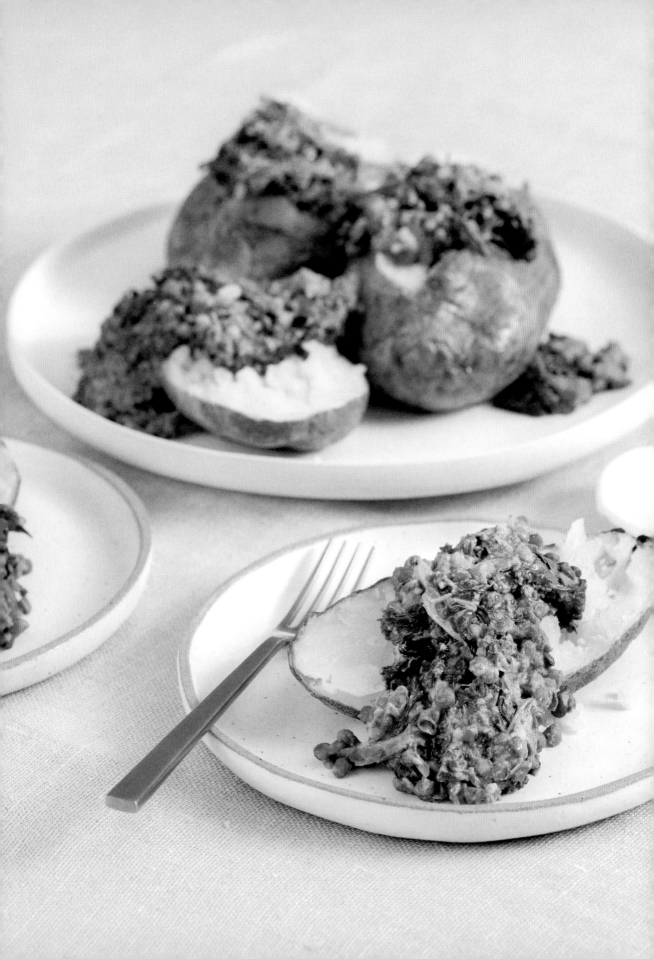

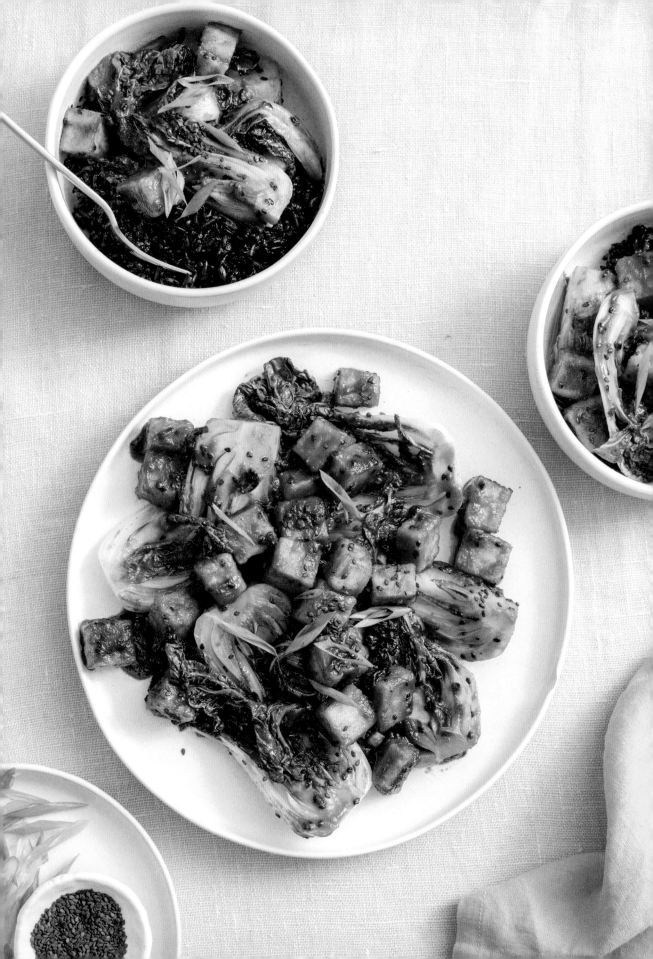

Sticky Sesame Tofu with Bok Choy Serves 4

There is something about a sweet and salty combination that makes any meal more delicious. Sticky sesame tofu is a big favourite in my family, so I wanted to create a simple low-FODMAP version that keeps it flavourful and nutrient-dense. Tomato paste is packed with lycopene to help fight inflammation, and bok choy adds an easy-to-digest dose of greens. This is a filling meal served with antioxidant-rich black rice, but you might have a little room left for some Ginger Vanilla Rice Pudding (page 285).

This recipe makes enough sauce for the tofu; if you want more for the rice, be sure to double it.

DAIRY-FREE • GLUTEN-FREE • LOW-FODMAP • NUT-FREE • VEGAN

1. In a medium bowl, mix together the cornstarch and salt. Add the tofu cubes and toss to coat.

2. In a small bowl, mix together the tomato paste, tamari, maple syrup, rice vinegar, sesame oil, sesame seeds, and hot sauce. Set aside.

3. In a large nonstick skillet, heat 1 tablespoon (15 mL) of the avocado oil over medium-high heat. Working in batches, place the bok choy, cut side down, in the pan, cover with a lid, and cook until browned on the bottom, 3 to 4 minutes. Transfer to a medium bowl.

4. In the same skillet, heat the remaining 1 tablespoon (15 mL) avocado oil over medium heat. Add the tofu and cook until browned and crisp on all sides, 1 to 2 minutes per side. Remove the pan from the heat. Add the sauce and toss to coat the tofu. Add the bok choy back into the pan and toss again. Serve with black rice.

Tip In this recipe, you cannot use arrowroot powder as a substitute for cornstarch. If you use arrowroot, the tofu will be slimy instead of crispy.

FODMAP Note 1⅓ cups (325 mL) per serving of bok choy is high-FODMAP, so be sure to measure out your greens.

¼ cup (60 mL) cornstarch (see Tip)

¼ teaspoon (1 mL) salt

1 package (12 ounces/340 g) extra-firm tofu, cut into 1-inch (2.5 cm) cubes

¼ cup (60 mL) tomato paste

3 tablespoons (45 mL) gluten-free tamari

2 tablespoons (30 mL) pure maple syrup

1 tablespoon (15 mL) rice vinegar

1 tablespoon (15 mL) sesame oil

1 tablespoon (15 mL) sesame seeds

2 to 3 teaspoons (10 to 15 mL) hot sauce

2 tablespoons (30 mL) avocado oil, divided

⅔ pound (300 g) bok choy, sliced in half lengthwise (see FODMAP Note)

Cooked black rice, for serving

Roasted Spaghetti Squash with Chickpeas, Red Peppers, and Kale Pesto Serves 4

There is almost nothing more comforting than roasted spaghetti squash. This dish layers sweet, savoury, earthy, and tart flavours to create a super satisfying and filling meal. Hemp hearts in the pesto boost low-FODMAP protein while adding anti-inflammatory omega-3 fatty acids, and the green onion tops lend a garlicky flavour that is FODMAP-friendly. Do not let the multiple steps deter you—the three components of the dish come together in the time it takes to roast the squash. This is a terrific dish for casual entertaining, served with the Kohlrabi Chopped Salad (page 219), or whenever you are craving comfort food.

DAIRY-FREE • GLUTEN-FREE • GRAIN-FREE • LOW-FODMAP • NUT-FREE • VEGAN

ROASTED SPAGHETTI SQUASH

2 small spaghetti squash
(about 3¼ pounds/1.465 kg total)

2 tablespoons (30 mL) extra-virgin
olive oil

¼ teaspoon (1 mL) salt

Freshly cracked black pepper

KALE PESTO

¼ peel-on lemon, seeded and
roughly chopped

3 cups (750 mL) packed curly kale

½ cup (125 mL) hemp hearts

2 tablespoons (30 mL) nutritional yeast

1 tablespoon (15 mL) sliced green onion
(dark green parts only)

¾ teaspoon (3 mL) salt

⅓ cup (75 mL) extra-virgin olive oil

CHICKPEA SAUTÉ

1 tablespoon (15 mL) extra-virgin
olive oil

1 clove garlic

1 cup (250 mL) canned chickpeas,
rinsed and drained

2 medium sweet red peppers, seeded
and thinly sliced

¼ teaspoon (1 mL) dried thyme

¼ teaspoon (1 mL) salt

1. **Roast the spaghetti squash:** Preheat the oven to 400°F (200°C). Line a small baking sheet with parchment paper.

2. Cut the spaghetti squash in half lengthwise and scoop out the seeds. Rub the cut side of the squash with the olive oil, salt, and pepper. Place cut side down onto the prepared baking sheet. Roast until the squash is fork-tender and strands easily form when you drag a fork across the flesh, 40 to 50 minutes.

3. **Meanwhile, make the kale pesto:** In a food processor, add the lemon and pulse until finely diced. Add the kale, hemp hearts, nutritional yeast, green onion, and salt. Process while drizzling in the olive oil until a uniform and thick pesto forms. Taste and adjust salt or add a squeeze of lemon, if needed. Set aside.

4. **Make the chickpea sauté:** In a medium nonstick skillet, heat the olive oil over medium-low heat. Add the whole garlic clove and cook, stirring occasionally, for 5 minutes. Remove and discard the garlic. This is your low-FODMAP garlic-infused oil.

5. Increase the heat to medium, then add the chickpeas, red peppers, thyme, and salt. Cook, stirring occasionally, until the red peppers have softened but retain some crispness, 7 to 8 minutes.

6. To serve, divide the squash halves among plates. Using a fork, gently scrape the flesh of the squash and fluff the strands. Top the squash with the chickpea sauté and then the kale pesto.

FODMAP Note If you are not following a low-FODMAP diet, you can use 1 clove of garlic in place of the green onion in the pesto. I also encourage you to increase the chickpeas to 1½ cups (375 mL) to make it a more protein-rich meal.

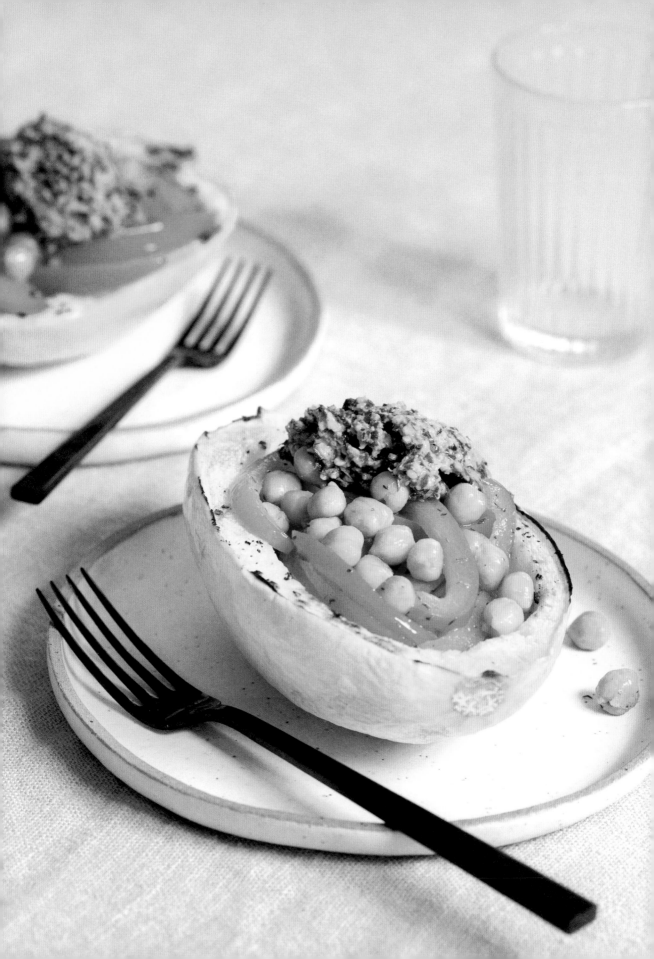

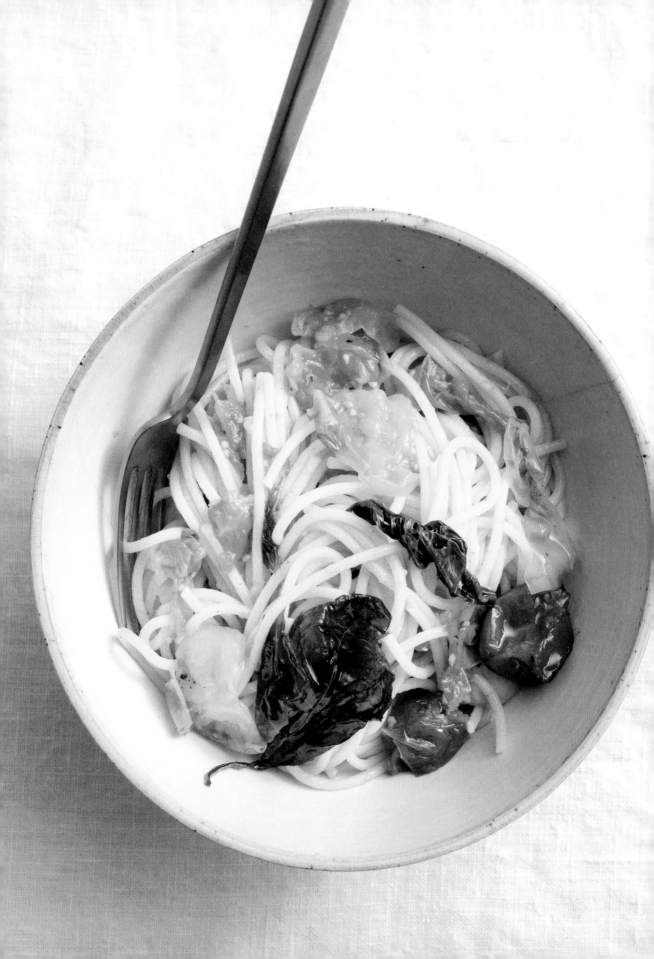

Pasta with Tomato Garlic Confit Serves 4

This is a simple and luxurious dish. Your kitchen will smell fantastic as the tomatoes, in all their lycopene-rich glory, slow-roast in extra-virgin olive oil with fragrant herbs and anti-inflammatory garlic to feed your gut microbiota. The olive oil even helps improve the bioavailability of the phytochemicals in the tomatoes. You will have an extra head of garlic and plenty of infused olive oil left over, which is wonderful for dressing salads or drizzling over bread. If you like, toss warmed white beans with the pasta to add more fibre and protein or use chickpea pasta. Because it takes five minutes to pull together and then an hour of hands-off time, this is the perfect dish to make while babies nap or when people come for dinner, so you can focus on enjoying the company instead of sweating over a stove. This pasta is delicious served alongside a light salad like the Shaved Fennel, Apple, and Celery Salad (page 200).

DAIRY-FREE • GLUTEN-FREE • HIGH-FODMAP • NUT-FREE • VEGAN

1. Preheat the oven to 350°F (180°C).

2. Remove any loose skin from the garlic bulbs. Using a sharp knife, trim about ¼ inch (5 mm) off of the heads of garlic to expose the cloves; keep the heads intact. Place the garlic in a 9-inch (2.5 L) square baking dish, cut side up.

3. Add the cherry tomatoes to the baking dish. Place the thyme and basil leaves around the tomatoes. Pour enough olive oil into the dish to cover the vegetables. Sprinkle the salt overtop and finish with plenty of cracked black pepper. Slide the dish into the oven and bake for 1 hour.

4. When the tomatoes and garlic are almost finished baking, bring a large pot of water to a boil. Cook the pasta according to package directions. Drain in a colander and rinse under cool running water. Return the pasta to the pot off the heat.

5. Remove the tomato and garlic mixture from the oven. Using a large spoon, carefully transfer the garlic to a small plate. Using the same spoon, add the tomatoes and basil to the pasta. Discard the thyme sprigs. Carefully remove the garlic cloves from 1 bulb and add to the pasta, reserving the garlic cloves from the other bulb for another use. Pour ¼ cup (60 mL) of the olive oil mixture into the pasta and toss everything together. Add more olive oil as desired so the pasta looks glossy. Divide among shallow bowls.

6. Store the roasted olive oil in an airtight container on the counter for up to 1 week and use it to cook or flavour any dish that goes well with herbs and garlic. Roasted garlic can be stored in an airtight container in the fridge for up to 5 days.

2 heads garlic

2 pints (1 L) cherry tomatoes

2 to 3 sprigs fresh thyme

1 large handful of fresh basil leaves

Extra-virgin olive oil, for cooking (about 2 cups/500 mL)

1 teaspoon (5 mL) salt

Freshly cracked black pepper

1 package (12 ounces/340 g) of your favourite gluten-free long pasta, such as spaghetti

Baked Eggplant Rolls with Kale and Cauliflower Ricotta Serves 4

Lasagna is a lifelong favourite of mine. This is my plant-powered homage to that transcendent dish—eggplant wrapped around a ricotta that has cauliflower and kale for a double-dose of anti-inflammatory brassicas plus calcium and vitamin E-rich almonds. It takes a bit of effort, sure, but it is still very doable even for a quieter weeknight. It would also be perfect for Sunday dinner alongside the Kohlrabi Chopped Salad (page 219) or Brussels Sprouts Caesar with Garlicky Walnuts (page 204) and a nice loaf of sourdough.

DAIRY-FREE • GLUTEN-FREE • GRAIN-FREE • HIGH-FODMAP • VEGAN

BAKED EGGPLANT ROLLS

2 medium Italian eggplants, cut lengthwise into ¼-inch (5 mm) slices (at least 16 slices)

Coarse salt

1 bunch fresh basil, leaves only

1 jar (24 ounces/750 mL) store-bought pasta sauce

KALE AND CAULIFLOWER RICOTTA

1 tablespoon (15 mL) extra-virgin olive oil, plus more for the baking dish

1 bunch curly kale, destemmed and torn into large pieces

2 cups (500 mL) chopped cauliflower florets

Freshly cracked black pepper

1 cup (250 mL) raw almonds, soaked in water for 4 hours or overnight

¼ cup (60 mL) water

3 tablespoons (45 mL) freshly squeezed lemon juice

1 clove garlic, chopped

1 teaspoon (5 mL) salt, plus more for seasoning

Shredded vegan cheese, for topping (optional)

1. **Start the baked eggplant rolls:** Preheat the oven to 375°F (190°C).

2. Place the eggplant slices on a wire rack set on a baking sheet. Generously salt both sides of the eggplant with coarse salt and let sit for 15 minutes.

3. **Meanwhile, make the kale and cauliflower ricotta:** In a large skillet, heat the olive oil over medium heat. Add the kale and cauliflower and cook, stirring occasionally, until softened, about 5 minutes. Season with salt and pepper.

4. In a food processor, combine the kale and cauliflower mixture with the drained almonds, water, lemon juice, garlic, and salt. Pulse until it looks like ricotta cheese. You should be able to press the mixture together with your fingers. If it looks too dry, drizzle in some water, 1 tablespoon (15 mL) at a time, as you pulse.

5. **Finish the baked eggplant rolls:** Rinse the eggplant slices and pat dry with a clean kitchen towel. You'll need the 16 best slices of the eggplant for this dish. If you have more, you can see how much you can fit into your dish at the end. Lightly grease a 9-inch (2.5 L) square baking dish with olive oil.

6. Lay a slice of eggplant on a clean surface with the short end in front of you. Place a few basil leaves on the eggplant and a dollop of the kale and cauliflower ricotta at the end closest to you, about 1 inch (2.5 cm) from the edge. Lift the edge that is closest to you up and over the filling and roll. Place the rolled eggplant, seam side down, into the prepared baking dish. Continue to fill and roll the remaining slices of eggplant. Pour the pasta sauce over the eggplant rolls. Sprinkle the vegan cheese overtop, if using. Cover the baking dish with foil and bake for 30 minutes. Uncover and bake until the sauce is thick and bubbling, 10 to 15 minutes more. Let cool for 10 minutes before serving. Leftovers can be stored in an airtight container in the fridge for up to 3 days or in the freezer for up to 1 month.

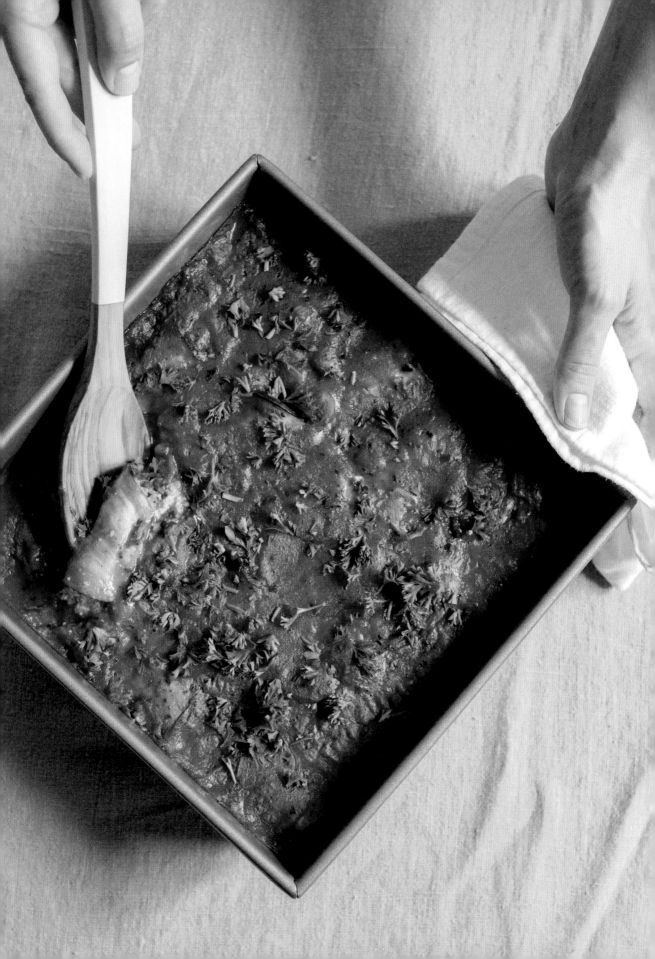

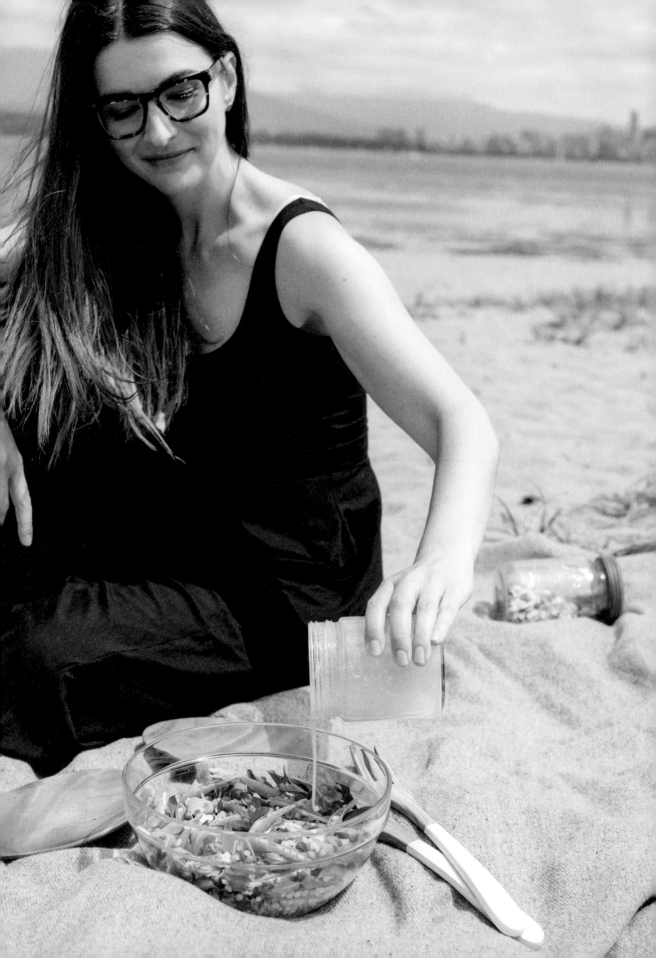

Soups and Salads

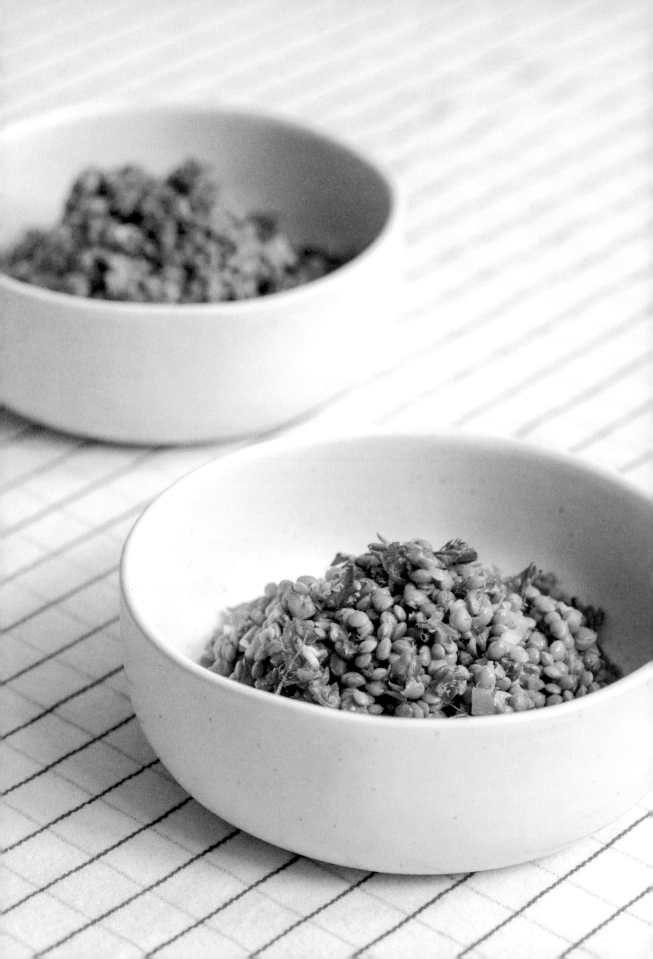

Marinated Lentil Salad Serves 4

Meet your new batch cook hero! Having this lentil salad in the fridge will make it easy to add filling and flavourful plant-based protein to your plate. Lentils and shallot team up to feed your gut microbiota and keep it thriving. Coriander, seed of the cilantro plant, has long been used as a traditional digestive remedy; it is thought to stimulate the production of stomach acid and reduce intestinal spasms.

DAIRY-FREE • GLUTEN-FREE • GRAIN-FREE • HIGH-FODMAP • NUT-FREE • VEGAN

1. **Cook the lentils:** In a medium pot, add the lentils, garlic, and bay leaves. Cover with water and bring to a boil over high heat. When the water is boiling, reduce the heat to medium to maintain a gentle boil. Cook, covered with the lid slightly ajar, until the lentils are cooked but still firm, 15 to 30 minutes. Drain and rinse under cool running water. Discard the garlic and bay leaves. Transfer the lentils to a medium salad bowl. If using cooked lentils, omit the garlic and bay leaves and simply add lentils to the salad bowl.

2. **Make the dressing:** Meanwhile, in a small skillet, toast the coriander seeds over medium heat until fragrant, 2 to 3 minutes. Let cool slightly, then using the back of a wooden spoon or a mortar and pestle, gently crush the seeds. Add the crushed seeds to a small mason jar with the apple cider vinegar, shallot, olive oil, mustard, maple syrup, and salt. Place the lid on tightly and shake to blend.

3. **Assemble the salad:** Add the carrots, parsley, sun-dried tomatoes, and dill to the lentils along with the dressing. Stir gently to combine and serve. Store in an airtight container in the fridge for up to 5 days.

Tip This salad would be delicious with any firm lentil such as Puy or beluga. Red lentils will not work, as they break down in cooking. The cooking time will depend on the type of lentils you use. Follow the directions on the package and keep an eye on them while cooking.

LENTIL SALAD

1½ cups (375 mL) dry French or green lentils, rinsed (or about 3½ cups/875 mL cooked lentils; see Tip)

2 cloves garlic

2 bay leaves

2 medium carrots, diced

½ cup (125 mL) lightly packed curly parsley, minced

¼ cup (60 mL) sun-dried tomatoes, diced

2 tablespoons (30 mL) minced fresh dill

DRESSING

1 teaspoon (5 mL) coriander seeds

⅓ cup (75 mL) apple cider vinegar

2 tablespoons (30 mL) minced shallot

1 tablespoon (15 mL) extra-virgin olive oil or avocado oil

1 tablespoon (15 mL) Dijon mustard

1 tablespoon (15 mL) pure maple syrup

¾ teaspoon (3 mL) salt

Plum and Radicchio Salad with Tahini Yogurt Dressing Serves 4

This salad is full of flavourful Mediterranean ingredients like bitter radicchio, tart plums, crunchy walnuts, and creamy yogurt. We really do not eat enough bitter vegetables because our palettes tend to be overly used to salty and sweet foods. Bitter greens such as radicchio and rapini stimulate digestion and are a wonderful balm for someone who craves sweets. Mint adds another layer of flavour to this special salad and helps to soothe the gut.

DAIRY-FREE • GLUTEN-FREE • GRAIN-FREE • HIGH-FODMAP • VEGAN

TAHINI YOGURT DRESSING

½ cup (125 mL) coconut yogurt

2 tablespoons (30 mL) tahini

1 tablespoon (15 mL) freshly squeezed lemon juice

1 small clove garlic, grated with a microplane

½ teaspoon (2 mL) salt

½ teaspoon (2 mL) organic cane sugar

½ teaspoon (2 mL) ground sumac

¼ teaspoon (1 mL) red chili flakes

PLUM AND RADICCHIO SALAD

1 small head red radicchio, finely shredded

4 firm black or red plums, pitted and sliced

¼ cup (60 mL) raw walnuts, chopped

¼ cup (60 mL) Medjool dates, pitted and chopped

¼ cup (60 mL) fresh mint leaves, thinly sliced into ribbons

1. **Make the tahini yogurt dressing:** In a small bowl, whisk together the coconut yogurt, tahini, lemon juice, garlic, salt, cane sugar, sumac, and chili flakes. If needed, add 1 to 2 tablespoons (15 to 30 mL) water for desired consistency. Store in an airtight container in the fridge for up to 4 days. (It makes a great veggie dip.)

2. **Make the plum and radicchio salad:** In a medium bowl, toss the radicchio with half of the dressing. Layer the plums, walnuts, dates, and mint overtop of the radicchio. Serve with the remaining dressing on the side.

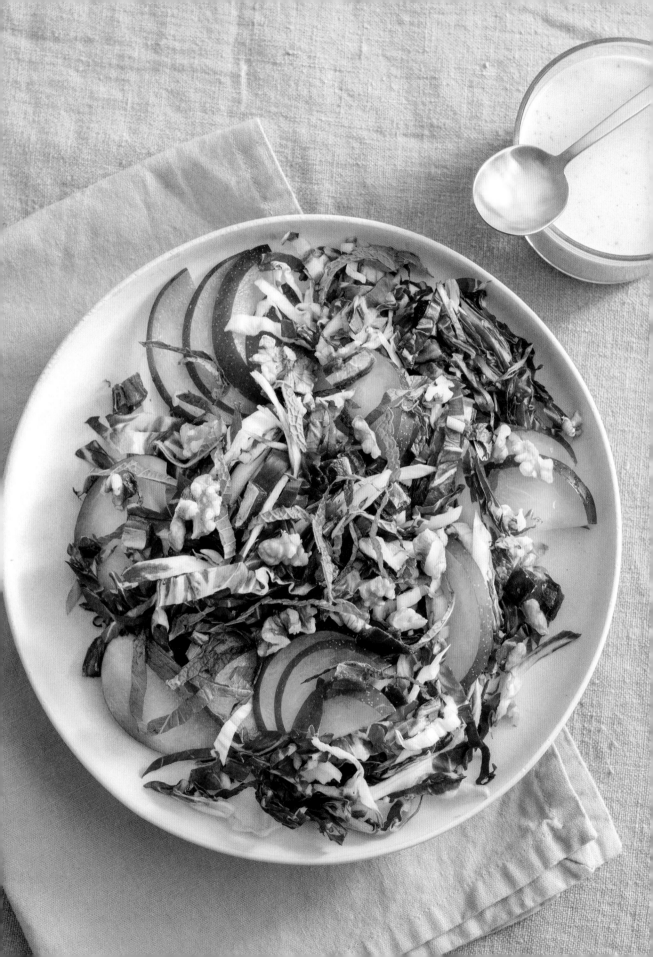

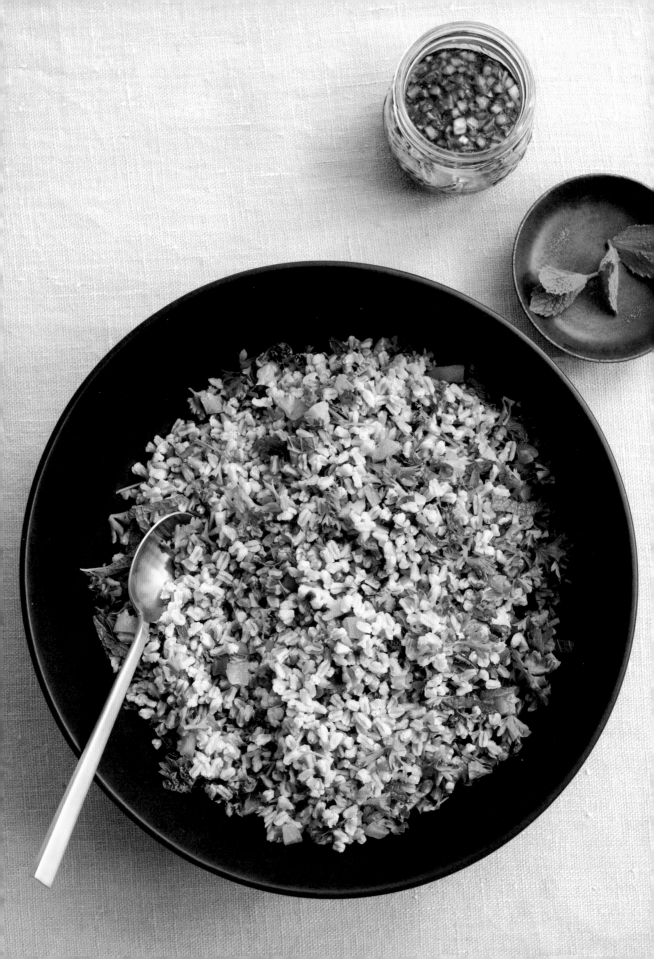

Farro, Apricot, and Walnut Salad Serves 3 to 4

Farro is a chewy, nutty, and satisfying ancient grain with major nutrition benefits. A serving of farro boasts the same protein as an egg, 7 grams of fibre, and plenty of gut-friendly zinc and magnesium. It makes this hearty salad—spiked with walnuts rich in omega-3 fatty acids, sweet apricots, and tangy pomegranate molasses—a filling, flavourful, and energizing lunch or a lovely side for dinner.

DAIRY-FREE • GLUTEN-FREE OPTION • HIGH-FODMAP • VEGAN

1. **Make the dressing:** In a small bowl or mason jar, mix together the olive oil, pomegranate molasses, shallot, white wine vinegar, maple syrup, and salt. Set aside.

2. **Make the salad:** In a medium pot, add the dry farro, water, and salt. Bring to a boil over high heat. When the water is boiling, reduce the heat to medium and simmer, covered with the lid slightly ajar, and cook until the farro is chewy but tender, 45 to 60 minutes. Drain any excess water and set aside.

3. Meanwhile, in a dry medium skillet, toast the walnuts, stirring occasionally, over medium heat, until fragrant and starting to turn golden, 2 to 3 minutes. Transfer the walnuts into a large bowl and let cool.

4. Place the apricots in a small bowl, cover with hot water, and let sit for 5 minutes to soften. Drain the apricots, discard the water, and chop. Add the apricots to the bowl with the cooled walnuts.

5. Add the cooked farro, parsley, and mint to the bowl. Drizzle the dressing over the salad and toss to coat. Store in an airtight container in the fridge for up to 4 days.

DRESSING

2 tablespoons (30 mL) extra-virgin olive oil

2 tablespoons (30 mL) pomegranate molasses (see Tip)

½ medium shallot, minced

1 tablespoon (15 mL) white wine vinegar

2 teaspoons (10 mL) maple syrup

¾ teaspoon (3 mL) salt

FARROW, APRICOT, AND WALNUT SALAD

1 cup (250 mL) uncooked whole-grain farro (or 3 cups/750 mL cooked; see Tip)

3 cups (750 mL) water

¼ teaspoon (1 mL) salt

¾ cup (175 mL) chopped raw walnuts

½ cup (125 mL) dried apricots

1½ cups (375 mL) lightly packed chopped fresh curly parsley

½ cup (125 mL) lightly packed fresh mint leaves, thinly sliced

Tips 1. **Pomegranate molasses is a tangy, flavourful reduction of pomegranate juice. You can find it in many grocery stores and in Middle Eastern and gourmet food shops. You can also make your own pomegranate molasses, but it takes time, so plan ahead. To make your own, in a small pot, combine 2 cups (500 mL) pomegranate juice with ¼ cup (60 mL) sugar over medium-low heat and simmer, stirring occasionally, until it looks like a thick molasses syrup, about 1 hour.**

2. I like to make a big batch of farro or other grains on weekends. When cooked, drain and spread the farro on a parchment-lined baking sheet to cool slightly. Then place the baking sheet in the freezer for 2 hours to freeze. When the farro is frozen, toss it into a freezer bag or divide it into several bags (3 cups/750 mL cooked for this recipe). To reheat the farro for this salad, bring a medium pot of water to a boil over high heat. When the water is boiling, reduce the heat to medium, remove the farro from the bag, then add the frozen farro to the pot and simmer for 3 minutes. Drain the farro and add to the bowl.

3. For gluten-free option, use millet, brown rice, or quinoa instead of farro.

Shaved Fennel, Apple, and Celery Salad Serves 4

This deceptively simple salad is crunchy, bright, and energizing. Whenever you find bright green celery at the market with beautiful leaves attached, be sure to grab it. Celery leaves are antioxidant-rich and have a special flavour, but flat-leaf parsley is a great nutrient-dense substitute in a pinch. This salad will put you in a spring mood, even though the ingredients are easily available year-round.

DAIRY-FREE • GLUTEN-FREE • GRAIN-FREE • HIGH-FODMAP • VEGAN

DRESSING

2 tablespoons (30 mL) freshly squeezed lemon juice

2 tablespoons (30 mL) Dijon mustard

1 tablespoon (15 mL) extra-virgin olive oil

1 teaspoon (5 mL) pure maple syrup

½ clove garlic, grated

½ teaspoon (2 mL) salt

Pinch of red chili flakes

FENNEL, APPLE, AND CELERY SALAD

2 ribs celery, thinly sliced

1 tablespoon (15 mL) freshly squeezed lemon juice

⅛ teaspoon (0.5 mL) salt

¼ cup (60 mL) chopped raw almonds or slivered almonds

1 cup (250 mL) thinly sliced fennel bulb (about ½ small bulb)

1 cup (250 mL) thinly sliced English cucumber

1 cup (250 mL) lightly packed celery leaves or flat-leaf parsley

1 Pink Lady apple, cored and thinly sliced

1. **Make the dressing:** In a small mason jar, add the lemon juice, mustard, olive oil, maple syrup, garlic, salt, and chili flakes. Place the lid on tightly and shake.

2. **Make the salad:** In a medium bowl, toss the celery with the lemon juice and salt. Let sit.

3. In a small skillet, toast the almonds, stirring often, over medium heat until fragrant and starting to turn golden, 3 to 4 minutes. Remove from the heat.

4. Add the fennel, cucumber, celery leaves, apple, and almonds to the celery and lemon juice mixture. Toss to combine. Pour half of the dressing over the salad and toss again. Taste and add more dressing or adjust the seasoning, if needed. Serve with remaining dressing on the side.

Tip Thinly slice the fennel, apple, and celery with a mandoline to ensure the salad has a pleasant crunch without being overly difficult to chew.

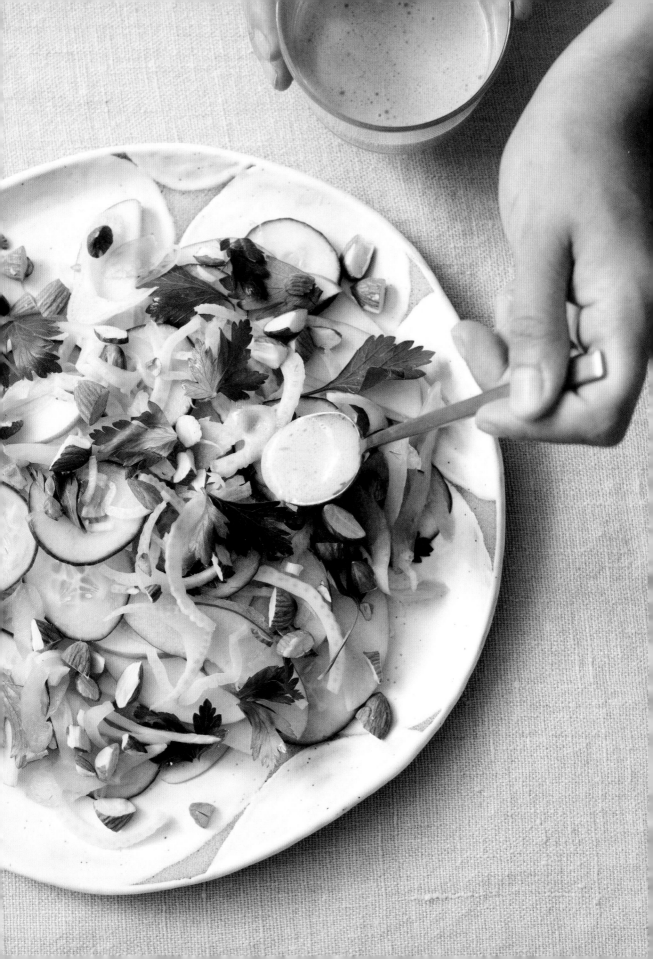

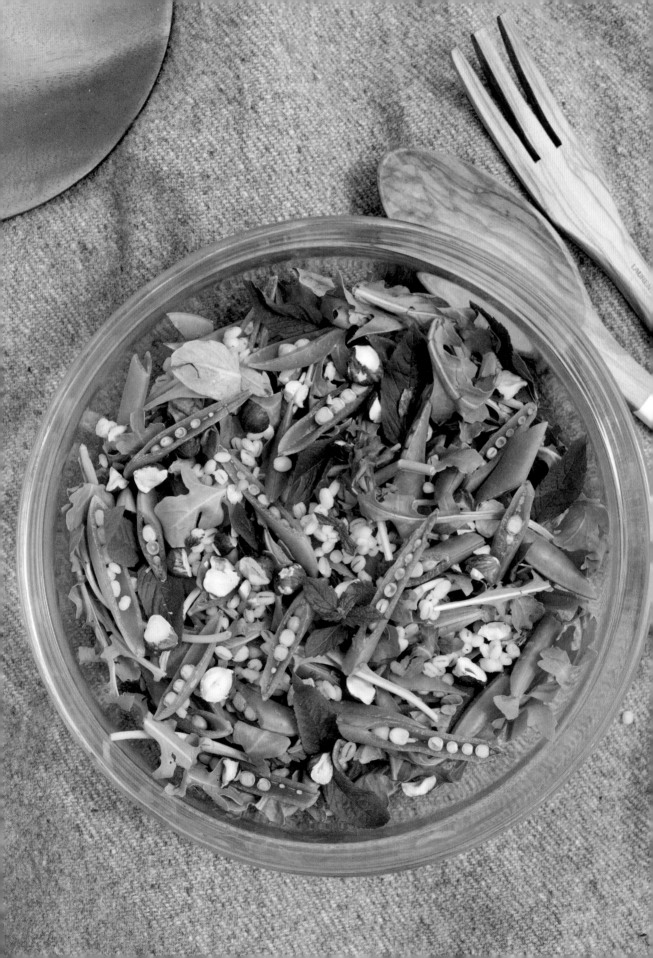

Snap Pea Salad with Hazelnuts and Barley Serves 4

Snap peas make a gentle, sweet base for this salad that is crunchy, chewy, and fresh all at the same time. We don't always think of snap peas as being super nutritious, but they actually contain a lot of vitamins A, C, and K along with fibre and protein. Barley is rich in soluble fibre, which helps to regulate digestion and support the growth of beneficial bacteria in the gut, while mint is gut-soothing. This salad makes a lovely side dish or a light meal topped with some grilled tofu.

DAIRY-FREE • HIGH-FODMAP • VEGAN

1. In a medium bowl, combine the snap peas, arugula, barley, hazelnuts, and mint. Toss together.

2. In a small mason jar, add the lemon juice, olive oil, mustard, salt, and garlic. Place the lid on tightly and shake.

3. Drizzle the dressing over the salad and toss to combine.

1 pound (450 g) snap peas, sliced lengthwise or on the diagonal

4 cups (1 L) packed baby arugula

1 cup (250 mL) cooked barley

⅓ cup (75 mL) raw hazelnuts, chopped

¼ cup (60 mL) packed fresh mint, sliced into thin ribbons

3 tablespoons (45 mL) freshly squeezed lemon juice

2 tablespoons (30 mL) extra-virgin olive oil or avocado oil

2 teaspoons (10 mL) Dijon mustard

½ teaspoon (2 mL) salt

½ clove garlic, grated or crushed

Brussels Sprouts Caesar with Garlicky Walnuts Serves 4

If you want to show people how addictively delicious health food can be, serve them this salad. Even if you think you do not like Brussels sprouts, this salty, crunchy salad will make you a believer. Cruciferous veggies like Brussels sprouts are a food I try to eat daily; crucifers contain unique sulfur-based phytochemicals that are well researched for their anti-inflammatory properties. I have topped this salad with cheesy, garlicky walnuts as croutons and an omega-3-packed hemp dressing because one can never have too many plants.

DAIRY-FREE • GLUTEN-FREE • GRAIN-FREE • HIGH-FODMAP • VEGAN

GARLICKY WALNUTS

1 cup (250 mL) raw walnuts

2 tablespoons (30 mL) nutritional yeast

2 teaspoons (10 mL) extra-virgin olive oil

½ teaspoon (2 mL) garlic powder

½ teaspoon (2 mL) salt

HEMP CAESAR DRESSING

6 tablespoons (90 mL) freshly squeezed lemon juice

¼ cup (60 mL) hemp hearts

2 tablespoons (30 mL) nutritional yeast

2 tablespoons (30 mL) drained capers

2 tablespoons (30 mL) Dijon mustard

2 tablespoons (30 mL) water

1 clove garlic, grated

1 teaspoon (5 mL) salt

1 teaspoon (5 mL) extra-virgin olive oil

½ teaspoon (2 mL) garlic powder

SALAD

1 pound (450 g) Brussels sprouts, trimmed and shredded (see Tip; or 2 bunches Tuscan kale, thick rib and stems removed and cut into thin ribbons)

1. **Make the garlicky walnuts:** Preheat the oven to 350°F (180°C). Line a small baking sheet with parchment paper.

2. In a small bowl, toss together the walnuts, nutritional yeast, olive oil, garlic powder, and salt. Spread evenly on the prepared baking sheet and bake for 10 minutes until the coating looks golden. Let cool, then roughly chop the walnuts.

3. **Meanwhile, make the hemp Caesar dressing:** In a small food processor or using a large wide-mouthed jar with a handheld immersion blender, combine the lemon juice, hemp hearts, nutritional yeast, capers, mustard, water, garlic, salt, olive oil, and garlic powder. Blend until smooth. Taste and adjust the salt or lemon juice, if needed, so it is salty and tangy.

4. **Assemble the salad:** In a large bowl, toss the Brussels sprouts with half of the hemp Caesar dressing. Add more dressing to the salad to make it as creamy as you want. I like to use about three-quarters of the dressing. Any remaining dressing can be stored in an airtight container in the fridge for up to 3 days. Sprinkle the chopped garlicky walnuts on top.

Tip Shred the Brussels sprouts in a food processor and you'll have the salad made in less than 5 minutes.

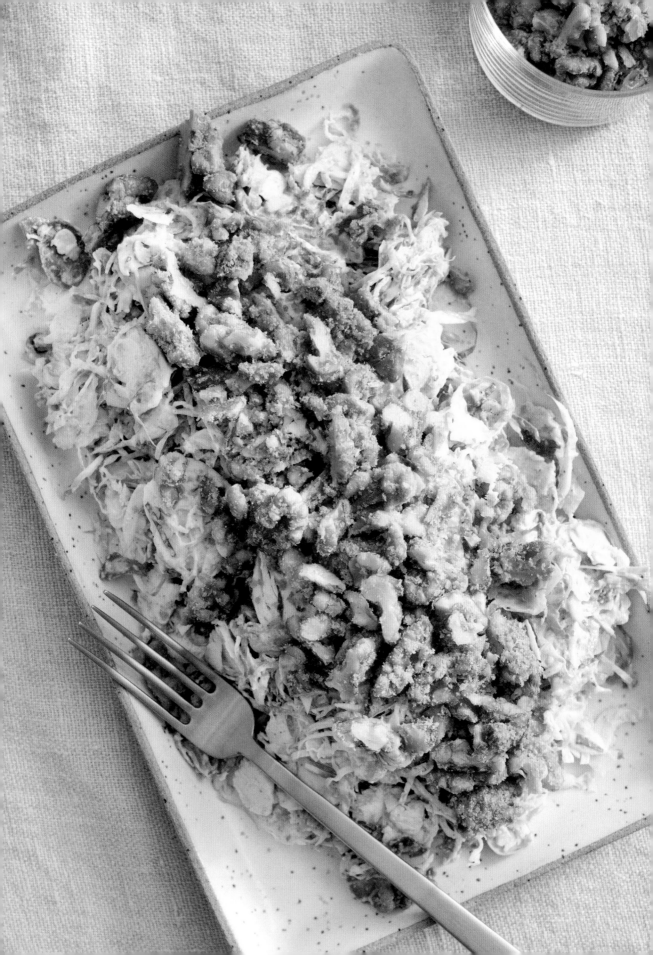

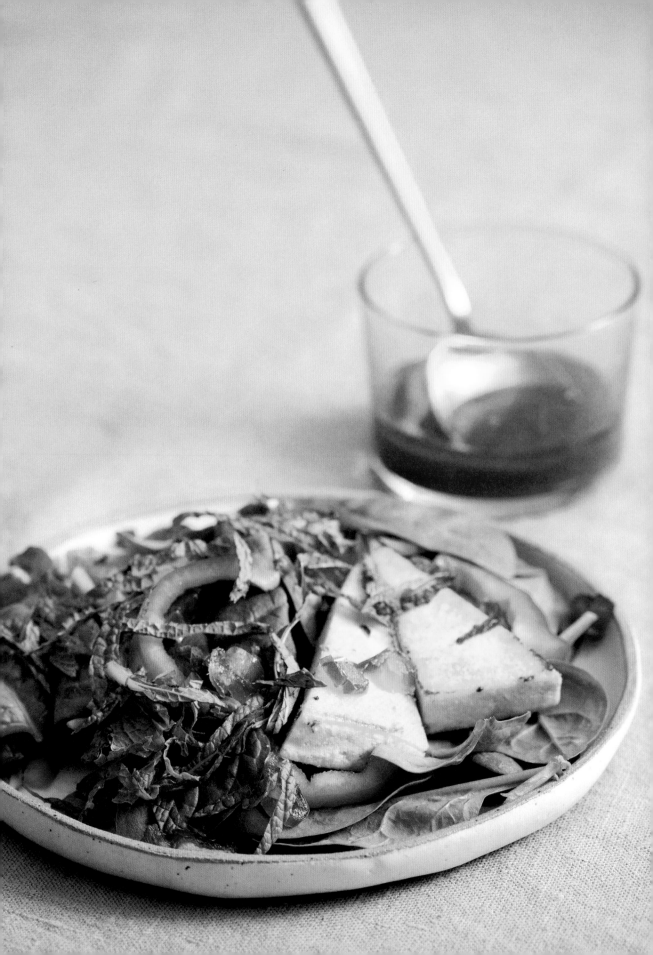

Harissa Spinach Salad with Marinated Tofu Serves 3 to 4

Harissa, a paste made from chilies, oil, and spices, is thought to hail from Tunisia, but is popular throughout North Africa and the Middle East. Capsaicin, a compound found in chili peppers, is anti-inflammatory and being researched for its pain-fighting abilities. I have used harissa to create a garlicky, spicy dressing that transforms spinach into one of those salads you crave and want to eat all of the time.

Note the instruction to use thawed frozen tofu. Freezing and thawing the tofu alters the structure to make it almost meaty in texture. It will soak up more of the marinade too! In a pinch, you can skip the freezing, but the tofu will not absorb as much flavour from the marinade. Plan ahead and thaw the tofu overnight in the fridge, then cut and marinate it in the morning for maximum flavour.

DAIRY-FREE • GLUTEN-FREE • GRAIN-FREE • HIGH-FODMAP • NUT-FREE • VEGAN

1. **Marinate the tofu:** Slice the thawed tofu into 4 squares, then slice each square diagonally into 4 triangles. In a medium airtight container, marinate the tofu in the lemon juice, mint, nutritional yeast, apple cider vinegar, maple syrup, and salt for at least 15 minutes or up to 12 hours in the fridge.

2. **Cook the tofu:** In a large nonstick skillet, heat the olive oil over medium-high heat. Reduce the heat to medium, add the marinated tofu, and cook until golden on the bottom, 4 to 5 minutes. Flip and cook until golden on the other side, 3 to 4 minutes. Remove from the heat.

3. **Make the salad:** In a large bowl, whisk together the lemon juice, avocado oil, harissa paste, garlic, salt, and maple syrup. Add the spinach, mint, red pepper, and dates. Toss to combine. Divide the salad among bowls and top with the tofu.

Tip Harissa paste comes in a variety of different blends and spice levels. It is important to use a flavourful, spicy harissa or the dressing will end up a bit flat.

FODMAP Note To make this salad low-FODMAP, ensure the harissa paste contains no garlic. Omit the garlic from the dressing and omit the dates from the salad.

MARINATED TOFU

1 package (12 ounces/340 g) thawed frozen extra-firm tofu

¼ cup (60 mL) freshly squeezed lemon juice (about 1½ lemons)

2 tablespoons (30 mL) minced fresh mint leaves

2 tablespoons (30 mL) nutritional yeast

1 tablespoon (15 mL) apple cider vinegar

1 teaspoon (5 mL) pure maple syrup

1 teaspoon (5 mL) salt

1 tablespoon (15 mL) avocado oil

HARISSA SPINACH SALAD

2 tablespoons (30 mL) freshly squeezed lemon juice

1 tablespoon (15 mL) avocado oil

1 tablespoon (15 mL) harissa paste (see Tip)

½ clove garlic, grated with a microplane

½ teaspoon (2 mL) salt

½ teaspoon (2 mL) pure maple syrup

½ pound (225 g) baby spinach

¼ cup (60 mL) shredded fresh mint leaves

1 sweet red pepper, thinly sliced

2 Medjool dates, pitted and thinly sliced

Kale Salad with Spiced Corn and Jicama Serves 4

I could eat a kale salad every day. I love dreaming up new variations, like this one inspired by a classic taco salad. The spiced corn and red onion mix packs a lot of flavour as well as microbiome-boosting FODMAPs for a healthier gut. To make this a complete meal, serve with pan-fried smoked tempeh, add black beans to the corn mixture, or enjoy it alongside my Chickpea Umami Burgers (page 142) or Roasted Eggplant and Tempeh Tacos with Cumin Lime Mayonnaise (page 154).

DAIRY-FREE • GLUTEN-FREE • GRAIN-FREE • HIGH-FODMAP • VEGAN

DRESSING

¼ cup (60 mL) freshly squeezed lime juice (about 2 limes)

2 tablespoons (30 mL) avocado oil

¼ teaspoon (1 mL) organic cane sugar

¼ teaspoon (1 mL) ground cumin

¼ teaspoon (1 mL) salt

KALE SALAD

1 tablespoon (15 mL) avocado oil

½ red onion, diced

1½ cups (375 mL) fresh or frozen corn kernels

1 teaspoon (5 mL) chili powder

½ teaspoon (2 mL) ground cumin

½ teaspoon (2 mL) salt

1 bunch curly kale, destemmed and torn into bite-size pieces

½ jicama, peeled and chopped into ½-inch (1 cm) cubes

¼ cup (60 mL) chopped raw walnuts or pumpkin seeds

½ avocado, pitted, peeled, and diced

1 lime, cut into wedges, for garnish

1. **Make the dressing:** Combine the lime juice, avocado oil, cane sugar, cumin, and salt in a small mason jar. Place the lid on tightly and shake.

2. **Make the salad:** In a medium nonstick skillet, heat the avocado oil over medium heat. Add the red onion and cook, stirring occasionally, until soft and glossy, 5 to 7 minutes.

3. Add the corn kernels and cook, stirring occasionally, until the mixture begins to brown, 5 to 7 minutes. Sprinkle the chili powder, cumin, and salt over the mixture and stir to combine. Remove from the heat, squeeze a lime wedge overtop, and set aside.

4. Place the kale and jicama in a large bowl. Drizzle the dressing over the salad and toss to coat. (If you want to soften the kale a bit, using your hands, massage the dressing into the leaves.) Top the salad with the spiced corn mixture, walnuts, and avocado. Garnish with lime wedges.

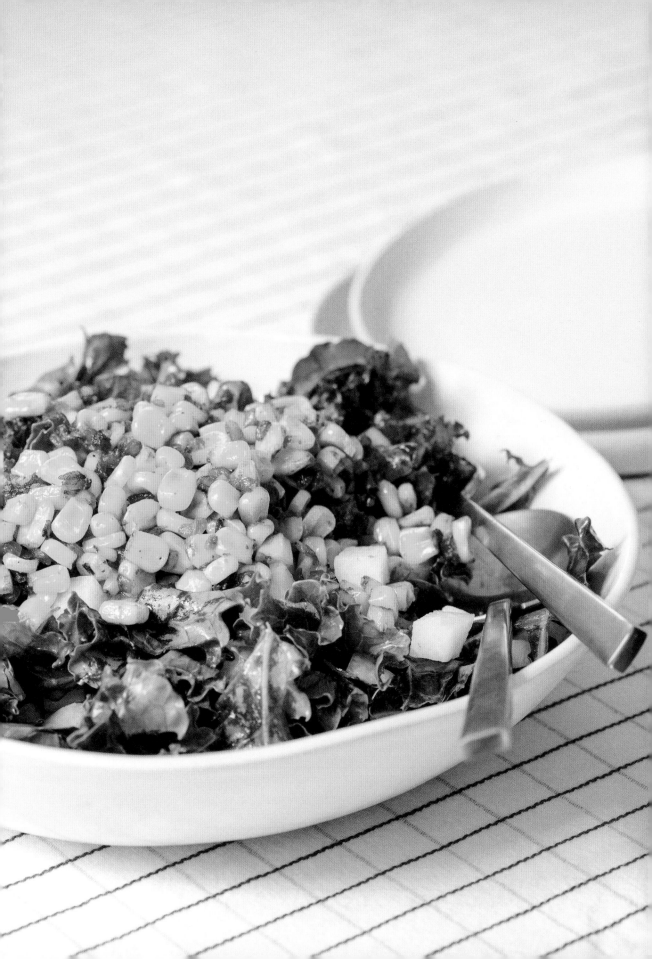

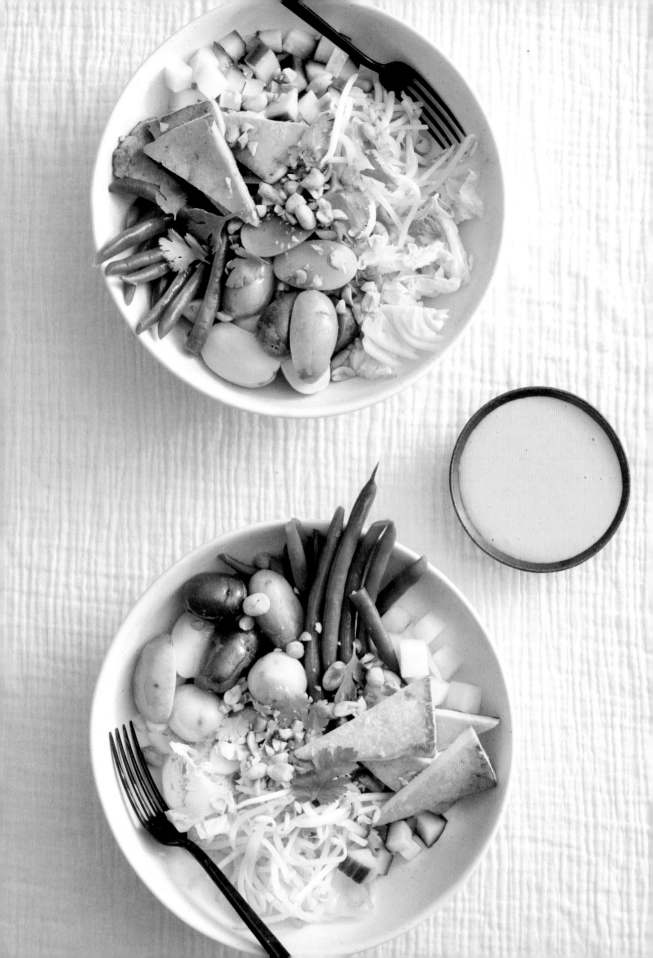

Gado Gado Serves 4

Gado gado is a traditional Indonesian salad of cooked vegetables. While most of us know it with peanut sauce, it was originally made with cashews. Gado gado is the perfect introduction to tempeh, a fermented soybean cake that is denser and more flavourful than tofu. (You can replace the tempeh with extra-firm tofu as shown in the photo, but I encourage you to try tempeh.) This has long been a favourite dish of mine while travelling, so I decided to create a low-FODMAP version so you can take a mini vacation any day of the week. Watch your portions here exactly, as some of these ingredients can be high-FODMAP in larger servings.

DAIRY-FREE • GLUTEN-FREE • GRAIN-FREE • LOW-FODMAP • VEGAN

1. **Marinate the tempeh:** Slice the tempeh crosswise into 12 pieces. (If using tofu, cut into 4 squares, then each square sliced diagonally into 4 triangles. You should have 16 triangles, total.) In a medium airtight container, combine the tamari, sesame oil, and hot sauce. Add the tempeh. Secure the lid and gently shake to coat the tempeh. Set aside to marinate while you cook the vegetables.

2. **Start the salad:** Bring a large pot of salted water to a boil. Add the potatoes. Cook for 15 minutes, until almost tender. Add the green beans to the pot and continue to boil for 3 minutes more. Drain and quickly rinse with cool water. Set aside.

3. **Meanwhile, make the peanut sauce:** In a small food processor or using a large wide-mouthed jar with a handheld immersion blender, combine the peanut butter, coconut milk, tamari, lime juice, cane sugar, salt, and hot sauce. Process until well blended. Adjust the lime juice or sugar, to taste.

4. **Cook the tempeh:** Heat the coconut oil in a medium nonstick skillet over medium heat. Place the marinated tempeh in the pan and cook until browned, 3 to 4 minutes per side.

5. **Assemble the salad:** Divide the potatoes, green beans, kale, kohlrabi, and cucumber among bowls. Add the tempeh and a drizzle of peanut sauce to each bowl. Top with bean sprouts, cilantro, and chopped peanuts. Serve with remaining sauce on the side.

TEMPEH

2 tablespoons (30 mL) gluten-free tamari

1 tablespoon (15 mL) sesame oil

1 teaspoon (5 mL) hot sauce

1 package (8 ounces/225 g) tempeh or 1 package (12 ounces/340 g) extra-firm tofu

1 tablespoon (15 mL) refined coconut oil

SALAD

1 pound (450 g) baby potatoes, halved

½ pound (225 g) green beans, trimmed and halved

2 cups (500 mL) shredded Tuscan kale or cabbage

1 cup (250 mL) thinly sliced kohlrabi

½ English cucumber, diced

1 cup (250 mL) bean sprouts

½ cup (125 mL) chopped fresh cilantro

¼ cup (60 mL) chopped unsalted peanuts

PEANUT SAUCE

½ cup (125 mL) natural peanut butter

½ cup (125 mL) canned full-fat coconut milk

2 tablespoons (30 mL) gluten-free tamari

2 tablespoons (30 mL) freshly squeezed lime juice (1 or 2 limes)

1 teaspoon (5 mL) organic cane sugar

Pinch of salt

Hot sauce, to taste

Silky Broccoli Soup with Sesame Oil Serves 4 as a starter

I really wanted to create a low-FODMAP cream of broccoli soup. To keep the starch low so it's easier on the tummy, I use a blend of celeriac (one of my favourite veggies), tahini, and hemp hearts instead of high-FODMAP cashews to create a silky smooth texture. It is important to use only the broccoli florets because the stalks are higher in FODMAPs. If you are not following a low-FODMAP diet, this makes a nice light meal for two.

DAIRY-FREE • GLUTEN-FREE • GRAIN-FREE • LOW-FODMAP • NUT-FREE • VEGAN

2 tablespoons (30 mL) extra-virgin olive oil

3 cups (750 mL) chopped broccoli florets

1 cup (250 mL) celeriac, peeled and cut into ½-inch (1 cm) cubes (about 1 small celeriac)

Salt and freshly cracked black pepper, to taste

3 cups (750 mL) water

1 tablespoon (15 mL) low-FODMAP vegetable-based bouillon (see FODMAP Note)

2 large handfuls of baby spinach

¼ cup (60 mL) nutritional yeast

2 tablespoons (30 mL) hemp hearts

2 tablespoons (30 mL) tahini

1 teaspoon (5 mL) freshly squeezed lemon juice

Red chili flakes, to taste

Toasted sesame oil, for serving

1. In a large pot, heat the olive oil over medium heat. Add the broccoli and celeriac and cook, stirring occasionally, until the vegetables brown a bit, 5 to 7 minutes. Do not stir too much to let the browning occur. Season well with salt and pepper.

2. Add the water and bouillon. Bring the soup to a gentle boil and cook until the celeriac is soft, 7 to 8 minutes. Remove from the heat. Add the spinach, nutritional yeast, hemp hearts, and tahini to the soup. Using an immersion blender, purée until smooth. Stir in the lemon juice and a pinch of chili flakes. Taste and adjust the salt, if needed. Ladle into soup bowls and drizzle with a bit of sesame oil. Leftovers can be stored in an airtight container in the fridge for up to 3 days.

FODMAP Note Low-FODMAP bouillon can be found in some specialty and health food stores or online. I use Fody Vegetable Soup Base powder. If not following a low-FODMAP diet, this soup is also delicious made with Better Than Bouillon Seasoned Vegetable Base.

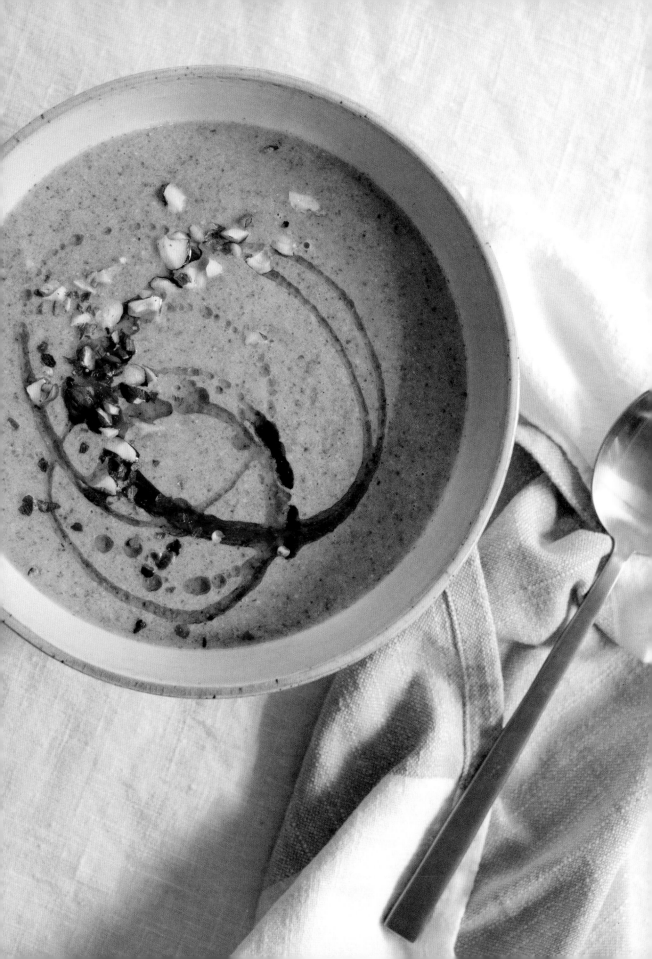

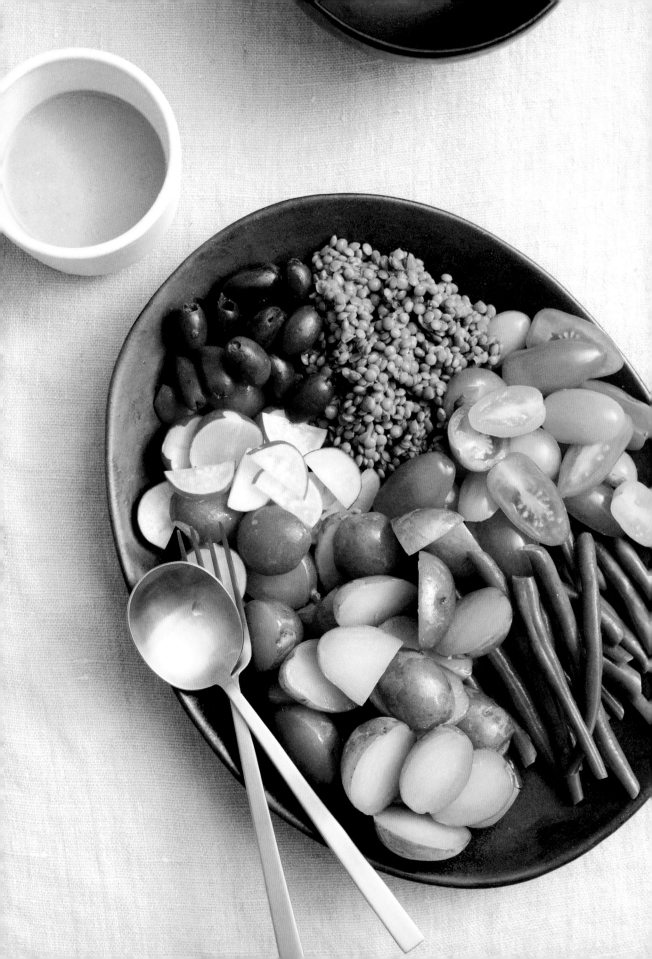

Lentil Niçoise Serves 4

We typically think of a low-FODMAP diet as being free of legumes, but keeping low-FODMAP portions of legumes in the diet means that you'll reap the long-term benefits of their fibre and mineral content. This classic, crunchy and colourful Provençal salad makes a beautiful lunch or a light meal to linger over with a glass of wine on a warm summer evening. If following a low-FODMAP diet, be sure to portion carefully as this recipe is calculated in precise low-FODMAP amounts.

DAIRY-FREE • GLUTEN-FREE • GRAIN-FREE • LOW-FODMAP • NUT-FREE • VEGAN

1. **Make the salad:** Bring a large pot of salted water to a boil over high heat. Add the potatoes and cook until for fork-tender, 13 to 15 minutes. Add the green beans in the last 3 to 5 minutes of cooking, depending on thickness of the beans. Drain and rinse the vegetables under cold running water to stop the cooking process.

2. In a small bowl, toss the lentils in the olive oil, white wine vinegar, and salt.

3. **Make the vinaigrette:** In a small mason jar, add the white wine vinegar, olive oil, capers, mustard, cane sugar, salt, and pepper. Place the lid on tightly and shake.

4. To serve, arrange the lentil mixture, potatoes, beans, tomatoes, radishes and leaves (if using), and olives on a platter. Drizzle half of the vinaigrette over the salad. Serve the remaining vinaigrette on the side.

FODMAP Notes 1. If you are not following a low-FODMAP diet, feel free to use more tomatoes, beans, or freshly cooked Puy lentils.

2. Adding 1 tablespoon (15 mL) of minced shallot is a nice zippy addition to the dressing too.

SALAD

1½ pounds (675 g) baby potatoes, halved

½ pound (225 g) green beans, trimmed

2 cups (500 mL) canned lentils, rinsed and drained

1 teaspoon (5 mL) extra-virgin olive oil

1 teaspoon (5 mL) white wine vinegar or freshly squeezed lemon juice

Pinch of salt

20 cherry tomatoes, halved

1 bunch radishes, halved (use the leaves if fresh)

Heaping ½ cup (125 mL) pitted Kalamata olives

VINAIGRETTE

¼ cup (60 mL) white wine vinegar or freshly squeezed lemon juice

2 tablespoons (30 mL) extra-virgin olive oil

1 tablespoon (15 mL) drained capers, chopped

1 tablespoon (15 mL) Dijon mustard

2 teaspoons (10 mL) organic cane sugar or pure maple syrup

½ teaspoon (2 mL) salt

Freshly cracked black pepper

Cabbage and Fennel Slaw with Jalapeño Grapefruit Dressing Serves 6 as a side

I really love a good slaw. Not only is cabbage very affordable, it is also low-FODMAP and a Brassica vegetable, meaning that it comes packed with anti-inflammatory and gut-boosting indole compounds. In addition, cabbage is rich in l-glutamine, an amino acid that supports the health of the gut lining. I have created a zesty jalapeño grapefruit dressing that comes together quickly in the blender, so this is an easy salad to whip up on a weeknight. It is delicious with the Chickpea Umami Burgers (page 142) or Roasted Eggplant and Tempeh Tacos with Cumin Lime Mayonnaise (page 154). Keep the dressing separate from the slaw if you are planning to have leftovers, as it tends to separate in the fridge.

DAIRY-FREE • GLUTEN-FREE • GRAIN-FREE • LOW-FODMAP • NUT-FREE • VEGAN

CABBAGE AND FENNEL SLAW

6 cups (1.5 L) shredded cabbage or coleslaw mix

1 medium fennel bulb, finely shredded with a mandoline

1 cup (250 mL) cilantro, leaves and tender stems, roughly chopped

⅓ cup (75 mL) raw pumpkin seeds

JALAPEÑO GRAPEFRUIT DRESSING

1 red grapefruit, peel and pith removed and halved

1 jalapeño pepper, with or without seeds, roughly chopped

2 tablespoons (30 mL) vegan mayonnaise

4 teaspoons (20 mL) freshly squeezed lime juice

1 teaspoon (5 mL) avocado oil

1 teaspoon (5 mL) organic cane sugar

½ teaspoon (2 mL) salt

1. **Make the slaw:** In a large salad bowl, combine the shredded cabbage, fennel, cilantro, and pumpkin seeds.

2. **Make the dressing:** In a high-speed blender, add the grapefruit, jalapeño, vegan mayonnaise, lime juice, avocado oil, cane sugar, and salt. Blend until smooth.

3. If serving right away, toss the salad with half the dressing. Serve the remaining dressing on the side. Otherwise, store the dressing in a jar with a lid in the fridge for up to 2 days. Shake the jar before using.

FODMAP Notes 1. If you are buying pre-made coleslaw mix, watch for high-FODMAP ingredients such as beets or Brussels sprouts.

2. If you are not following a low-FODMAP diet, I recommend adding ¼ medium red onion, thinly sliced to the slaw and ½ clove minced garlic to the dressing.

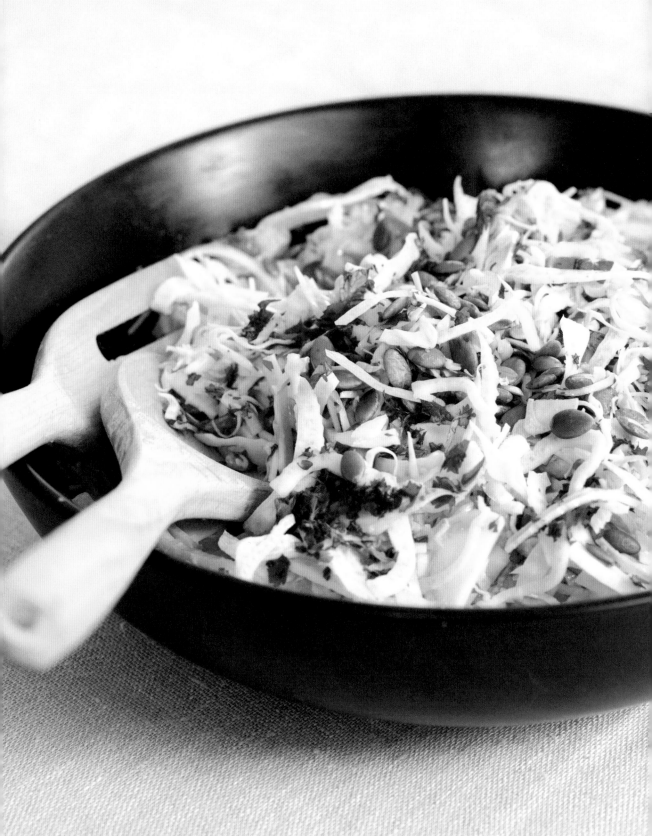

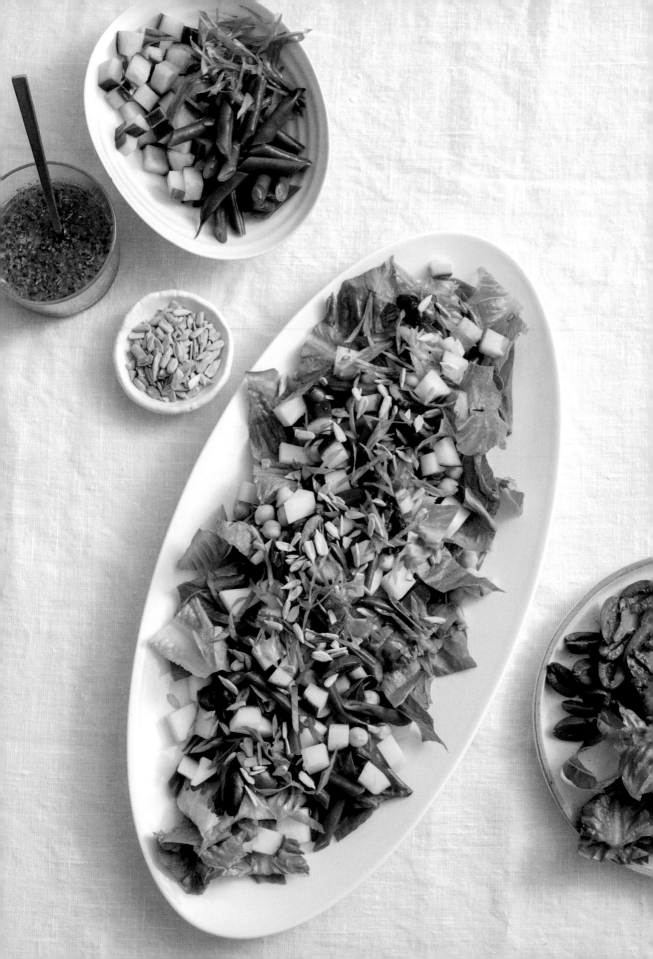

Kohlrabi Chopped Salad Serves 4

I always thought that a chopped salad was a salad with crunchy chopped-up veggies. Turns out that a chopped salad is very much a thing and it involves lettuce. Introducing my kohlrabi chop with plenty of crunchy, low-FODMAP veggies and, yes, chopped lettuce. This has a fun, throwback Italian-style dressing that I cannot get enough of. Be sure to keep to the exact measurements of kohlrabi, chickpeas, and green beans to keep it low-FODMAP. If you're not following a low-FODMAP diet, enjoy at least ½ cup (125 mL) of chickpeas per serving for more protein.

DAIRY-FREE • GLUTEN-FREE • GRAIN-FREE • LOW-FODMAP • NUT-FREE • VEGAN

1. **Blanch the green beans:** Bring a small pot of water to a boil over high heat. When the water is boiling, add the green beans and blanch for 2 minutes. Drain and rinse under cold running water.

2. **Make the dressing:** In a small mason jar, add the red wine vinegar, olive oil, nutritional yeast, cane sugar, salt, oregano, and pepper. Place the lid on tightly and shake.

3. **Assemble the salad:** In a large bowl, toss together the romaine, kohlrabi, green beans, cucumber, chickpeas, olives, green onions, and sunflower seeds. Drizzle the dressing over the salad and toss again.

SALAD

20 green beans, chopped into 1-inch (2.5 cm) pieces

1 heart of romaine, trimmed and chopped

2 cups (500 mL) peeled and cubed kohlrabi

1 cup (250 mL) cubed English cucumber

1 cup (250 mL) canned chickpeas, rinsed and drained

½ cup (125 mL) Kalamata olives, pitted and halved

4 green onions (dark green parts only), sliced into ½-inch (1 cm) pieces

2 tablespoons (30 mL) raw sunflower seeds

DRESSING

¼ cup (60 mL) red wine vinegar

2 tablespoons (30 mL) extra-virgin olive oil

1 tablespoon (15 mL) nutritional yeast

1 teaspoon (5 mL) organic cane sugar

1 teaspoon (5 mL) salt

½ teaspoon (2 mL) dried oregano

Freshly cracked black pepper

Summer Zucchini Salad with Hazelnuts Serves 4

This salad is inspired by a *Bon Appétit* recipe from a few years back and a dish I tried from my favourite local restaurant. It celebrates zucchini in all of its midsummer glory by pairing it with sweet and earthy hazelnuts and fragrant basil. Zucchini is low in fibre, making this a great raw vegetable option for when your gut is irritated, and it packs plenty of potassium and healing beta-carotene along with small amounts of vitamin C.

DAIRY-FREE • GLUTEN-FREE • GRAIN-FREE • HIGH-FODMAP • VEGAN

2 medium zucchini

2 tablespoons (30 mL) extra-virgin olive oil, divided

1 tablespoon (15 mL) freshly squeezed lemon juice

¼ teaspoon (1 mL) salt, plus more for seasoning

¼ cup (60 mL) raw hazelnuts

Freshly cracked black pepper

1 cup (250 mL) hummus

½ cup (125 mL) lightly packed fresh basil leaves, sliced into thin ribbons

1. Slice 1 zucchini in half lengthwise, then slice the halves into 2-inch (5 cm) wide pieces. Slice the other zucchini into thin ribbons with a mandoline or vegetable peeler.

2. In a medium bowl, add the zucchini ribbons, 1 tablespoon (15 mL) of the olive oil, lemon juice, and salt. Toss with your hands to ensure that the zucchini is well coated with the marinade. Set aside.

3. Heat a dry medium nonstick skillet over medium heat. When the pan is hot, add the hazelnuts. Toast, stirring often, until fragrant, 3 to 4 minutes. Transfer the hazelnuts to a small plate to cool.

4. In the same skillet, heat the remaining 1 tablespoon (15 mL) olive oil over medium-high heat. Add the zucchini pieces, cut side down, to the pan. Cover with a lid and let steam for 2 minutes. Remove the lid and cook until the zucchini is brown on the bottom, 3 to 4 minutes. Remove from the heat, flip the zucchini pieces over, and season well with salt and pepper.

5. To serve, spread the hummus on a serving plate or in a shallow bowl. Shake any excess marinade off the zucchini ribbons. Arrange the zucchini ribbons and the seared zucchini over the hummus. Top with the toasted hazelnuts and basil.

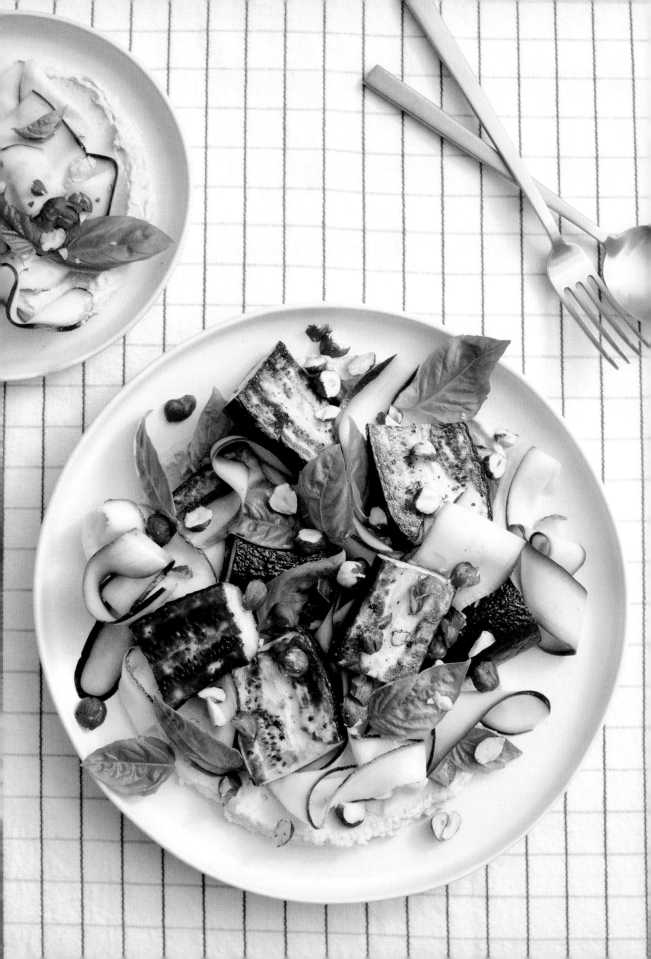

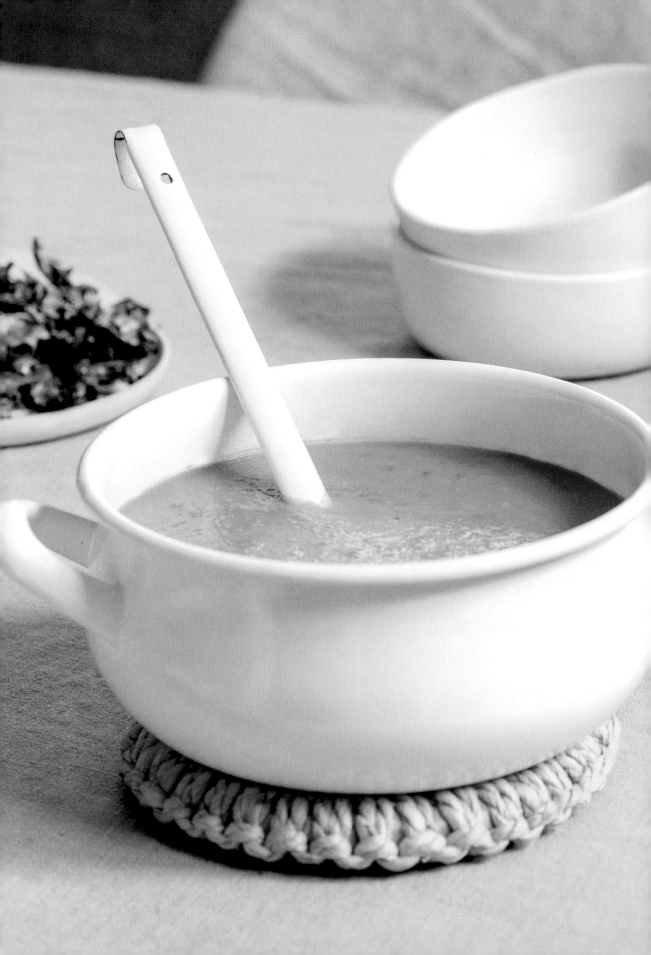

Creamy Tomato and White Bean Soup with Crispy Kale Serves 4

The secret to creating creamy vegan soups and dips is white beans. They are a staple in my home for their creamy texture and neutral, almost buttery flavour. Beans can be hard to tolerate for an irritated tummy, but blending them into a delicious tomato soup makes it easier to enjoy their soothing soluble fibre and gut-boosting minerals. Garlic and onion build flavour and offer prebiotic fibres to help feed beneficial bacteria in the gut.

While this soup is delicious and comforting on its own, do not skip the crispy kale topping. Its addictive crunch adds another layer of texture to this easy weeknight meal. In fact, I have been known to make a double batch of crispy kale because I have a tendency to eat most of it before it is time to serve the soup.

DAIRY-FREE • GLUTEN-FREE • GRAIN-FREE • NUT-FREE • HIGH-FODMAP • VEGAN

1. Preheat the oven to 400°F (200°C). Line a large baking sheet with parchment paper.

2. **Make the creamy tomato and white bean soup:** In a large pot, heat the olive oil over medium heat. Add the onion, fennel, and celery and cook, stirring occasionally, until the onions are soft and glossy, 5 to 7 minutes. Season with salt and pepper. Add the garlic and cook, stirring constantly, for 1 minute.

3. Add the tomatoes, either crushing them with your hands before adding them to the pot or using a spatula to crush them in the pot. Stir in the beans, vegetable broth, thyme, salt, and garlic powder. Bring to a boil, then reduce the heat to medium-low and simmer, uncovered, for 15 minutes.

4. **Meanwhile, make the crispy kale:** In a large bowl, toss the kale with the olive oil, salt, and chili flakes. Evenly spread the kale on the prepared baking sheet and bake for 5 minutes. Rotate the baking sheet and bake for 3 to 6 minutes more, watching carefully, as kale goes from crispy to burnt quickly.

5. Remove the soup from the heat. Using a handheld immersion blender, purée the soup. (I like to leave a bit of texture so it is not perfectly smooth.) Stir in the lemon zest and juice. Taste and adjust the salt and pepper, if needed. Ladle the soup into soup bowls and top with a few chili flakes and crispy kale. Leftover soup (without the crispy kale) can be stored in an airtight container in the fridge for up to 5 days. Store the crispy kale loosely covered on the counter for up to 3 days.

CREAMY TOMATO AND WHITE BEAN SOUP

¼ cup (60 mL) extra-virgin olive oil or avocado oil

1 medium yellow onion, diced

½ small fennel bulb, diced (about 1 cup/250 mL)

2 ribs celery, diced

Freshly cracked black pepper

4 cloves garlic, chopped

1 can (28 ounces/796 mL) whole plum tomatoes

1 can (14 ounces/398 mL) no-salt-added white beans (navy, cannellini, or butter)

2 cups (500 mL) low-sodium vegetable broth

6 sprigs fresh thyme, leaves only (1 tablespoon/15 mL) (or 1 teaspoon/ 5 mL dried thyme leaves)

1 teaspoon (5 mL) salt, plus more for seasoning

½ teaspoon (2 mL) garlic powder

Zest of 1 lemon

Juice of ½ lemon

Red chili flakes, for garnish

CRISPY KALE

1 large bunch curly kale, destemmed and torn into large pieces

1 tablespoon (15 mL) extra-virgin olive oil

¼ teaspoon (1 mL) salt

Pinch of red chili flakes

Blood Orange, Beet, and Pistachio Salad with Toasted Buckwheat Serves 4

This salad is a riot of deep velvety colours and different textures. Buckwheat is a gluten-free seed that adds plenty of crunch while being easy on digestion. Blood oranges contain soluble fibre, which is soothing to the gut while being packed, as are the beets, with anti-inflammatory pigments. This is a beautiful salad for entertaining. Try serving with Smoky Red Pepper Hummus (page 256) and the Amazing Seeded Grain-Free Bread (page 263) for a lovely appetizer spread.

DAIRY-FREE • GLUTEN-FREE • VEGAN

4 medium red beets

¼ cup (60 mL) raw buckwheat groats

2 tablespoons (30 mL) + 1 teaspoon (5 mL) extra-virgin olive oil, divided

Pinch of salt, plus more for seasoning

½ cup (125 mL) raw or roasted pistachios

3 blood oranges (or if unavailable, use navel or Cara Cara oranges)

½ medium shallot, finely diced or sliced with a mandoline

Juice of ½ lemon

1 teaspoon (5 mL) pure maple syrup

Freshly cracked black pepper

1. Preheat the oven to 400°F (200° C).

2. Scrub and trim the beets. Wrap the beets in a large piece of aluminum foil and place on a baking sheet. Roast until soft, about 1 hour. Remove from the oven and take off the foil. Set aside to cool slightly. Reduce the oven temperature to 350°F (180°C) for the buckwheat.

3. When the beets are cool enough to handle, peel and slice them into ¼-inch (5 mm) rounds and place on a platter or in a salad bowl.

4. Line a small baking sheet with parchment paper.

5. In a small bowl, toss the buckwheat with 1 teaspoon (5 mL) of the olive oil and salt. Spread the mixture onto the prepared baking sheet and roast until the buckwheat is golden brown, 12 to 16 minutes. Stir halfway through cooking time. Set aside to cool.

6. If the pistachios are raw, heat a dry small skillet over medium heat. When the pan is hot, add the pistachios and stir and shake them a few times until toasted, 3 to 4 minutes. Skip this step if the pistachios are roasted.

7. Carefully cut away all of the peel and pith from the blood oranges. Then, carefully run a paring knife between the flesh of the orange sections and the skin, until the section pops out. Place the orange sections onto the platter and squeeze out any extra juice from the remaining orange skins overtop.

8. Arrange the shallot, pistachios, and buckwheat over the blood oranges.

9. In a small bowl, mix together the remaining 2 tablespoons (30 mL) olive oil, lemon juice and maple syrup. Drizzle over the salad. Finish with a generous sprinkling of salt and pepper.

Tips 1. You can roast the beets and toast the buckwheat a day in advance. Store the roasted beets covered in the fridge. Store the toasted buckwheat in an airtight container on the counter.

2. If storing leftovers, I recommend keeping the pistachios and buckwheat separate on the counter, so they don't go soft in the fridge.

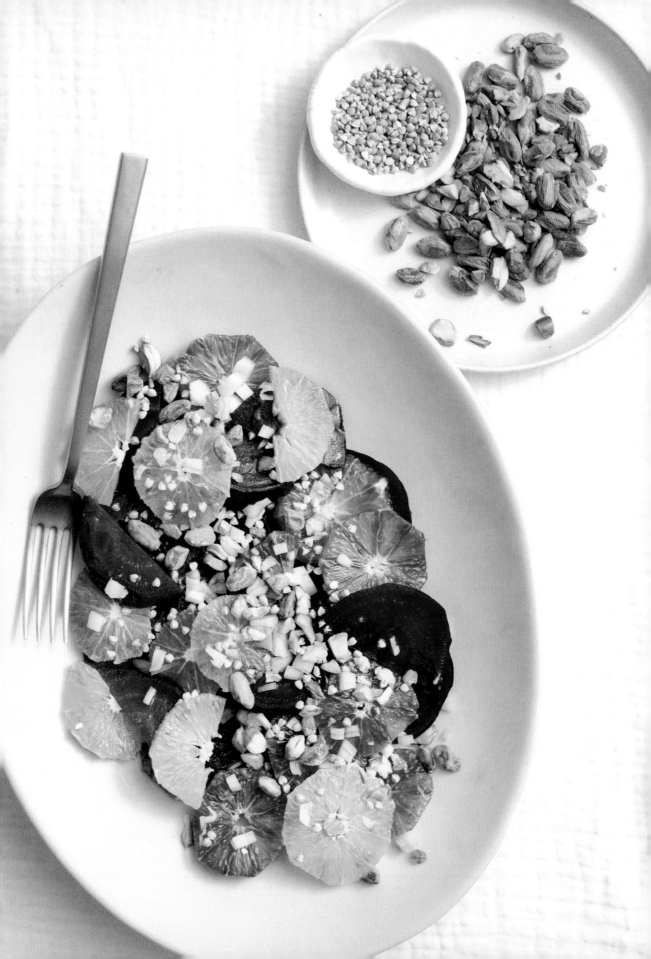

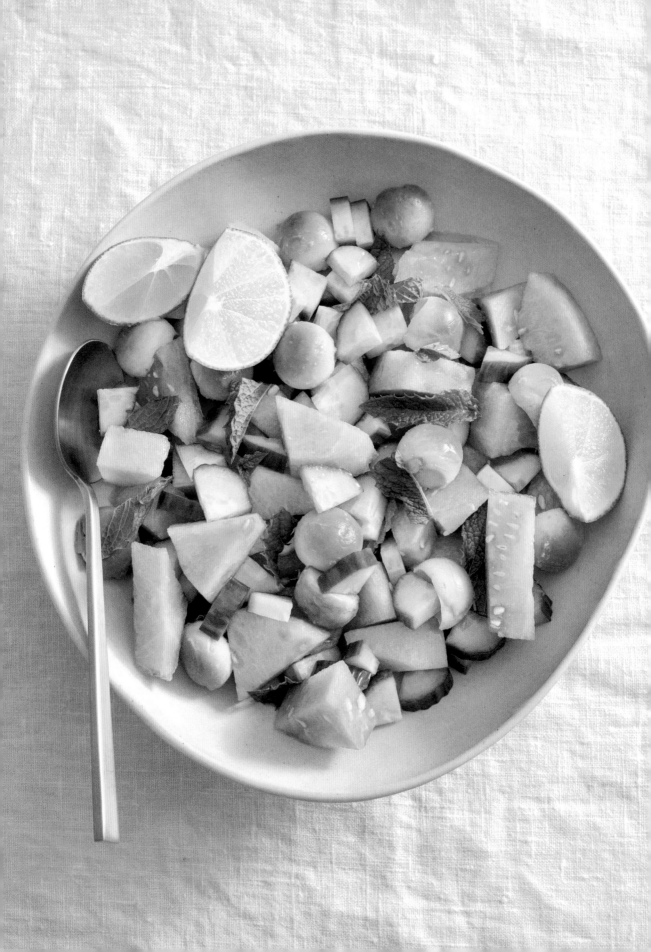

Watermelon Salad with Avocado and Mint Serves 4

This salad screams summer to me—juicy, crunchy, and sweet and made with minimal effort. Full of microbiome-boosting FODMAPs, these fruit and vegetables are relatively easy on an irritated gut because they are not high in insoluble fibres. Mint is also soothing and relaxing to the smooth muscle lining the gut, but if you are super reflux-y, you might want to skip the mint for now. Perfect on those days when it is too hot to cook, this salad is delicious served alongside Mediterranean Artichoke Burgers (page 161) or on its own with some grilled tofu.

DAIRY-FREE • GLUTEN-FREE • GRAIN-FREE • HIGH-FODMAP • NUT-FREE • VEGAN

1. In a large bowl, toss the avocado with the lime juice, salt, and pepper. Add the watermelon, cucumber, mint, and avocado oil. Gently fold to combine.

1 avocado, peeled, pitted, and diced

Juice of 1 lime

Pinch each of salt and pepper

4 cups (1 L) diced watermelon

2 cups (500 mL) diced English cucumber (skin-on, if tolerated)

½ cup (125 mL) lightly packed fresh mint leaves, sliced into thin ribbons

1 tablespoon (15 mL) avocado oil

Thai Mushroom and Tofu Laab Serves 4

My first taste of tofu laab at Night and Market restaurant in Los Angeles, when I was on the book tour for *Eat More Plants*, inspired this salad. Laab is a spicy, tart, meat-based salad that hails from Laos and Thailand, where there are as many variations as there are cooks. My version is a decidedly non-traditional one, using tofu and mushroom. It is a tangy, salty, chewy combination packed with fresh herbs and even a bit of crunch from the toasted rice powder. Getting enough protein is essential for the healing process, and tofu tends to be easier on the gut and more concentrated in protein than beans. So this delicious salad is exactly what the gut-health dietitian ordered.

DAIRY-FREE • GLUTEN-FREE • HIGH-FODMAP • NUT-FREE • VEGAN

½ cup (125 mL) Thai jasmine rice (for the toasted rice powder; see Tip)

2 tablespoons (30 mL) avocado oil, divided

1 package (12 ounces/340 g) extra-firm tofu, cut into 4 squares

Salt

1 pound (450 g) mixed mushrooms (baby bella, cremini, shiitake, or enoki), chopped

2 tablespoons (30 mL) gluten-free tamari

1½ teaspoons (7 mL) organic cane sugar

¼ cup (60 mL) minced shallot

¼ cup (60 mL) freshly squeezed lime juice (about 2 limes)

½ to 1 teaspoon (2 to 5 mL) red chili flakes

1 cup (250 mL) fresh cilantro leaves, chopped

¼ cup (60 mL) packed fresh mint leaves, sliced into thin ribbons

1. In a small dry skillet, toast the rice, shaking the pan occasionally, until golden brown and fragrant, 15 to 20 minutes. Let cool for 5 minutes. Using either a clean coffee grinder or a mortar and pestle, grind the rice into a powder. Set aside. Store in an airtight container at room temperature for up to 1 month.

2. In a large nonstick skillet, heat 1 tablespoon (15 mL) of the avocado oil over medium-high heat. Add the tofu and cook until brown on the bottom and crisp, 4 to 5 minutes. Flip, season with salt, and cook until brown on the bottom and crisp, 3 to 4 minutes. Flip again, season with salt, and transfer to a plate.

3. In the same skillet, heat the remaining 1 tablespoon (15 mL) avocado oil over medium-high heat. Add the mushrooms, in 2 batches if needed so you do not crowd the pan. Cook, stirring occasionally, until browned and the water is evaporated, 4 to 5 minutes. Remove from the heat.

4. Tear the cooked tofu into bite-size pieces and add to the skillet with the mushrooms.

5. In a small bowl, blend together the tamari and cane sugar. Pour over the mushroom tofu mixture and stir to combine. Let cool for 10 minutes.

6. Add the shallot, lime juice, and chili flakes. Mix well. Taste and adjust the salt, if needed (I usually add about ¼ teaspoon/1 mL). Sprinkle 2 tablespoons (30 mL) of the toasted rice powder overtop and stir to combine. Toss the cilantro and mint with the mushroom tofu mixture.

Tip Omit the toasted rice powder or substitute it with 2 tablespoons (30 mL) gluten-free panko bread crumbs to add a bit of crunch without extra effort.

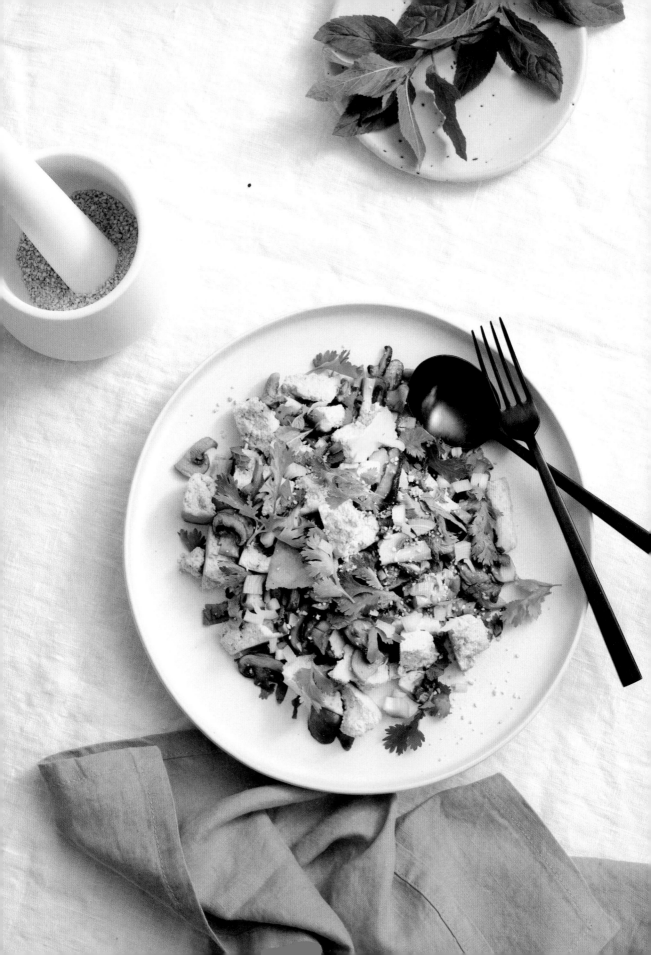

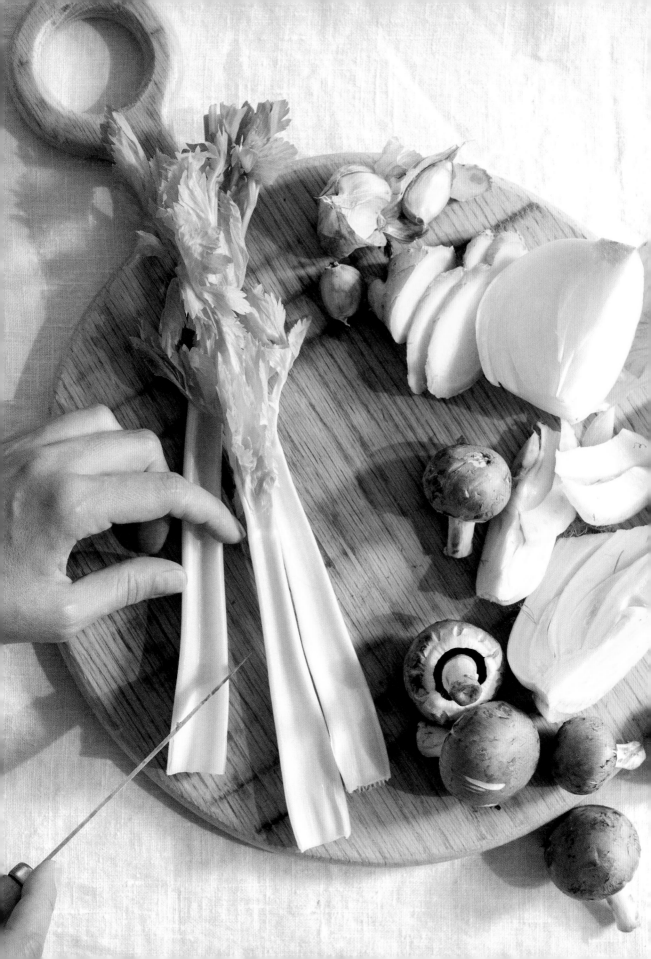

No-Bones Prebiotic Broth Makes about 2 quarts (2 L)

Regular bone broth isn't doing anything for your gut except giving it a rest from dietary fibre when you're feeling inflamed. This broth, on the other hand, is packed with prebiotic FODMAPs that are water soluble, which means they leach into the broth to feed your gut bacteria even when your gut is too inflamed and irritable to handle a lot of fibre. Consume the broth as is or use it as the base of a puréed soup for those times when you're ready for more plant goodness. If you like, leave in half of the vegetables (save the rest for later or compost) then purée with an immersion blender for a light blended soup to support healing.

DAIRY-FREE • GLUTEN-FREE • GRAIN-FREE • HIGH-FODMAP • NUT-FREE • VEGAN

1. Place the onion, celery, carrots, mushrooms, fennel, ginger, turmeric, garlic, and salt in a large pot and fill with enough water to cover the vegetables by 2 inches (5 cm). Bring to a boil over high heat. When the broth is boiling, reduce the heat to medium and let simmer, uncovered, for 1 hour.

2. Remove from the heat and, using a slotted spoon, scoop out all or half of the vegetables depending on whether you want a broth or light puréed soup. (Instead of throwing out the cooked vegetables, pulse in a food processor until finely chopped and use, or purée in a high-speed blender, pour into ice cube trays, and freeze for up to 1 month. Add to soups, veggie burgers, casseroles, or chilies.)

3. Store the broth in an airtight container in the fridge for up to 5 days or in the freezer for up to 1 month.

Tip If you are feeling under the weather, triple the ginger and turmeric for some major fire, then sip throughout the day.

1 onion, quartered

4 ribs celery, roughly chopped

3 carrots, scrubbed and roughly chopped

½ pound (225 g) cremini mushrooms, brushed

1 small fennel bulb, trimmed and quartered

3-inch (8 cm) piece of fresh ginger, peeled and cut into ¼-inch (5 mm) slices

1-inch (2.5 cm) piece of fresh turmeric, peeled and sliced in half lengthwise (or ½ teaspoon/2 mL ground turmeric)

3 skin-on cloves garlic

1½ teaspoons (7 mL) salt

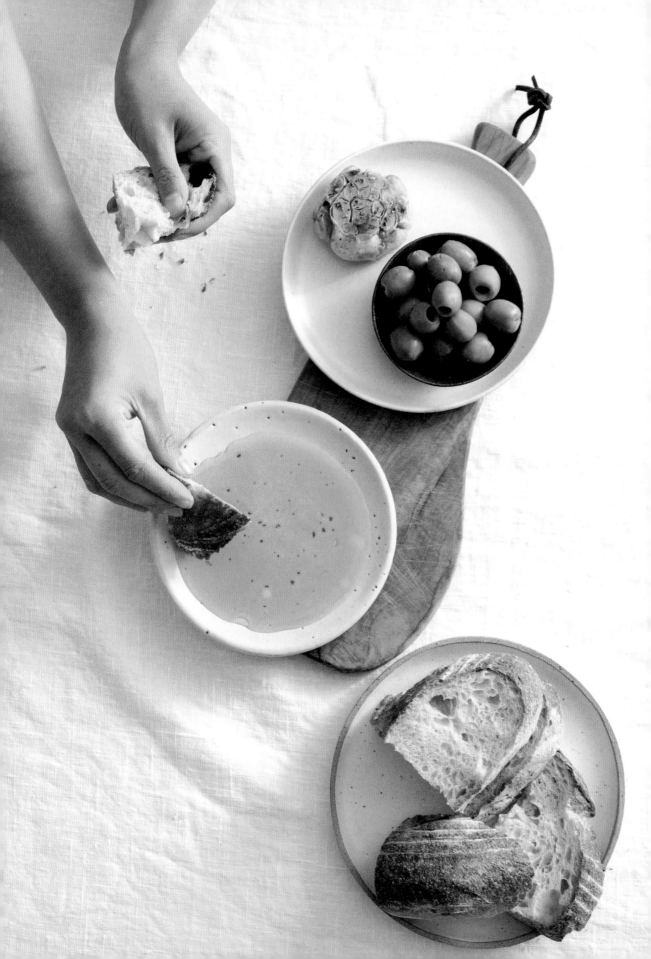

Snacks and Sides

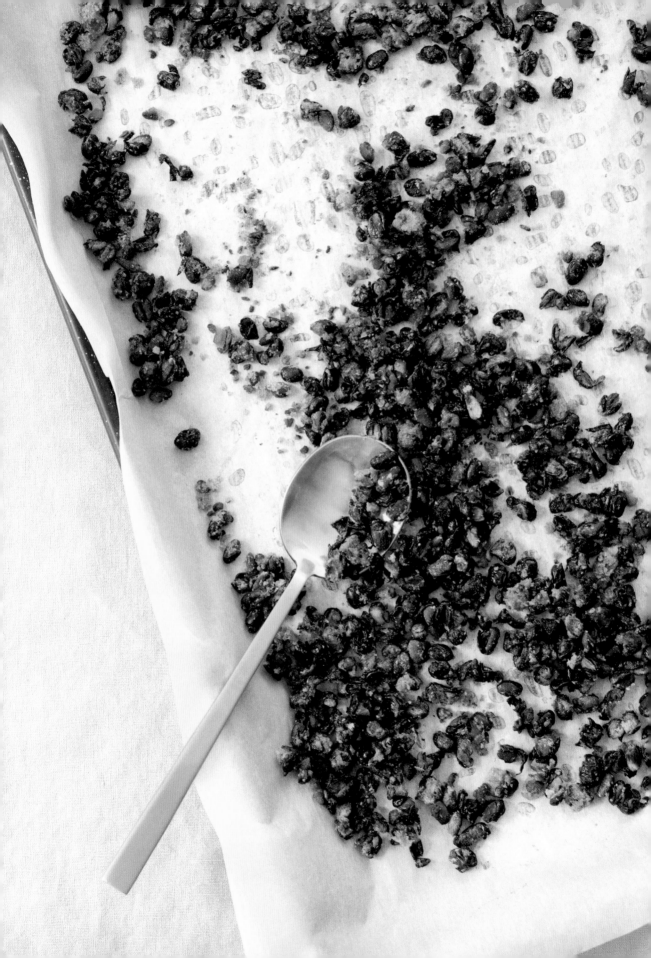

Nacho Roasted Black Beans Makes 1½ cups (375 mL)

Roasted beans are such a great snack because they contain slow burning carbs for lasting energy and plenty of fibre and protein to keep you going. I usually roast chickpeas, but black beans are a nice change of pace. Their black seed coats are rich in anti-inflammatory anthocyanin phytochemicals, giving them even more benefits. I recommend making a double or triple batch if you are serving friends. A deliciously addictive snack that disappears quickly.

DAIRY-FREE • GLUTEN-FREE • GRAIN-FREE • HIGH-FODMAP • NUT-FREE • VEGAN

1. Preheat the oven to 375°F (190°C). Line a baking sheet with parchment paper.

2. Evenly spread the black beans on the prepared baking sheet. Roast for 15 minutes. Do not stir. Roasting without oil helps the beans get crispier.

3. In a medium bowl, whisk together the avocado oil, nutritional yeast, salt, garlic powder, onion powder, chili powder, and paprika. Transfer the beans into the bowl and toss to coat with the seasoning paste. Evenly spread the coated beans back onto the baking sheet and bake until the beans start to blister, 10 to 15 minutes more. Do not stir. Let cool for 10 minutes before serving. Store uncovered on the counter for up to 2 days.

1 can (14 ounces/398 mL) black beans, drained and rinsed (or about 1½ cups/ 375 mL cooked beans)

2 tablespoons (30 mL) avocado oil

1 tablespoon (15 mL) nutritional yeast

½ teaspoon (2 mL) salt

½ teaspoon (2 mL) garlic powder

½ teaspoon (2 mL) onion powder

¼ teaspoon (1 mL) chili powder

⅛ teaspoon (0.5 mL) smoked paprika

Easy Asparagus Fritters Makes 7 to 8 fritters

Asparagus fritters are a common Italian treat, but they are usually made with eggs, not chickpea flour. Asparagus is high in prebiotics, making these fritters a tasty treat for you and your microbiome. Flavourful and satisfying, they're an energizing addition to any snack platter. You could also serve them alongside the Brussels Sprouts Caesar with Garlicky Walnuts (page 204) as a light but filling meal.

DAIRY-FREE • GLUTEN-FREE • GRAIN-FREE • HIGH-FODMAP • NUT-FREE • VEGAN

ASPARAGUS FRITTERS

1 pound (450 g) fresh asparagus, trimmed and cut into ½-inch (1 cm) pieces (about 2 cups/500 mL chopped)

¾ cup (175 mL) chickpea flour

¼ cup (60 mL) nutritional yeast

2 tablespoons (30 mL) ground flaxseed

2 cloves garlic, grated with a microplane

¾ teaspoon (3 mL) salt

¾ teaspoon (3 mL) onion powder

½ teaspoon (2 mL) garlic powder

½ teaspoon (2 mL) ground cumin

Freshly cracked black pepper

½ cup (125 mL) water

¼ cup (60 mL) grated yellow onion (about ¼ large onion); squeeze out excess moisture before measuring

¼ cup (60 mL) finely chopped fresh dill or basil leaves

Avocado oil, for frying

DIP

½ cup (125 mL) vegan mayonnaise

¼ cup (60 mL) Dijon mustard

1. **Make the asparagus fritters:** Bring a medium pot of water to a boil over high heat. Add the asparagus and parboil for 2 minutes. Drain and transfer to a plate.

2. In a medium bowl, whisk together the chickpea flour, nutritional yeast, flaxseed, garlic, salt, onion powder, garlic powder, cumin, and pepper. Stir in the water. Add the onion, dill, and asparagus and stir.

3. In a large nonstick skillet, heat 1 tablespoon (15 mL) avocado oil over medium-high heat. Add ⅓ cup (75 mL) of batter per fritter to the pan. Cook 3 or 4 fritters at a time. Fry until crisp and golden on the bottom, about 2 minutes per side. If the oil begins to smoke, reduce the heat to medium. Transfer the fritters to a plate lined with paper towel to absorb excess oil. Repeat to use the remaining batter.

4. **Make the dip:** In a small bowl, mix together the vegan mayonnaise and mustard. Serve alongside the fritters.

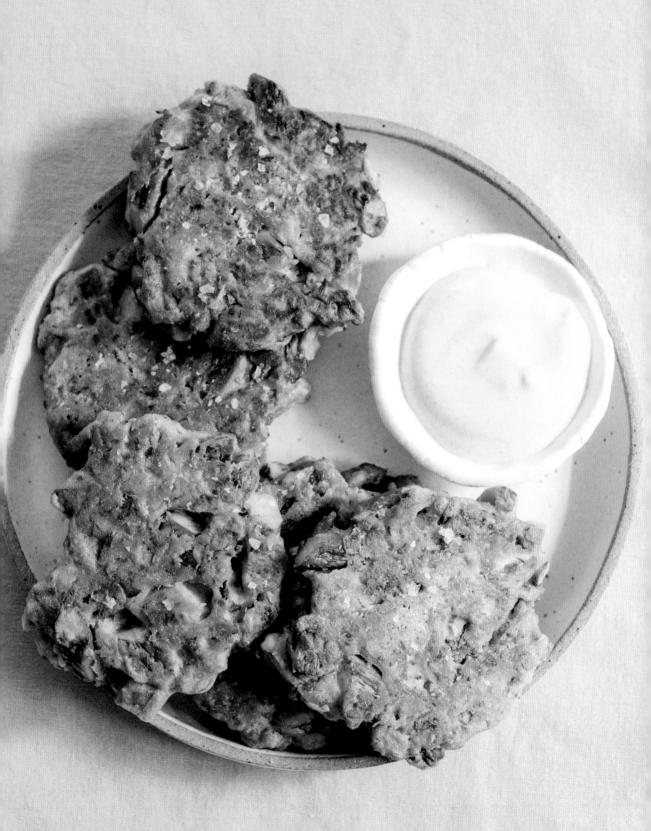

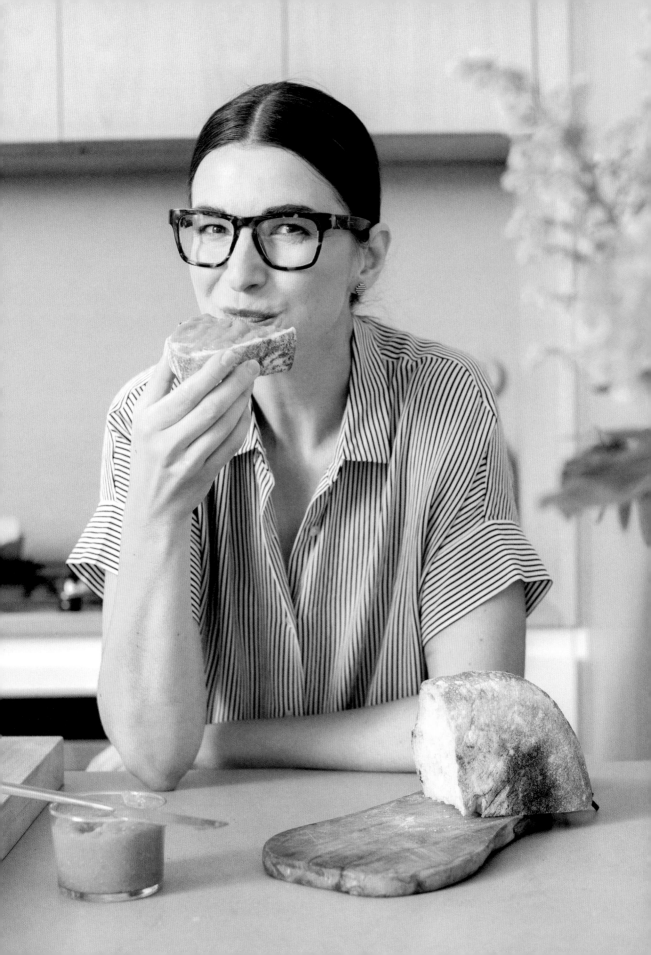

Carrot Apricot Jam Makes about 2 cups (500 mL)

This is not your average sugary spread. Vitamin A–rich carrots and FODMAP-packed apricots create a vibrantly hued jam that is delicious spread on your morning toast or as a condiment on a snack board. Digestion-soothing ginger and soluble fibre-rich ground chia seeds make this sweet, tart, spicy, and slightly earthy spread a very grown-up treat that is good for your gut too.

DAIRY-FREE • GLUTEN-FREE • GRAIN-FREE • HIGH-FODMAP • NUT-FREE • VEGAN

1. In a small pot, add the carrots and water. Cover with a lid and cook over medium heat until the carrots begin to soften, 5 minutes. Add the apricots, ginger, cane sugar, and lemon juice. Add 1 or 2 tablespoons (15 or 30 mL) more water if the mixture looks dry. Reduce the heat to medium-low and cook, uncovered, mashing occasionally with a spatula or wooden spoon, until the apricots and carrots have broken down and the moisture is mostly absorbed, about 15 minutes. When done, the mixture should be fairly thick. Remove from the heat and let cool for 5 minutes.

2. Using a handheld immersion blender, purée the mixture. Taste and add more sugar if the fruit is sour. Stir in the ground chia seeds. Let cool fully. Store in an airtight container in the fridge for up to 1 week.

2 medium carrots, peeled and grated (about 2 cups/500 mL)

¼ cup (60 mL) water, plus more if needed

1 pint (500 mL) ripe apricots, pitted and chopped (5 to 6 medium apricots)

1-inch (2.5 cm) piece of fresh ginger, peeled and grated with a microplane

3 tablespoons (45 mL) organic cane sugar, plus more to taste

1 tablespoon (15 mL) freshly squeezed lemon juice

2 tablespoons (30 mL) ground white chia seeds

Spicy Tofu Feta Dip Makes about 2 cups (500 mL)

I used to love eating tirokafteri, which is a Greek feta cheese dip. It's creamy, spicy, salty, and very addictive. But I think this tofu version is even better. It is inspired by the genius tofu feta recipe from the Vancouver restaurant Virtuous Pie that food writer Erin Ireland was allowed to share on her blog. It turned me into a tofu feta addict, and it was not long before I wondered if I could transform my favourite feta recipe into tirokafteri. Serve with seed crackers and sliced veggies or use as a sandwich spread.

DAIRY-FREE • GLUTEN-FREE • GRAIN-FREE • HIGH-FODMAP • LOW-FODMAP OPTION • NUT-FREE • VEGAN

1 package (12 ounces/340 g) firm tofu

2 to 3 pepperoncini peppers, patted dry, trimmed, and chopped

¼ cup (60 mL) pepperoncini pepper brine

¼ cup (60 mL) refined coconut oil, melted

3 tablespoons (45 mL) freshly squeezed lemon juice

2 tablespoons (30 mL) apple cider vinegar

1½ teaspoons (7 mL) salt

1 teaspoon (5 mL) onion powder (see FODMAP Note)

Pinch of red chili flakes

1. Crumble the tofu into a high-speed blender. Add the pepperoncini peppers, pepperoncini pepper brine, melted coconut oil, lemon juice, apple cider vinegar, salt, onion powder, and chili flakes. Blend until smooth, stopping to scrape down the sides of the blender jar as needed.

2. Transfer into an airtight container and refrigerate for at least 4 hours before using. The tofu needs time to soak up the flavours. The dip won't be as delicious if you eat it right away. Store in an airtight container in the fridge for up to 3 days. If it starts to taste a bit flat, refresh with more lemon juice.

FODMAP Note Omit the onion powder for a low-FODMAP dip. You may wish to use a bit of nutritional yeast to add some umami.

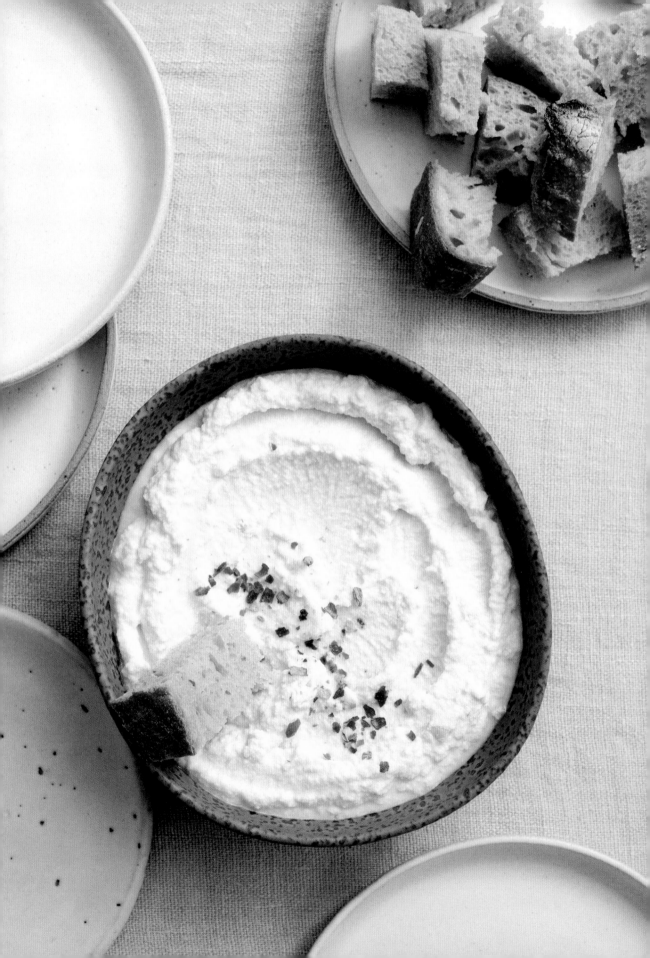

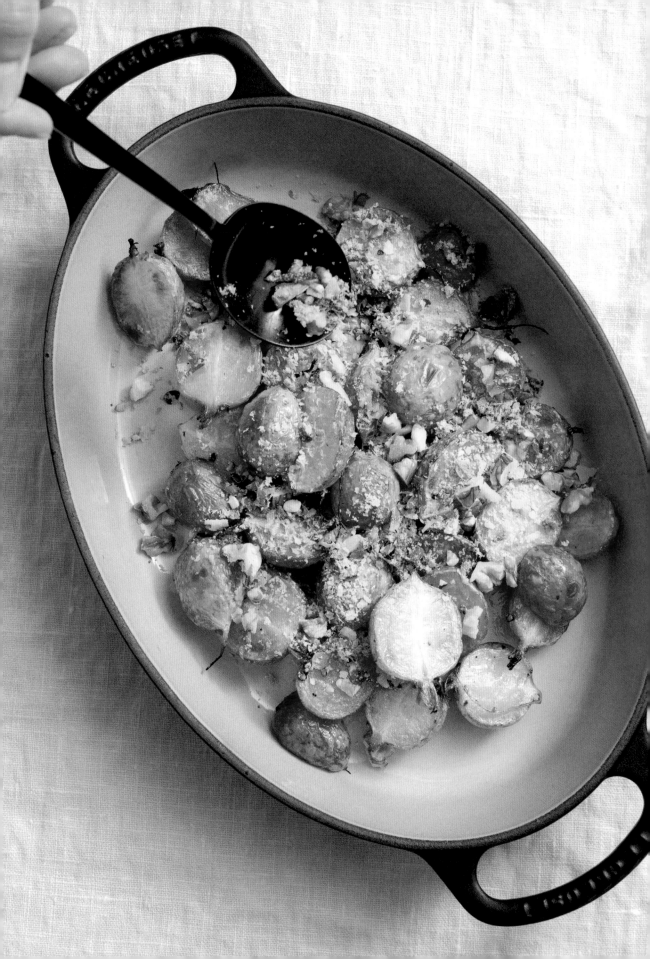

Roasted Radishes with Savoury Walnut Crumbles Serves 4

These radishes are insanely addictive! Roasting them softens the flavour and brings out their sweeter side. However, what really takes this dish over the top is the cheesy, salty, inexplicably delicious walnut topping. Radishes are a member of the cruciferous vegetable family, meaning they contain precursors to anti-inflammatory isothiocyanates that support well-being. Serve as a side dish or as part of a grazing board.

DAIRY-FREE • GLUTEN-FREE • GRAIN-FREE • HIGH-FODMAP • LOW-FODMAP OPTION • VEGAN

1. Preheat the oven to 450°F (230°C). Line a baking sheet with parchment paper.

2. In a small bowl, toss the radishes with the avocado oil, salt, and pepper. Place the radishes, cut side down, onto the prepared baking sheet. Do not crowd the pan. Roast until fork-tender and starting t o brown, 14 to 18 minutes.

3. Meanwhile, heat a small dry skillet over medium heat. When the pan is hot, add the walnuts. Stir and shake the nuts a few times until fragrant and toasted, 2 to 3 minutes. Transfer the nuts to a small plate to cool.

4. In a small bowl, mix together the walnuts, nutritional yeast, thyme, parsley, salt, and onion powder, if using.

5. Transfer the roasted radishes to a serving dish and toss with the walnut mixture. Serve warm.

FODMAP Note As an alternative to high-FODMAP onion powder, you can add a tiny pinch of asafoetida (hing) to lend an oniony flavour to the walnut crumble.

2 bunches radishes, trimmed and cut in half (about 20)

1 tablespoon (15 mL) avocado oil

¼ teaspoon (1 mL) salt

Freshly cracked black pepper

¼ cup (60 mL) chopped raw walnuts or walnut pieces

1 tablespoon (15 mL) nutritional yeast

1 tablespoon (15 mL) fresh thyme leaves

1 tablespoon (15 mL) minced curly parsley

½ teaspoon (2 mL) salt

½ teaspoon (2 mL) onion powder (see FODMAP Note)

Sweet Potato Broccoli Croquettes Makes about 30 croquettes

These croquettes have everything to do with me wanting to create a cheesy, salty, and sweet bundle of nutrient-dense plants. Vitamin A–rich sweet potato, anti-inflammatory broccoli, and mineral-rich hemp hearts make these a super nutritious treat for game night or any time. Great for using up leftover roasted or steamed sweet potatoes. It is worth making a double batch as they go quickly with both adults and children alike. To keep your serving low-FODMAP, enjoy no more than six croquettes per serving.

DAIRY-FREE • GLUTEN-FREE • LOW-FODMAP • NUT-FREE • VEGAN

SWEET POTATO AND BROCCOLI MIXTURE

2 cups (500 mL) riced broccoli (4 to 5 large florets)

2 cups (500 mL) cooked sweet potato cubes (about 2 medium sweet potatoes; see Tip)

4 green onions (dark green parts only), sliced

⅓ cup (75 mL) hemp hearts

3 tablespoons (45 mL) nutritional yeast

3 tablespoons (45 mL) pickled jalapeño pepper, drained and sliced

2 tablespoons (30 mL) ground flaxseed

2 tablespoons (30 mL) extra-virgin olive oil

1 tablespoon (15 mL) gluten-free bread crumbs

¾ teaspoon (3 mL) salt

½ teaspoon (2 mL) ground cumin

Freshly cracked black pepper

COATING

¼ cup (60 mL) nutritional yeast

3 tablespoons (45 mL) hemp hearts

2 tablespoons (30 mL) gluten-free bread crumbs

Salt and pepper

1. Preheat the oven to 425°F (220°C). Line a baking sheet with parchment paper.

2. **Prepare the sweet potato and broccoli mixture:** In a food processor, add the riced broccoli, sweet potato, green onions, hemp hearts, nutritional yeast, jalapeño slices, flaxseed, olive oil, bread crumbs, salt, cumin, and pepper. Pulse until it has the texture of mashed potato. The mixture will be quite soft but this is what you want so it stays moist during the baking process.

3. **Prepare the coating:** In a small bowl, mix together the nutritional yeast, hemp hearts, bread crumbs, and a big pinch each of salt and pepper.

4. **Assemble the croquettes:** Working with damp hands so the mixture doesn't stick, shape 1 tablespoon (15 mL) of the sweet potato and broccoli mixture into a 2-inch (5 cm) log and place it into the coating mixture. You don't want the logs too large or they won't hold together well. Use a spoon to coat the croquette and gently place the coated croquette onto the prepared baking sheet. Repeat until all the croquettes have been made. If the dough starts to stick to your fingers, rinse and re-wet your hands.

5. Bake the croquettes until their crusts turn golden on the bottom, 16 to 18 minutes. Let cool for 10 minutes on the pan before handling. Serve warm or at room temperature. The croquettes can be made up to 3 days in advance and stored in an airtight container in the fridge. Reheat in the oven at 350°F (180°C) for 10 to 15 minutes.

Tip If your sweet potato isn't already cooked, cut it into 1-inch (2.5 cm) chunks and toss with some olive oil and a pinch of salt. Roast until fork-tender, about 25 minutes. You can, however, use thawed frozen sweet potato chunks. Do not use canned sweet potato for this recipe; it has too much moisture.

FODMAP Note If not following a low-FODMAP diet, you can add 1 teaspoon (5 mL) onion powder and ½ teaspoon (2 mL) garlic powder to the sweet potato and broccoli mixture for even more flavour.

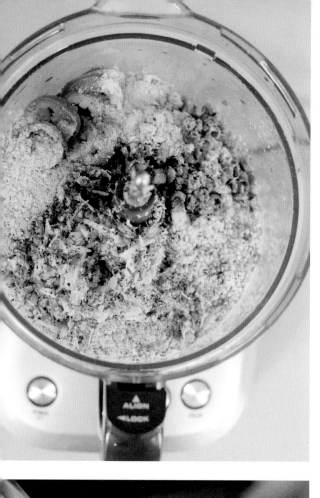
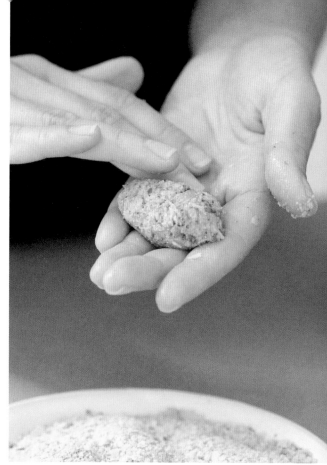
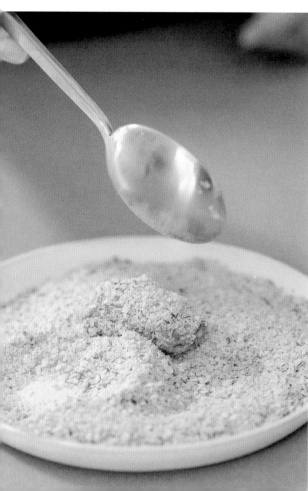
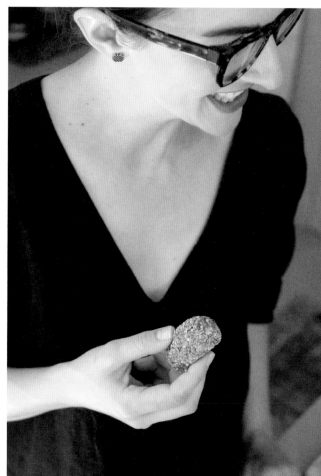

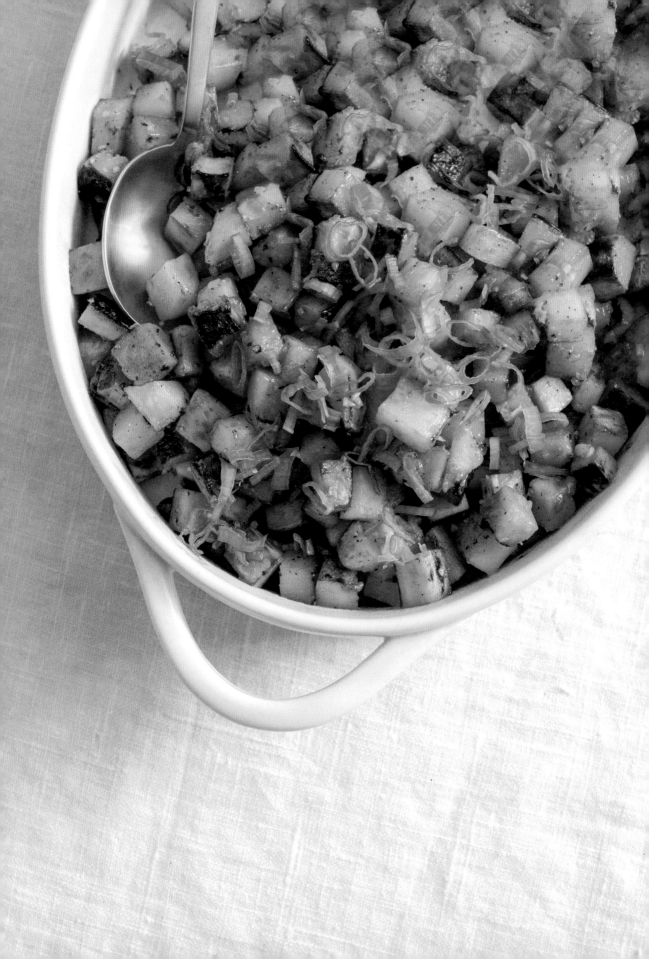

Miso-Glazed Root Veggie Hash Serves 4

When in doubt, roast it. However, sometimes it is even faster and easier to do it on the stovetop. Root vegetables are often overlooked as a satisfying, flavourful addition to any meal. With a miso-maple glaze as delicious as this one, I promise you will not make that mistake again! This hash would be wonderful alongside some grilled tofu and Blistered Dijon Green Beans with Almonds (page 248).

DAIRY-FREE • GLUTEN-FREE • GRAIN-FREE • LOW-FODMAP • NUT-FREE • VEGAN

1. In a large nonstick skillet, heat the avocado oil over medium heat. Add the sweet potato, parsnip, rutabaga, and celeriac. Stir to coat with the oil. Cover with a lid and cook, stirring once every 5 minutes, until the vegetables are soft and caramelized, 14 to 15 minutes.

2. Meanwhile, in a small bowl, mix together the miso, maple syrup, rice wine vinegar, and sesame oil.

3. When the vegetables are cooked, season generously with salt and pepper; remove from the heat. Pour the glaze over the vegetables, stirring continuously while the glaze bubbles and coats the vegetables, about 1 minute. Sprinkle with green onions and serve.

1 tablespoon (15 mL) avocado oil

1 cup (250 mL) sweet potato, unpeeled and cut into ½-inch (1 cm) cubes (about 1 small)

1 cup (250 mL) parsnip, peeled and cut into ½-inch (1 cm) cubes (about 1 medium)

1 cup (250 mL) rutabaga, peeled and cut into ½-inch (1 cm) cubes (about 1 small)

1 cup (250 mL) celeriac, peeled and cut into ½-inch (1 cm) cubes (about 1 small)

1 tablespoon (15 mL) white miso

1 tablespoon (15 mL) pure maple syrup

1 tablespoon (15 mL) rice wine vinegar

1 teaspoon (5 mL) sesame oil

Salt and freshly cracked black pepper

3 green onions (dark green parts only), very thinly sliced on the diagonal

Blistered Dijon Green Beans with Almonds Serves 6

Tangy, salty, and addictive, this dish will banish the idea that green beans are boring. Blistering the beans in the pan coaxes extra flavour from these humble veggies. Crunchy almonds add texture and a savoury Dijon dressing makes them totally crave-worthy. This is a delicious way to eat more green veggies when other greens are irritating your tummy. Take note of serving size if you're on a low-FODMAP plan, as green beans are high-FODMAP in larger portions. Delicious served with the Chickpea Umami Burgers (page 142) or Creamy Mushroom Lentil Toast (page 141).

DAIRY-FREE • GLUTEN-FREE • GRAIN-FREE • LOW-FODMAP • VEGAN

¼ cup (60 mL) raw almonds, chopped

2 tablespoons (30 mL) Dijon mustard

¼ teaspoon (1 mL) organic cane sugar

⅛ teaspoon (0.5 mL) salt

Red chili flakes, to taste

3 tablespoons (45 mL) avocado oil

1 pound (450 g) green beans, trimmed

1. Heat a small dry skillet over medium heat. When the pan is hot, add the almonds. Stir and shake the nuts a few times until fragrant and toasted, 2 to 3 minutes. Transfer the almonds to a small plate.

2. In a small bowl, whisk together the mustard, cane sugar, salt, and chili flakes.

3. In a large heavy skillet, heat the avocado oil over high heat. (You might need to cook the beans in 2 batches.) Add the green beans, reduce the heat to medium-high, and cook until the beans turn brown and shrivel, 5 to 10 minutes (depending on thickness). Flip the beans every 2 to 3 minutes so they cook evenly. Be careful, the oil will spatter as it heats up. Remove the pan from the heat and let cool for 1 minute.

4. Add the dressing to the pan and toss to coat the hot green beans. Sprinkle with the toasted almonds. Serve warm or at room temperature.

FODMAP Note Keep portion size in mind: the low-FODMAP serving size of green beans is 2.65 ounces (75 g), so 1 pound (450 g) serves 6 people. If you are not following a low-FODMAP diet, I recommend adding ½ clove grated or crushed garlic to the dressing.

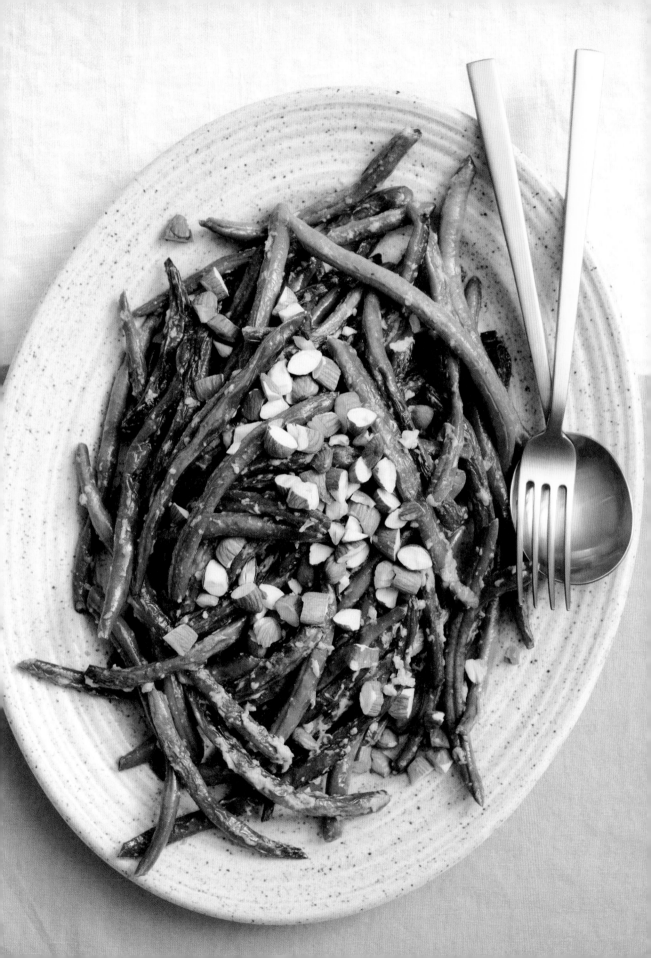

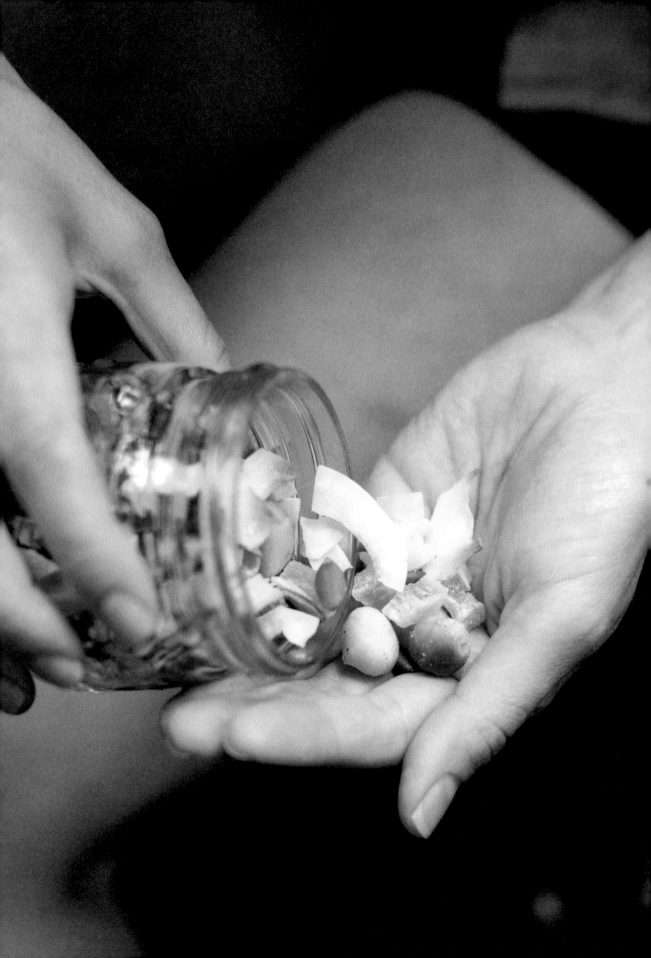

Tropical Coconut Trail Mix Makes 3 cups (750 mL)

Trail mix does not have to be boring. And, as luck would have it, most of the low-FODMAP trail mix options have a fun tropical vibe that you will want to keep eating day after day. Tummy-soothing ginger and zinc-rich pumpkin seeds have gut-healthy credentials, while Brazil nuts offer selenium, a critical anti-inflammatory mineral that is often depleted in those with digestive troubles. This trail mix keeps well so you will never be caught low-FODMAP hangry again.

DAIRY-FREE • GLUTEN-FREE • GRAIN-FREE • LOW-FODMAP • VEGAN

1. Preheat the oven to 350°F (180°C.) Line a baking sheet with parchment paper.

2. In a medium bowl, combine the macadamia nuts, pumpkin seeds, Brazil nuts, and crystallized ginger. Toss with the avocado oil and salt; evenly spread onto the prepared baking sheet. Toast until the nuts look lightly golden, 6 to 7 minutes. At the 5-minute mark, sprinkle the coconut on top of the mixture (it will toast quickly). Remove from the oven and cool completely on the baking sheet. Transfer the trail mix to an airtight container and store at room temperature for up to 2 weeks.

½ cup (125 mL) raw macadamia nuts

½ cup (125 mL) raw pumpkin seeds

½ cup (125 mL) raw Brazil nuts

¼ cup (60 mL) crystallized ginger, diced

1 teaspoon (5 mL) avocado or melted virgin or refined coconut oil

¼ teaspoon (1 mL) salt

1 cup (250 mL) unsweetened large flake coconut or unsweetened coconut chips

Tip If you prefer raw trail mix, you can skip the toasting and just mix the raw ingredients.

FODMAP Note Keep to a ⅓-cup (75 mL) serving to stay low-FODMAP. If you are not following a low-FODMAP diet, I highly recommend adding ½ cup (125 mL) diced unsweetened dried mango. You can also add cashews or substitute them for the macadamia nuts.

Spiced Tahini Roasted Squash Serves 4

When the weather turns chilly, there is nothing better than roasted squash—except maybe roasted squash lavished with richly spiced tahini. This warming dish is soft and easy on digestion while having a decent amount of fibre. Winter squash has lots of immune-supportive beta-carotene and is a surprisingly good source of calcium and magnesium too. This would be a perfect accompaniment to the Harissa Spinach Salad with Marinated Tofu (page 207) or a flavourful and unexpected side for the Lentil Walnut Loaf (page 177).

DAIRY-FREE • GLUTEN-FREE • GRAIN-FREE • NUT-FREE • VEGAN

1½ pounds (675 g) kabocha, acorn, or delicata squash, seeded and cut into 1-inch (2.5 cm) thick slices

2 tablespoons (30 mL) avocado oil, divided

¾ teaspoon (3 mL) ground cumin, divided

½ teaspoon (2 mL) salt, divided

Freshly cracked black pepper

3 tablespoons (45 mL) tahini

2 tablespoons (30 mL) freshly squeezed lemon juice

2 teaspoons (10 mL) pure maple syrup

½ teaspoon (2 mL) ground sumac

¼ teaspoon (1 mL) ground turmeric

1. Preheat the oven to 425°F (220°C). Line a large baking sheet with parchment paper.

2. In a large bowl, add the squash, 1 tablespoon (15 mL) of the avocado oil, ½ teaspoon (2 mL) of the cumin, ¼ teaspoon (1 mL) of the salt, and pepper. Toss to coat. Arrange the squash on the prepared baking sheet and roast for 15 minutes. Carefully flip the squash and roast until golden and fork-tender, 15 to 18 minutes more.

3. Meanwhile, in a small bowl, whisk together the tahini, lemon juice, remaining 1 tablespoon (15 mL) avocado oil, maple syrup, sumac, remaining ¼ teaspoon (1 mL) cumin, turmeric, and remaining ¼ teaspoon (1 mL) salt.

4. Brush both sides of the squash slices with the tahini sauce and serve.

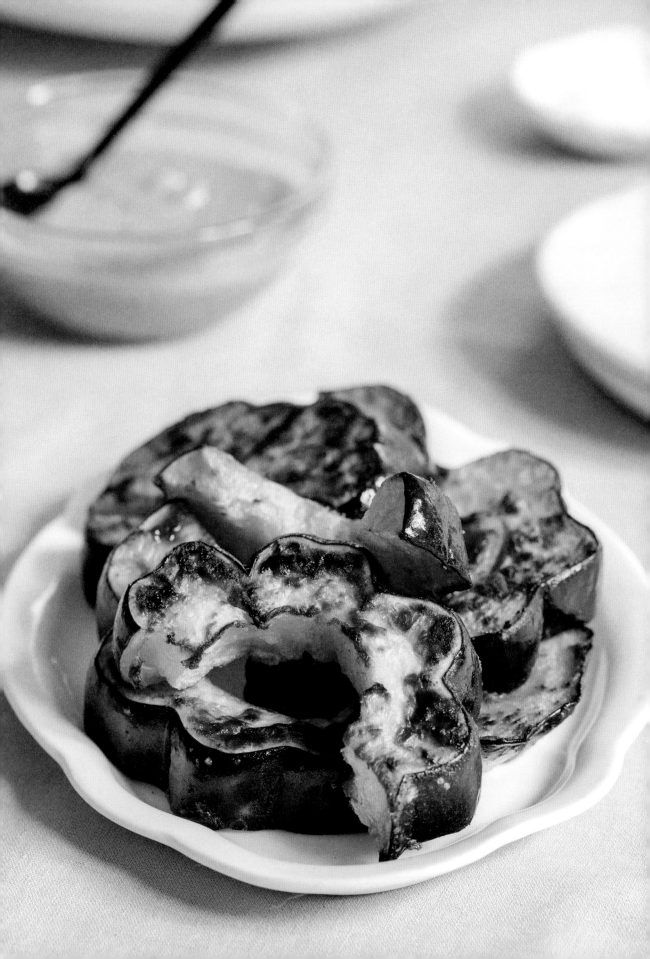

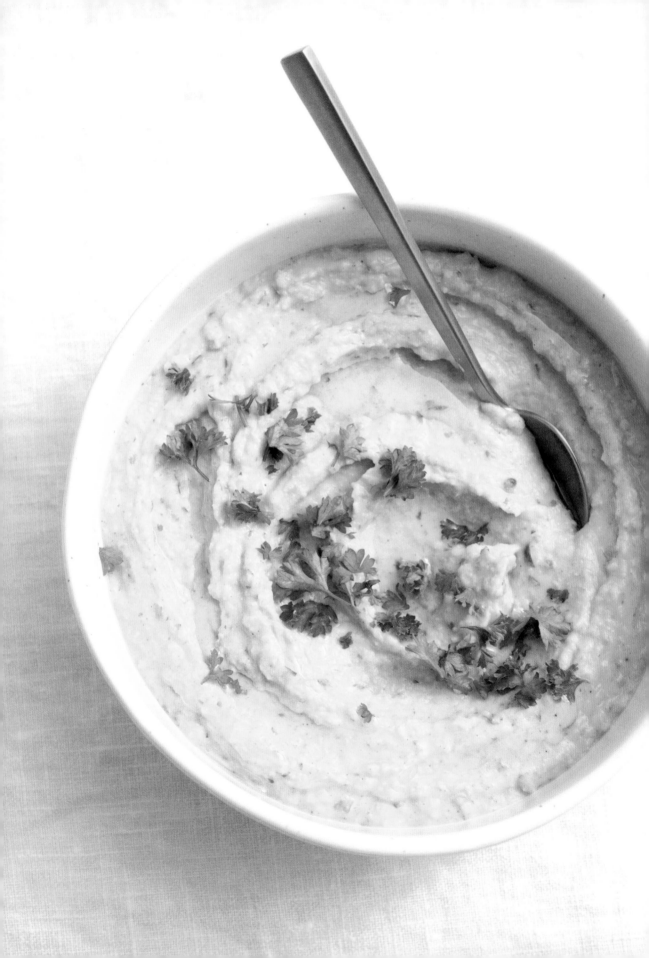

Curried White Bean Dip Makes about 2 cups (500 mL)

This easy-to-make dip packs a lot of flavour and makes a delicious sandwich spread or dip for fresh veggies. It is as golden as the sun and a fun way to get more legumes into your day. Legumes are such an important food for long-term gut health, but they can be difficult to digest for those with an irritated gut. Puréeing helps to break down the cell walls so they are easier to digest to help you get a little bit of these high-fibre, gut-bacteria-boosting beauties back into your diet. Because spices are the stars of this dip, use the freshest and best-quality ones you can find. If your spice drawer is looking a little stale, it's time for a refresh. It will make a big difference to the flavour of this dip.

DAIRY-FREE • GLUTEN-FREE • GRAIN-FREE • NUT-FREE • VEGAN

1. In a small food processor, add the white beans, avocado oil, lemon juice, curry powder, garlic, turmeric, salt, and cumin. Blend until smooth, 1 to 2 minutes. If the beans are a bit dry, drizzle in some water, 1 tablespoon (15 mL) at a time, with the processor running to achieve desired consistency.

2. Stir in the cilantro. Transfer the bean dip to an airtight container and refrigerate for at least 30 minutes to allow the flavours to blend. Serve or store in the fridge for up to 5 days.

1 can (14 ounces/398 mL) white beans (navy, cannellini, or white kidney beans; about 1½ cups/375 mL)

3 tablespoons (45 mL) avocado oil

2 tablespoons (30 mL) freshly squeezed lemon juice

2 teaspoons (10 mL) mild curry powder

1 clove garlic, crushed or grated with a microplane

½ teaspoon (2 mL) ground turmeric

½ teaspoon (2 mL) salt

¼ teaspoon (1 mL) ground cumin

¼ cup (60 mL) fresh cilantro or flat-leaf parsley, minced

Smoky Red Pepper Hummus Makes about 2½ cups (625 mL)

This light-textured dip is bursting with smoky, earthy flavour. Split red lentils cook down to make them much easier to digest than some other legumes, making this dip a perfect way to reintroduce iron-, protein-, and fibre-rich lentils into your diet. This is delicious as a sandwich spread or served with seeded crackers, sliced vegetables, or my Lentil Walnut Loaf (page 177).

DAIRY-FREE • GLUTEN-FREE • GRAIN-FREE • HIGH-FODMAP • NUT-FREE • VEGAN

¾ cup (175 mL) dry red lentils

½ cup (125 mL) jarred roasted red peppers, drained and patted dry

⅓ cup (75 mL) tahini

2 tablespoons (30 mL) freshly squeezed lemon juice

1 clove garlic, crushed or grated with a microplane

1 teaspoon (5 mL) salt

¼ teaspoon (1 mL) smoked paprika

1 teaspoon (5 mL) pure maple syrup (optional)

1. Place the lentils in a small pot and cover them with water by 3 inches (8 cm). Bring to a boil over medium heat. Cook, uncovered, until the lentils are soft, 4 to 6 minutes. Reduce the heat if necessary to avoid boiling over.

2. Using a fine-mesh sieve, strain the lentils and rinse under cool running water. Drain well. Place the lentils in a food processor with the roasted red peppers, tahini, lemon juice, garlic, salt, and paprika. Blend until silky smooth, about 1 minute. Taste and adjust the salt, if needed. If you need to tone down any bitterness, add the maple syrup. Store in an airtight container in the fridge for up to 5 days.

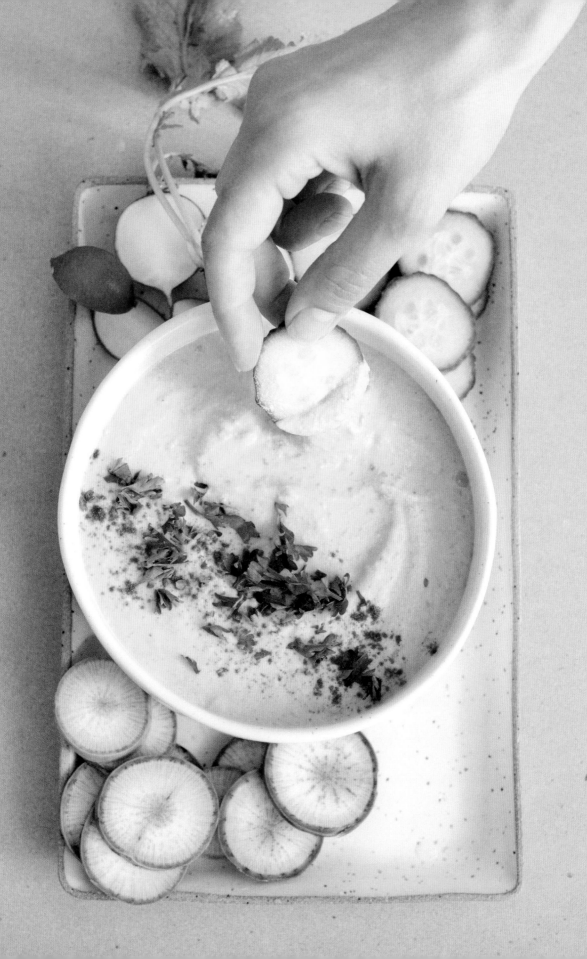

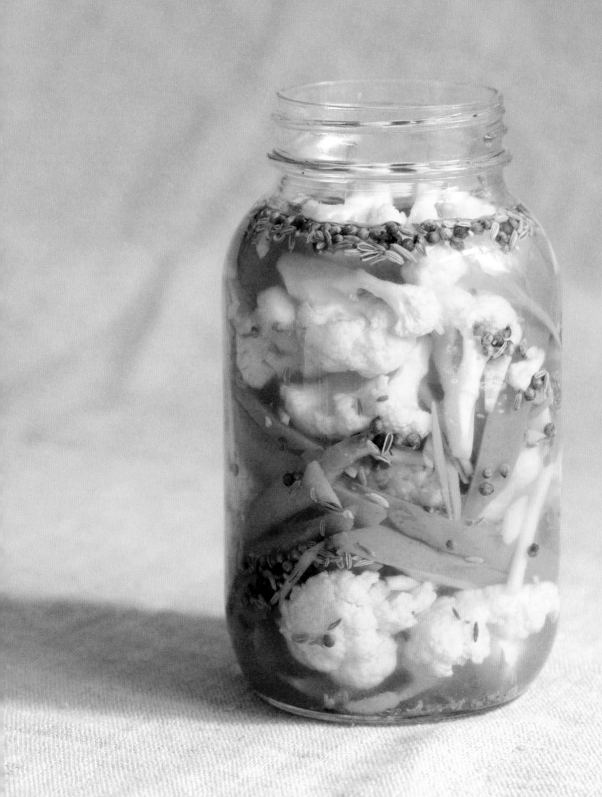

Lacto-Fermented Carrots and Cauliflower Makes about 1 quart (1 L)

There's nothing like fermenting at home to make you feel like a mad scientist. It just does not get old to me—watching over your ferment every day and seeing it bubbling away. Lacto-fermentation makes use of the naturally occurring bacteria on vegetables and in the environment. All you need is a little brine to discourage the growth of bad bugs. I have packed this full of gut-friendly spices and aromatics to help soothe your gut.

DAIRY-FREE • GLUTEN-FREE • GRAIN-FREE • NUT-FREE • VEGAN

1. Bring 4 cups (1 L) of water to a boil in a medium pot over high heat and let it continue boiling for 5 minutes. Remove from the heat and let cool for 10 minutes. This step helps remove the chlorine from the water so it doesn't interfere with fermentation.

2. Place 2 cups (500 mL) dechlorinated water in a clean 1-quart (1 L) mason jar. Using a non-metal spoon, stir in the salt and let it come to room temperature. Add the carrots, cauliflower, ginger, turmeric, garlic, coriander seeds, and cumin seeds. Press down the vegetables to make sure they are fully submerged. Cover the jar with a double layer of cheesecloth or single layer of paper towel and secure with an elastic band. Place the jar in a warm spot in your kitchen out of direct sunlight or inside a cold oven with the door closed (on top of the fridge is often a great spot if your home is cool). You can also wrap the jar in a clean kitchen towel for added warmth.

3. Check your ferment every day. Use a chopstick or wooden spoon to submerge the vegetables and release air pockets. Bubbles mean it is fermenting. You will also notice a very slight cloudiness from the cauliflower. After 3 days, taste the vegetables to see if they are fermented to your taste. In summer, 3 days of fermentation time might be enough, but 7 to 8 days might be required in the winter. When fully fermented, seal with a lid and store in the fridge for up to 3 weeks.

Tip **If you are pregnant or on immunosuppressive medications, I do not recommend you consume home ferments.**

1 tablespoon (15 mL) salt

2 medium carrots, scrubbed and cut on the diagonal in ¼-inch (5 mm) slices

2 cups (500 mL) small (1-inch/2.5 cm pieces) cauliflower florets

2-inch (5 cm) piece of fresh ginger, peeled and cut into matchsticks

2-inch (5 cm) piece of fresh turmeric, peeled and cut into matchsticks

3 cloves garlic, peeled and halved

2 teaspoons (10 mL) coriander seeds

1 teaspoon (5 mL) cumin seeds

Fermented Turmeric Sunflower Seed Cheese Serves 6

It's easier than you think to make your own plant-based cheese. Sunflower seeds are a nice change from cashew, both in cost and in flavour. Soaking and fermenting the seeds improves digestibility and adds live beneficial bacteria to your diet. This tangy, richly flavoured cheese is packed with minerals like iron, zinc, and magnesium while giving you a boost of B vitamins, thanks to my favourite umami ingredient, nutritional yeast.

DAIRY-FREE • GLUTEN-FREE • GRAIN-FREE • NUT-FREE • VEGAN

1 cup (250 mL) raw sunflower seeds, soaked in water for at least 6 hours or overnight

3 tablespoons (45 mL) freshly squeezed lemon juice

1 tablespoon (15 mL) nutritional yeast

1 tablespoon (15 mL) avocado oil

¾ teaspoon (3 mL) salt

½ teaspoon (2 mL) onion powder

½ teaspoon (2 mL) garlic powder

½ teaspoon (2 mL) ground turmeric (optional)

2 tablespoons (30 mL) water

Two 50 billion CFU probiotic capsules (I use Bio-K+)

1. Drain and rinse the sunflower seeds and place them in a small food processor. Add the lemon juice, nutritional yeast, avocado oil, salt, onion powder, garlic powder, turmeric (if using), and water. Blend until creamy, 1 to 2 minutes, scraping down the sides of the bowl if necessary.

2. Cut a double-thick piece of cheesecloth at least 12 inches (30 cm) square and lay it over a colander. Carefully break open the probiotic capsules and stir the contents into the sunflower mixture. Discard the capsules. Scoop the sunflower seed cheese into the centre of the cheesecloth and use the cheesecloth to shape it into a 4-inch (10 cm) disc. Tie the top of the cheesecloth with a twist tie or elastic. Place the wrapped cheese in the colander set over a bowl. Let ferment at room temperature for 48 hours.

3. Remove the cheese from the cheesecloth and serve or store it in an airtight container in the fridge for up to 4 days.

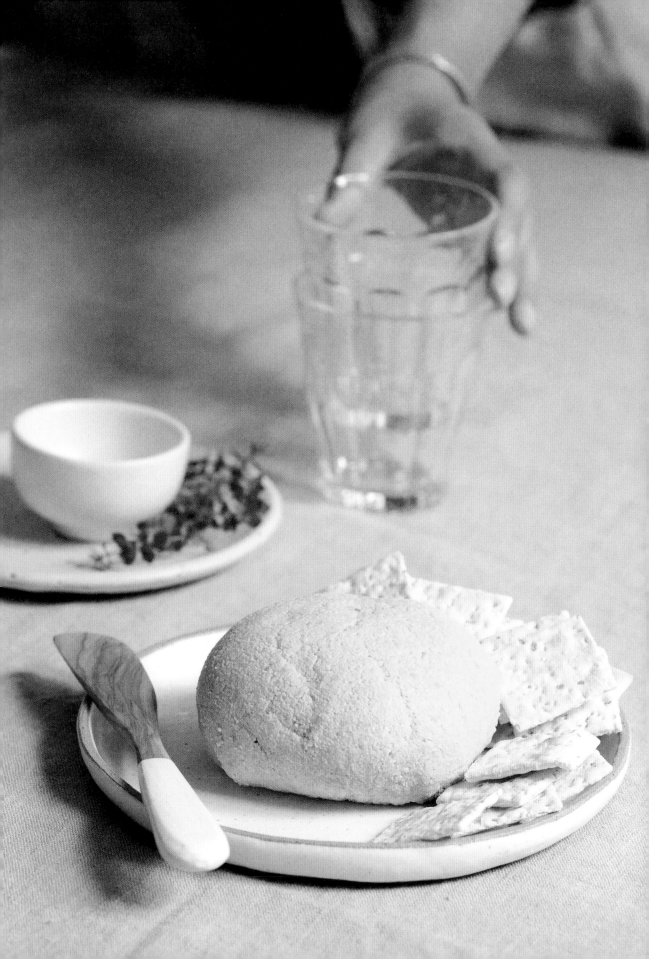

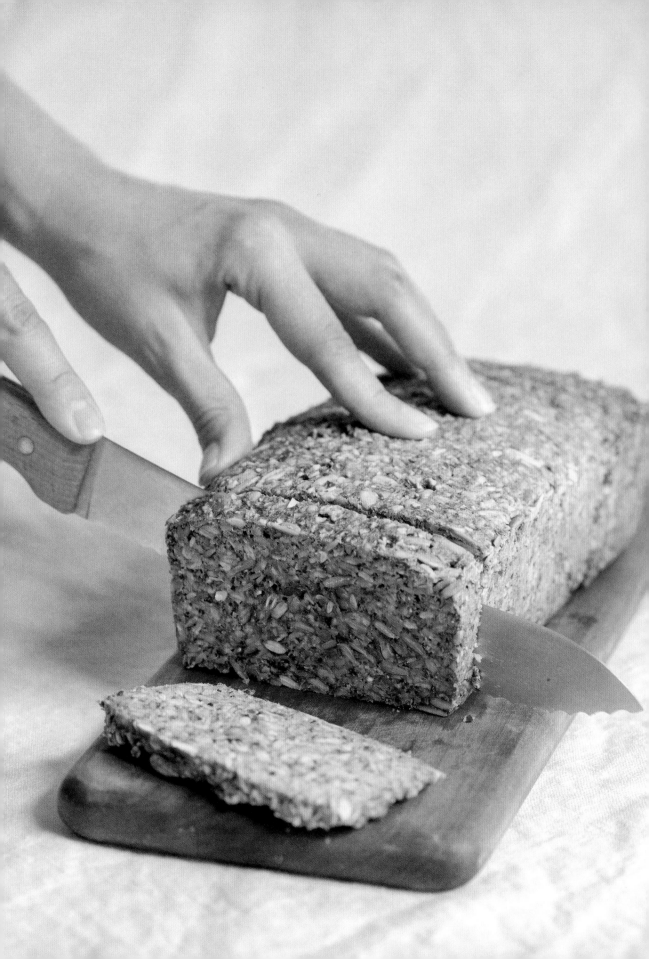

Amazing Seeded Grain-Free Bread Makes 1 loaf

This loaf—and all seed loaves like it—is inspired by incredible plant-based chef Sarah Britton's The Life-Changing Loaf of Bread. I wanted to try my hand at creating a version that was not only grain-free but also made 100 percent from seeds. Seeds are such a high-fibre, nutrient-dense addition to our diet, but many of us don't eat enough of them. This amazing bread—which has the taste and texture of a traditional German rye vollkornbrot—is packed with gut-friendly minerals and a lot of soluble fibre. It's very nutrient-dense and super filling. A thin slice is all you need!

DAIRY-FREE • GLUTEN-FREE • GRAIN-FREE • HIGH-FODMAP • NUT-FREE • VEGAN

1. Grease an 8 × 4-inch (1.5 L) loaf pan with a bit of tahini or coconut oil. Line the pan with parchment paper with extra hanging over the sides.

2. In a high-speed blender or small food processor, add 1 cup (250 mL) of the sunflower seeds and 1 cup (250 mL) of the pumpkin seeds. Pulse until the mixture resembles panko crumbs.

3. In a large bowl, stir together the pulsed seed flour with the remaining 1 cup (250 mL) sunflower seeds and remaining ½ cup (125 mL) pumpkin seeds, buckwheat flour, chia seeds, flaxseed, psyllium, salt, and caraway seeds, if using.

4. Add the tahini, maple syrup, and water. Mix well. Scrape the mixture into the prepared pan and let sit for 30 minutes.

5. Meanwhile, preheat the oven to 350°F (180°F).

6. Place the loaf pan on the middle rack and bake for 55 to 60 minutes. The bread is done when it is golden brown on top and the sides have pulled away from the edges of the pan. Let the bread cool in the pan for 10 minutes, then carefully lift it onto a rack using the parchment paper overhang. Let cool completely before slicing. Store the bread in a loosely covered container on the counter for up to 3 days or sliced and tightly wrapped in the freezer for up to 1 month. Toast from frozen.

2 cups (500 mL) raw sunflower seeds, divided

1½ cups (375 mL) raw pumpkin seeds, divided

½ cup (125 mL) buckwheat flour

¼ cup (60 mL) chia seeds

¼ cup (60 mL) ground flaxseed

¼ cup (60 mL) psyllium husks or psyllium powder (see Tip)

1 teaspoon (5 mL) salt

½ teaspoon (2 mL) caraway seeds (optional)

¼ cup (60 mL) tahini, plus more for greasing the pan (or grease the pan with coconut oil)

¼ cup (60 mL) pure maple syrup

2 cups (500 mL) water

Tip Psyllium husk and powder have different gelling abilities. Sometimes they are not interchangeable, but here they are. Psyllium husk will result in a softer loaf; powder will give you a firmer one.

Glorious Grain-Free Buns Makes 4 buns

These grain-free buns are so yummy, you might not want to go back to regular buns. They make eating grain-free easy. Made from almond flour and cauliflower, these buns are rich in protein and healthy fats to keep blood sugars on an even keel. Psyllium is packed with soluble fibre to help regulate digestion. So simple to make, these would make a delicious side for your favourite soup or stew, or base for a weekend tofu benny. Try them with my Chickpea Umami Burgers (page 142).

DAIRY-FREE • GLUTEN-FREE • GRAIN-FREE • VEGAN

1 cup (250 mL) almond flour

¼ cup (60 mL) arrowroot powder

¼ cup (60 mL) psyllium husk (see Tip)

1 tablespoon (15 mL) nutritional yeast

1 tablespoon (15 mL) everything bagel seasoning, divided (optional)

2 teaspoons (10 mL) baking powder

½ teaspoon (2 mL) salt

1 cup (250 mL) riced or grated cauliflower

2 tablespoons (30 mL) extra-virgin olive oil

2 tablespoons (30 mL) unsweetened non-dairy milk of your choice (I use almond)

1 tablespoon (15 mL) apple cider vinegar

1 teaspoon (5 mL) pure maple syrup

1. Preheat the oven to 400°F (200°C). Line a baking sheet with parchment paper.

2. In a medium bowl, whisk together the almond flour, arrowroot powder, psyllium, nutritional yeast, 2 teaspoons (10 mL) of the everything bagel seasoning (if using), baking powder, and salt.

3. Add the cauliflower, olive oil, non-dairy milk, apple cider vinegar, and maple syrup. Blend well with your hands to form a dough. If the mixture seems dry, add 1 to 2 tablespoons (15 to 30 mL) water.

4. Divide the dough into 4 portions and shape into 3-inch (8 cm) round buns, ⅓ inch (8 mm) thick. Place the buns on the prepared baking sheet. Pat the remaining 1 teaspoon (5 mL) everything bagel seasoning (if using) on the patties. Bake until uniformly golden brown on top, 20 to 22 minutes. Let the buns cool for 10 minutes on the baking sheet. If using as a sandwich bun, let cool fully before using, as the bun will firm up further as it cools. Buns can be stored loosely covered on the counter for up to 3 days.

Tip To make these buns, it is important to use psyllium husk. Do not substitute with psyllium powder.

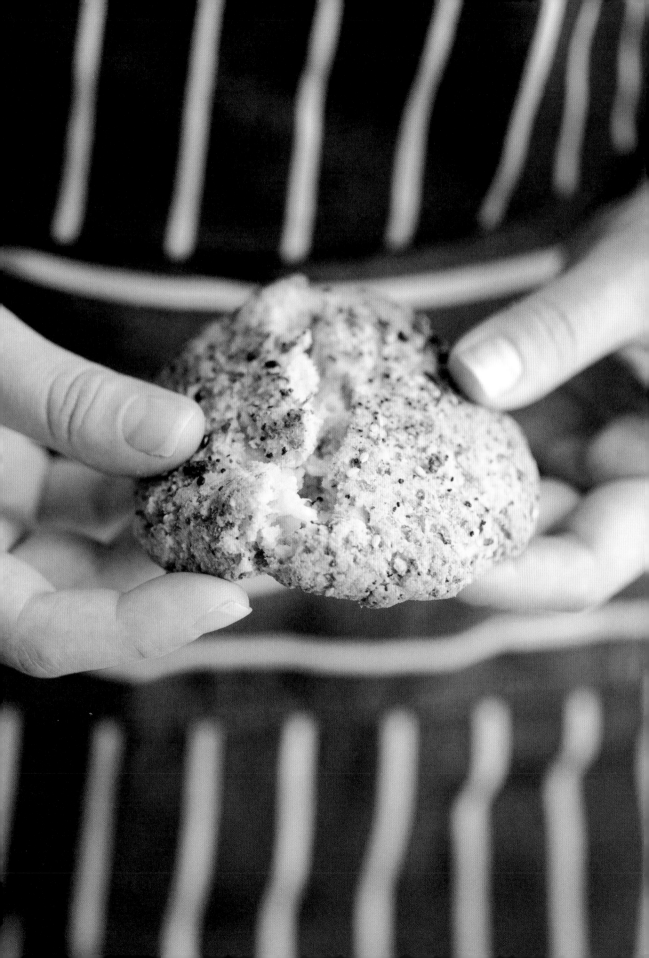

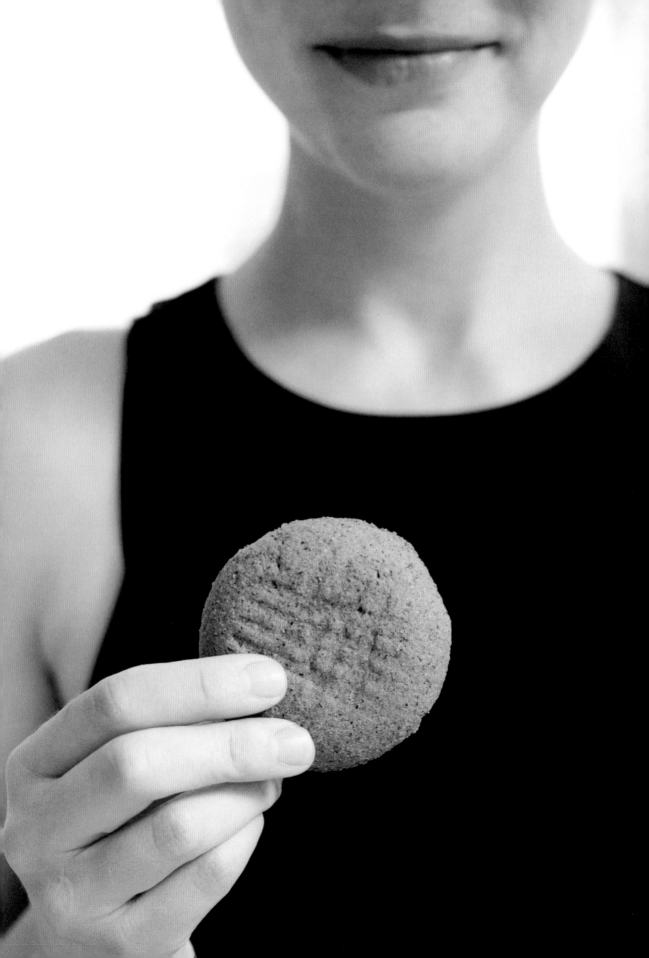

Baking and Sweets

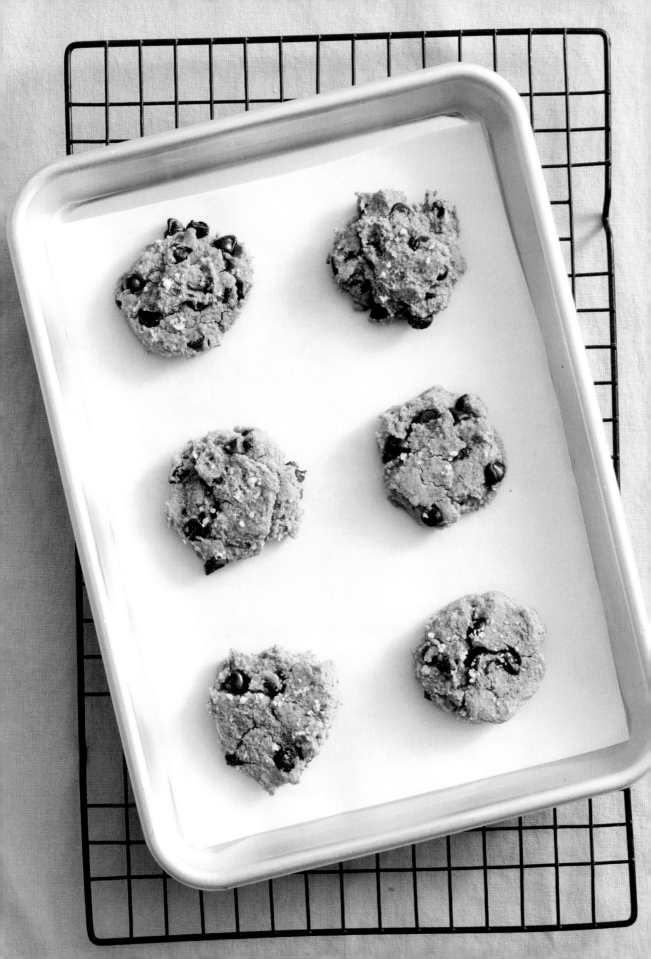

Chickpea Chocolate Chip Cookies Makes 18 cookies

This is my first chocolate chip cookie recipe ever, so I'm settling for nothing less than perfection. These chocolatey brownie-like cookies made from a chickpea base are high in fibre, grain-free, lightly sweetened, and packed with healthy fats. They are the perfect microbiome-friendly treat that keeps blood sugars stable and your gut microbes full and happy.

They're easy to make, with a food processor doing most of the work. A family staple in our house, these cookies are incredibly delicious and no one will suspect they are "healthy."

DAIRY-FREE • GLUTEN-FREE • GRAIN-FREE • HIGH-FODMAP • VEGAN

1. Preheat the oven to 375°F (190°C). Line a baking sheet with parchment paper.

2. In a food processor, pulse the chickpeas until finely chopped. Add the almond flour, maple syrup, olive oil, almond butter, flaxseed, vanilla, baking powder, salt, and almond extract. Process until well combined, scraping down the sides of the bowl, if necessary.

3. Remove the blade from the food processor and mix in the chocolate chips by hand. The batter will seem very sticky, but this is the correct consistency of the cookie dough.

4. Spoon eighteen 2-tablespoon (30 mL) portions of cookie dough onto the prepared baking sheet, leaving 2 inches (5 cm) between them. (The dough is sticky, so use a small spatula or another spoon to release the dough onto the baking sheet.) Gently press the dough with the palm of a damp hand to flatten to ½ inch (1 cm) thick. Sprinkle each cookie with a pinch of flaky sea salt, if using. Bake until the edges are firm to the touch, 14 to 15 minutes. Allow the cookies to cool on the baking sheet for 5 minutes before transferring to a rack to cool completely. Store in an airtight container on the counter for up to 3 days or in the freezer for up to 1 month.

1 can (14 ounces/398 mL) chickpeas, rinsed and drained (1½ cups/375 mL cooked chickpeas)

1 cup (250 mL) almond flour

½ cup (125 mL) pure maple syrup

⅓ cup (75 mL) olive oil

¼ cup (60 mL) natural almond butter

2 tablespoons (30 mL) ground flaxseed

1 tablespoon (15 mL) pure vanilla extract

1 teaspoon (5 mL) baking powder

½ teaspoon (2 mL) salt

½ teaspoon (2 mL) pure almond extract

¾ cup (175 mL) dairy-free dark chocolate chips (I use mini chips)

Flaky sea salt, for garnish (optional)

Matcha Chocolate Cups Makes 12 cups

Rich cacao and green tea are a match made in heaven—high in anti-inflammatory flavonoids, richly flavoured, and super satisfying. Made with a base of coconut oil and coconut butter, these chocolate treats have a melt-in-your-mouth texture and are sure to become a favourite treat. Low in sugar, they are great any time. Keep a batch in the fridge or freezer for whenever a chocolate craving strikes.

DAIRY-FREE • GLUTEN-FREE • GRAIN-FREE • HIGH-FODMAP • NUT-FREE • VEGAN

CHOCOLATE CUPS

½ cup (125 mL) + 1 tablespoon (15 mL) refined coconut oil

½ cup (125 mL) raw cacao or cocoa powder

2 tablespoons (30 mL) pure maple syrup

1 teaspoon (5 mL) pure vanilla extract

Pinch of salt

MATCHA FILLING

½ cup (125 mL) coconut butter (manna), warmed to liquid consistency and well stirred (see Tip)

2 tablespoons (30 mL) pure maple syrup

2 teaspoons (10 mL) pure vanilla extract

1½ teaspoons (7 mL) matcha powder

Pinch of salt

1. Line a 12-cup muffin tin with mini paper liners.

2. **Make the chocolate cup mixture:** In a small pot, melt the coconut oil over medium-low heat. Remove from the heat and whisk in the cacao powder, maple syrup, vanilla, and salt.

3. Add 1 teaspoon (5 mL) of the melted chocolate mixture to each of the lined muffin cups. Place the muffin tin in the freezer for 5 minutes to harden the chocolate.

4. **Meanwhile, make the matcha filling:** In a small bowl, mix together the coconut butter, maple syrup, vanilla, matcha, and salt. The mixture will thicken and be a bit tough to mix.

5. Remove the muffin tin from the freezer. Portion 2 teaspoons (10 mL) of the matcha mixture and, using your hands, gently form into a small patty. Place the formed matcha on top of the chocolate layer in the muffin cup. Use the tips of your fingers to flatten slightly. Repeat to fill the remaining muffin cups.

6. If the remaining chocolate mixture has started to harden, gently reheat over medium-low heat. Pour a scant 1 tablespoon (15 mL) of the chocolate mixture over the matcha mixture in each muffin cup. Place in the freezer until set, about 15 minutes, before serving. Store in an airtight container in the fridge for up to 1 week or in the freezer for up to 1 month.

Tip Coconut butter (also called coconut manna) is essentially a nut butter made from whole coconut. It has a very different texture and flavour profile than coconut oil. If it is not available, substitute with cashew butter.

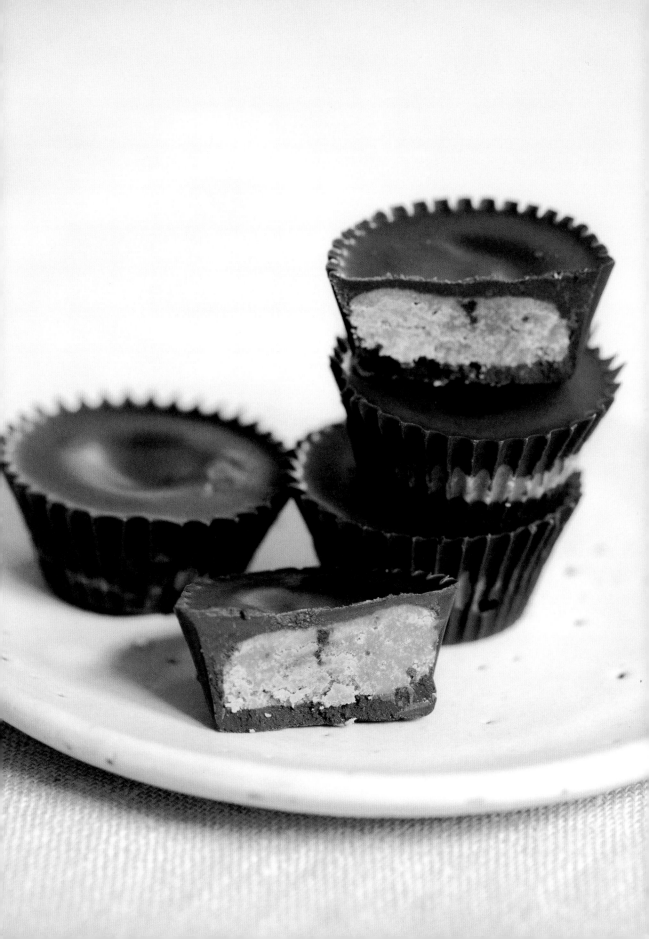

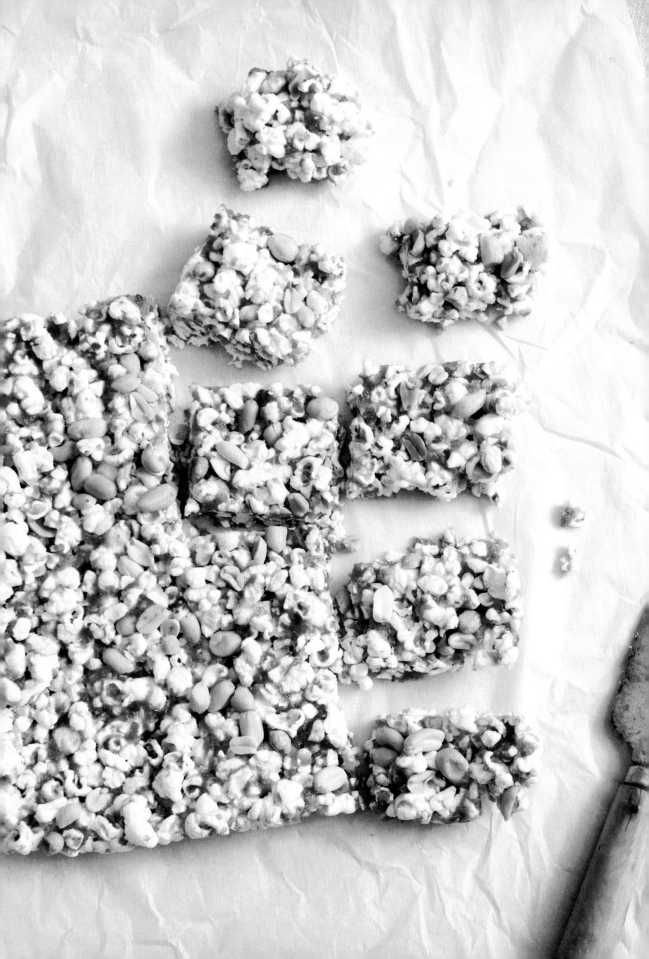

Salted Tahini Caramel Popcorn Bars Makes 8 bars

Think grown up Rice Krispies Treats, but microbiome-friendly. High-fibre popcorn and prebiotic-rich dates help feed your beneficial microbes while you feed your soul with salted tahini caramel. These bars have a soft and chewy texture, with plenty of crunch from the peanuts.

DAIRY-FREE • GLUTEN-FREE • HIGH-FODMAP • VEGAN

1. Line an 8-inch (2 L) square baking dish with parchment paper.

2. In a small pot, melt the coconut oil over medium-low heat.

3. In a small blender or using a wide-mouthed blending cup with a handheld immersion blender, combine the melted coconut oil, dates, tahini, vanilla, and salt. Pulse until the mixture is mostly smooth.

4. In a large bowl, stir together the popcorn and salted tahini caramel by hand so the popcorn is well coated. Stir in the peanuts. Using damp hands, firmly press the popcorn mixture into the prepared dish. Place in the fridge for at least 1 hour to firm up, then cut into bars. Store in an airtight container in the fridge for up to 1 week.

Tip I recommend using store-bought popcorn instead of homemade popcorn. Store-bought has a lighter texture and makes these bars less dense.

⅓ cup (75 mL) refined coconut oil

1 cup (250 mL) packed pitted Medjool dates

⅓ cup (75 mL) tahini, well stirred

1 tablespoon (15 mL) pure vanilla extract

¼ teaspoon + ⅛ teaspoon (1.5 mL) salt

6 cups (1.5 L) store-bought salted popcorn (see Tip)

⅓ cup (75 mL) chopped salted peanuts

Cherry Pie Nice Cream Serves 4

There are many healthy swaps that do not satisfy, but nice cream does it for me every time. Watching bananas transform into a soft-serve confection in the food processor feels like magic. Bananas are surprisingly soothing to an irritated gut and filled with microbiome-boosting FODMAPs. This simple dessert is perfect for whipping up for company in just five minutes. I like to make a batch and store it in the freezer for whenever the craving strikes.

DAIRY-FREE • GLUTEN-FREE • GRAIN-FREE • HIGH-FODMAP • VEGAN

1 cup (250 mL) fresh or frozen pitted cherries, chopped

2 teaspoons (10 mL) pure vanilla extract

6 frozen overripe medium bananas

¼ cup (60 mL) raw pecan pieces

1. In a small bowl, toss the cherries with the vanilla.

2. Break the frozen bananas into pieces and toss them into a food processor. Process until the bananas form a soft-serve consistency, 1 to 2 minutes. You might need to scrape down the sides of the bowl once or twice. Stir in the vanilla-soaked cherries and pecans. Serve immediately or place in an airtight container in the freezer for 30 minutes for a firmer consistency. Store in the freezer for up to 3 days.

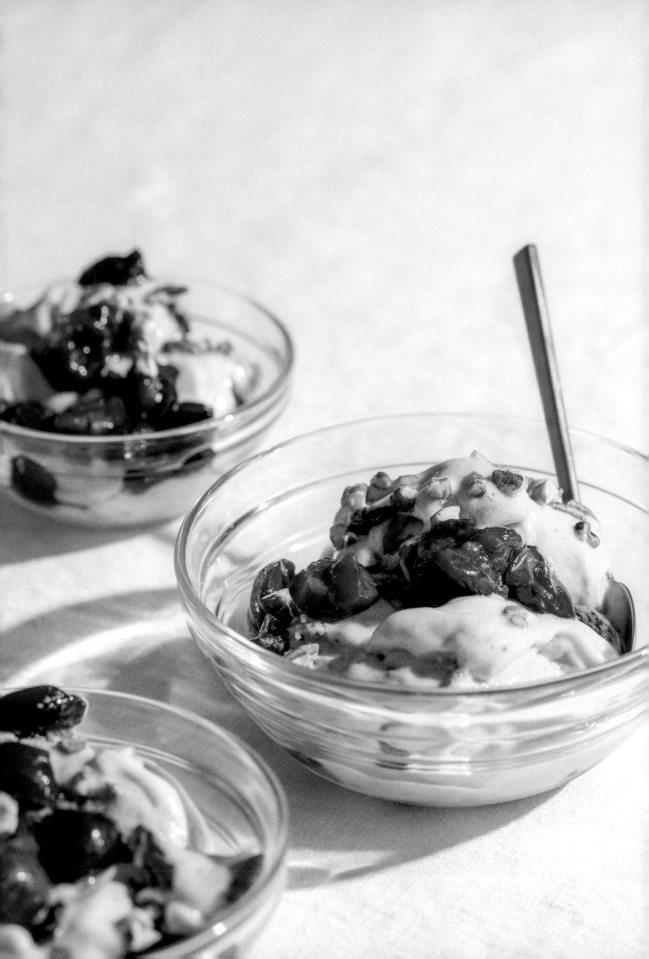

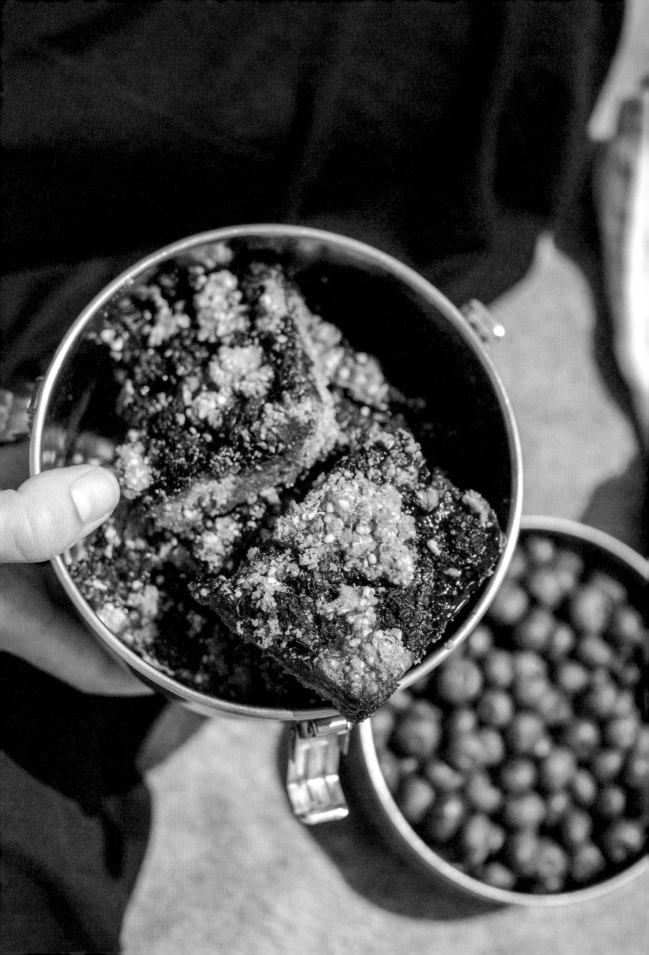

Blackberry Crumble Bars Makes 9 bars

Blackberries run wild all over Vancouver, so these jewel-like treats are synonymous with summer to me. Blackberries are high in fibre, at 4 grams per cup. In addition, they are high in FODMAPs, which feed your gut bacteria. Not too sweet, and satisfyingly hearty, they are a real crowd-pleaser. Paired with microbiome-friendly rye flour and anti-inflammatory hemp hearts, these healthy bars will put you in a summer state of mind. No matter what time of year it is.

DAIRY-FREE • HIGH-FODMAP • NUT-FREE • VEGAN

1. Preheat the oven to 350°F (180°C). Grease a 9-inch (2.5 L) square baking dish and line with parchment paper.

2. **Make the rye layer:** In a medium bowl, whisk together the rye flour, hemp hearts, baking powder, and salt. Add the olive oil, maple syrup, and vanilla. Stir together. It will look like thick, wet sand. Reserve ½ cup (125 mL) for the crumble topping. Press the remaining rye mixture firmly into the pan. Bake until still soft to the touch but set, 14 to 16 minutes.

3. **Meanwhile, make the blackberry layer:** In a medium bowl, stir together the blackberries, cane sugar, arrowroot powder, lemon zest, and salt. Toss to coat the berries evenly with the mixture.

4. Let the rye layer cool for 5 minutes before topping. Spread the blackberry mixture evenly over the rye layer. Crumble the reserved ½ cup (125 mL) rye mixture evenly over the blackberry layer. Bake until the blackberry mixture looks thick and bubbly and the crumble topping is golden brown, 38 to 40 minutes. Let cool for 15 minutes before cutting into bars. Store loosely wrapped on the counter for up to 4 days.

RYE LAYER

2 cups (500 mL) rye flour

¾ cup (175 mL) hemp hearts

¾ teaspoon (3 mL) baking powder

Rounded ¼ teaspoon (1 mL) salt

¾ cup (175 mL) extra-virgin olive or avocado oil

⅓ cup (75 mL) pure maple syrup

1 teaspoon (5 mL) pure vanilla extract

BLACKBERRY LAYER

4 cups (1 L) fresh or frozen blackberries

¼ cup (60 mL) organic cane sugar

¼ cup (60 mL) arrowroot powder

Zest of 1 lemon

Pinch of salt

Chocolate and Peanut Butter Caramel Shortbread Bars Makes 16 bars

These bars are a decadent, satisfying treat made from wholesome ingredients like almond flour and peanut butter. Inspired by millionaire bars, the cookie base is made from protein-packed almond flour and the caramel layer is melt-in-your-mouth decadence. Even with the three layers, these bars are quite simple to make and well worth the bit of extra effort. Yes, low-FODMAP treats can be zero compromise.

DAIRY-FREE • GLUTEN-FREE • GRAIN-FREE • LOW-FODMAP • VEGAN

SHORTBREAD BASE

2 cups (500 mL) almond flour

½ cup (125 mL) refined coconut oil

¼ cup (60 mL) pure maple syrup

1 teaspoon (5 mL) pure vanilla extract

¼ teaspoon (1 mL) salt

CARAMEL LAYER

1 cup (250 mL) natural peanut butter

¼ cup (60 mL) pure maple syrup

¼ cup (60 mL) refined coconut oil, melted

1 tablespoon (15 mL) pure vanilla extract

Pinch of salt

CHOCOLATE LAYER

¾ cup (175 mL) dairy-free dark chocolate chips (at least 70% cocoa)

1 tablespoon (15 mL) coconut oil

Flaky sea salt (optional)

1. Preheat the oven to 350°F (180°F). Lightly grease the bottom and sides of an 8-inch (2 L) square baking pan with coconut oil. Cut a length of parchment paper long enough to line the bottom of the pan with extra hanging over the sides.

2. **Make the shortbread base:** In a medium bowl, whisk together the almond flour, coconut oil, maple syrup, vanilla, and salt. Evenly press the mixture into the baking pan and lightly prick the base all over with a fork. Bake until the edges start to firm up and turn golden, 13 to 15 minutes. Remove from the oven and let cool for 10 minutes while you prepare the caramel layer.

3. **Make the caramel layer:** In a small bowl, whisk together the peanut butter, maple syrup, coconut oil, vanilla, and salt. Spread the caramel mixture over the shortbread base, then place the baking pan in the fridge while you prepare the chocolate layer.

4. **Make the chocolate layer:** In a small pot, bring 2 inches (5 cm) of water to a simmer over medium heat. Stir the chocolate chips with the coconut oil in a small heatproof bowl. Set the bowl over the simmering water. Ensure that the bottom of the bowl is not touching the water. Gently and continuously stir until the chocolate and coconut oil are melted and smooth. Remove from the heat and let sit for a few minutes to thicken slightly. Pour the melted chocolate mixture over the caramel layer. Sprinkle some flaky sea salt over the chocolate, if using. Place the pan in the fridge until firm, about 30 minutes. Remove from the pan using the parchment paper overhang. Cut into bars. Store in an airtight container in the fridge for up to 1 week.

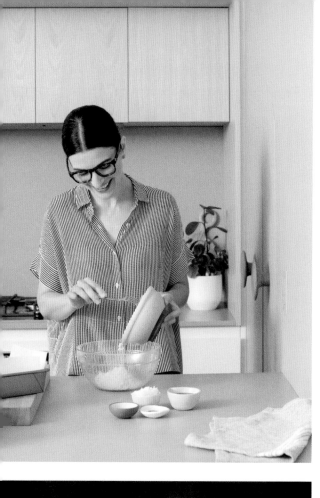

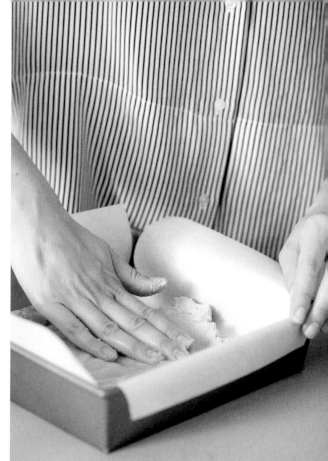

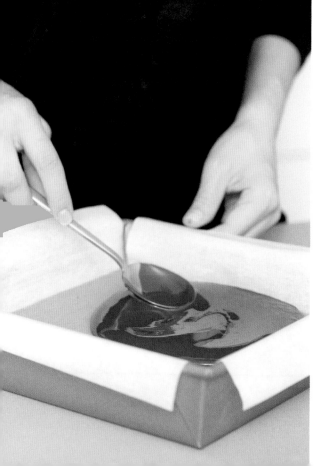

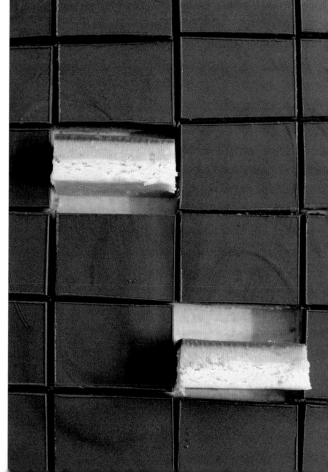

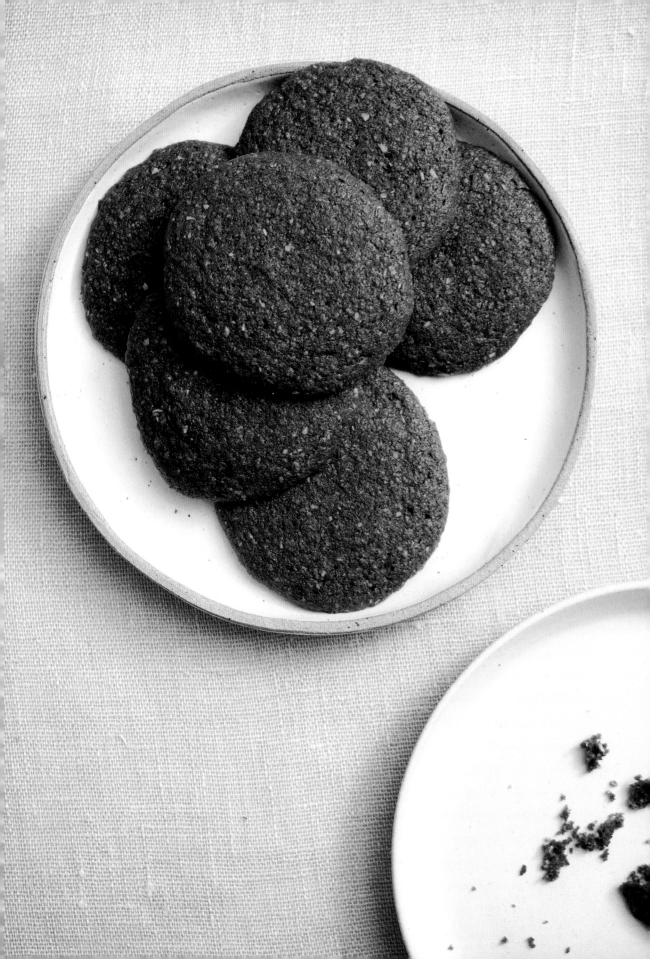

Ginger Snaps Makes about 12 cookies

Dark, flavourful molasses and ginger are a match made in cookie heaven. Blackstrap molasses is high in calcium and iron, making it a great addition to a plant-based diet, but it is high-FODMAP in large portions, so is usually off limits on a low-FODMAP diet. These cookies use just a bit of molasses; when you stick to a single cookie, it will keep you well under the FODMAP limit. Oat and buckwheat flour create a soft and tender texture. Don't worry when the batter looks like molasses; you're on the right track.

DAIRY-FREE • GLUTEN-FREE • LOW-FODMAP • NUT-FREE • VEGAN

1. Preheat the oven to 350°F (180°C). Line a baking sheet with parchment paper.

2. In a medium bowl, beat the coconut oil, molasses, and maple syrup.

3. Add the oat flour, buckwheat flour, ginger, cinnamon, and salt. Mix until combined. Let sit for 10 minutes to thicken.

4. Spoon twelve 1-tablespoon (15 mL) portions of cookie dough onto the prepared baking sheet, leaving 2 inches (5 cm) between them. (The dough is sticky, so use a small spatula or another spoon to release the dough onto the baking sheet.) Bake until the edges are firm to the touch, about 7 minutes. Let the cookies cool completely on the baking sheet. Store in an airtight container on the counter for up to 5 days or in the freezer for up to 1 month.

⅓ cup (75 mL) solid refined coconut oil

3 tablespoons (45 mL) blackstrap molasses

3 tablespoons (45 mL) pure maple syrup

½ cup (125 mL) gluten-free oat flour

½ cup (125 mL) buckwheat flour

2 teaspoons (10 mL) ground ginger

½ teaspoon (2 mL) cinnamon

¼ teaspoon (1 mL) salt

Peanut Ginger Macaroons Makes about 36 macaroons

I love these chewy, soft coconutty bites that are so easy to make. I put my own spin on this traditional treat with one of my favourite flavour combinations—peanut and ginger. A little ginger and turmeric give these cookies a special flavour without being overpowering. Coconut is healthier than you might think; it is high in potassium, and just ¼ cup (60 mL) has almost 4 grams of gut-friendly fibre. You can even enjoy two to three macaroons as a low-FODMAP serving. They freeze well and are perfect whenever you need a little pick-me-up.

DAIRY-FREE • GLUTEN-FREE • GRAIN-FREE • LOW-FODMAP • VEGAN

1 cup (250 mL) natural smooth or crunchy peanut butter

⅔ cup (150 mL) pure maple syrup

¼ cup (60 mL) water

1 teaspoon (5 mL) grated fresh ginger

1 teaspoon (5 mL) pure vanilla extract

½ teaspoon (2 mL) ground turmeric

¼ teaspoon (1 mL) salt

4 cups (1 L) unsweetened shredded coconut

1. Preheat the oven to 350°F (180°F). Line a large baking sheet with parchment paper.

2. In a medium bowl, whisk together the peanut butter, maple syrup, water, ginger, vanilla, turmeric, and salt until blended. Add the coconut and stir to combine. Using damp hands, work the mixture a bit to make sure the coconut is well coated and sticky.

3. Roll thirty-six 1-tablespoon (15 mL) portions of macaroon dough into balls using damp hands or use a cookie scoop to portion the dough. Place the balls onto the prepared baking sheet. The macaroons do not spread, so they can be placed close together. Bake until lightly golden on the bottom, about 15 minutes. Let the macaroons cool completely on the baking sheet. They will firm up when cool. If you notice any cracks on the surface, you can carefully press them together while still warm. Store lightly covered on the counter for up to 5 days or in the freezer for up to 1 month. If freezing, let the macaroons sit at room temperature for 1 to 2 minutes before serving for best flavour and texture.

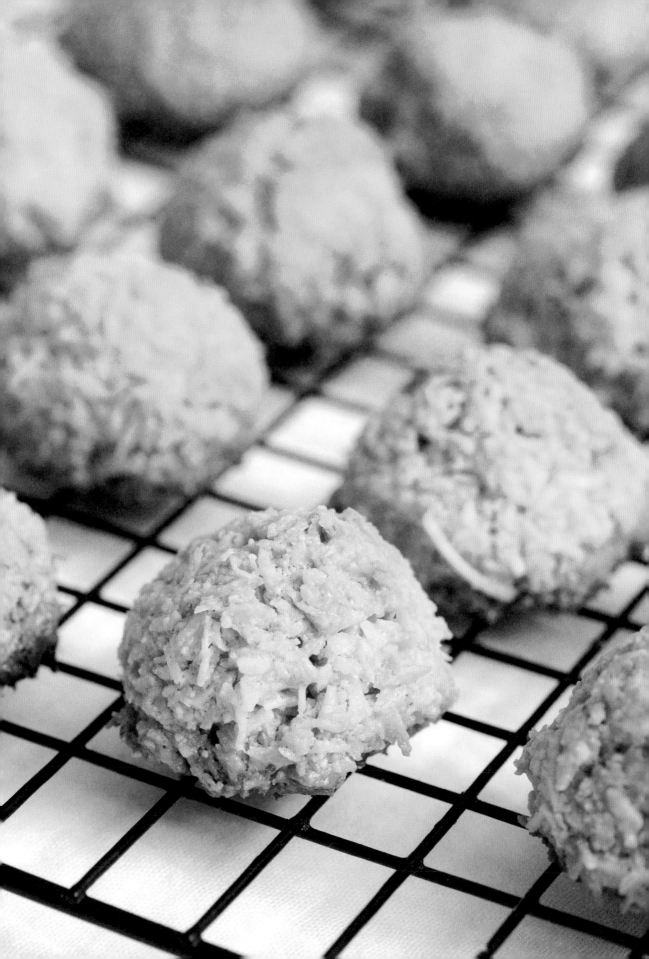

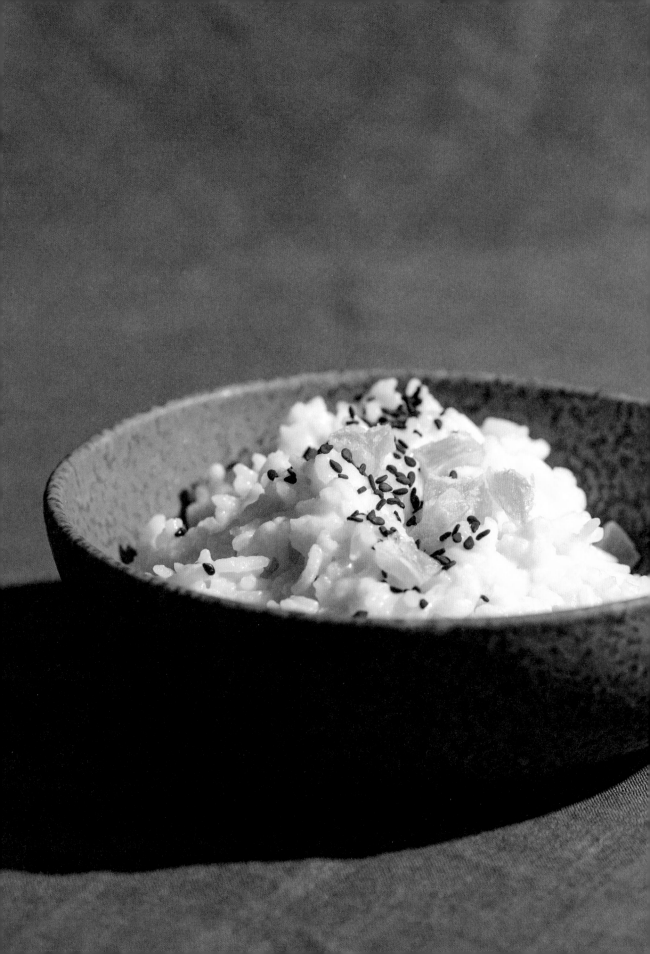

Ginger Vanilla Rice Pudding Serves 6

I grew up eating arroz doce, a Portuguese sweet rice pudding that is a lot different from the North American variety. Its texture is more like a sweet and silky risotto. I wanted to recreate that texture with one of my favourite gut-healing plants, ginger. Ginger contains anti-inflammatory compounds known as gingerols. It is also prokinetic, meaning that it helps with stomach emptying—in fact, ginger is used to ease nausea in pregnancy. This pudding is warm, easy on the tummy, and intoxicatingly fragrant.

DAIRY-FREE • GLUTEN-FREE • NUT-FREE OPTION • LOW-FODMAP • VEGAN

1. In a medium pot, add the almond milk, rice, coconut milk, cane sugar, ginger, vanilla, and salt. Bring to a boil over medium heat. When the mixture reaches a boil, reduce the heat to medium-low and cook, stirring occasionally, until it resembles a thick porridge, 20 to 25 minutes. Adjust the temperature, if needed, to maintain a gentle simmer so the rice cooks properly.

2. Divide the rice pudding among bowls and top with a sprinkle of diced candied ginger and sesame seeds, if using.

Tips 1. This pudding is best served within an hour of cooking. As it chills, the rice tends to absorb and dull the flavours. If you have leftovers, you can reheat them over medium-low heat with a bit of water and a dash of extra vanilla and sugar to revive the intensity of flavour. It's nice, but not quite as good as just-made.

2. For nut-free option, use water instead of almond milk.

3 cups (750 mL) unsweetened almond milk or water (see Tip)

1 cup (250 mL) uncooked white basmati rice

1 cup (250 mL) canned full-fat coconut milk

¼ cup (60 mL) organic cane sugar

2 tablespoons (30 mL) grated fresh ginger

1 tablespoon (15 mL) pure vanilla extract

¼ teaspoon (1 mL) salt

FOR SERVING

¼ cup (60 mL) crystallized ginger, diced

Black sesame seeds (optional)

Magic Turmeric Truffles Makes 12 truffles

One of my favourite holiday treats in the past were always those melty chocolate truffles that looked like actual (non-chocolate) truffles. They would melt on your fingers on their way to your mouth and had such an intense chocolate flavour. I hope I have done them justice! These truffles are so simple to make, and I have snuck a bit of anti-inflammatory turmeric into them. You could make these with any nut or seed butter, but cashew and sunflower have particularly silky textures that really do add to the melt factor. Keep it to one truffle to stay low-FODMAP.

Turmeric will stain your hands and clothing, so be careful when handling the dough.

DAIRY-FREE • GLUTEN-FREE • GRAIN-FREE • NUT-FREE OPTION • LOW-FODMAP • VEGAN

1 cup (250 mL) dairy-free dark chocolate chips (at least 70% cocoa)

1 tablespoon (15 mL) coconut oil

¼ cup (60 mL) cashew or sunflower seed butter (see Tip)

¼ cup (60 mL) canned full-fat coconut milk

1 tablespoon (15 mL) pure maple syrup

2 teaspoons (10 mL) pure vanilla extract

½ teaspoon (2 mL) cinnamon

½ teaspoon (2 mL) ground turmeric

Pinch of salt

COATING (OPTIONAL)

2 tablespoons (30 mL) cocoa powder

2 tablespoons (30 mL) cinnamon

1. In a medium pot, bring 2 inches (5 cm) of water to a simmer over medium heat. Place the chocolate chips and coconut oil in a heatproof medium bowl and set the bowl over the simmering water. Ensure that the bottom of the bowl is not touching the water. Gently and continuously stir until the chocolate and coconut oil are melted and smooth.

2. When the chocolate is melted, remove the bowl from the heat and whisk in the cashew butter, coconut milk, maple syrup, vanilla, cinnamon, turmeric, and salt until smooth. Pour the chocolate mixture into a shallow, rimmed 2-cup (500 mL) glass container and place in the fridge for 60 minutes until firm.

3. Line a baking sheet or dinner plate with parchment paper. Roll 1-tablespoon (15 mL) portions of dough into balls using your hands or a cookie scoop to portion the dough. Place 12 truffles onto the prepared baking sheet. Work quickly so the dough doesn't get too warm. If the dough is not chilled enough to scoop, place it back into the fridge for 15 minutes more until firm enough to continue rolling the balls.

4. Place the truffles in the fridge for 15 minutes to firm up.

5. If coating the truffles, combine the cocoa and cinnamon in a shallow, small bowl. Roll the truffles, one at a time, in the mixture to coat. Store in an airtight container in the fridge for up to 1 week.

Tip For a nut-free option, use sunflower butter instead of cashew butter.

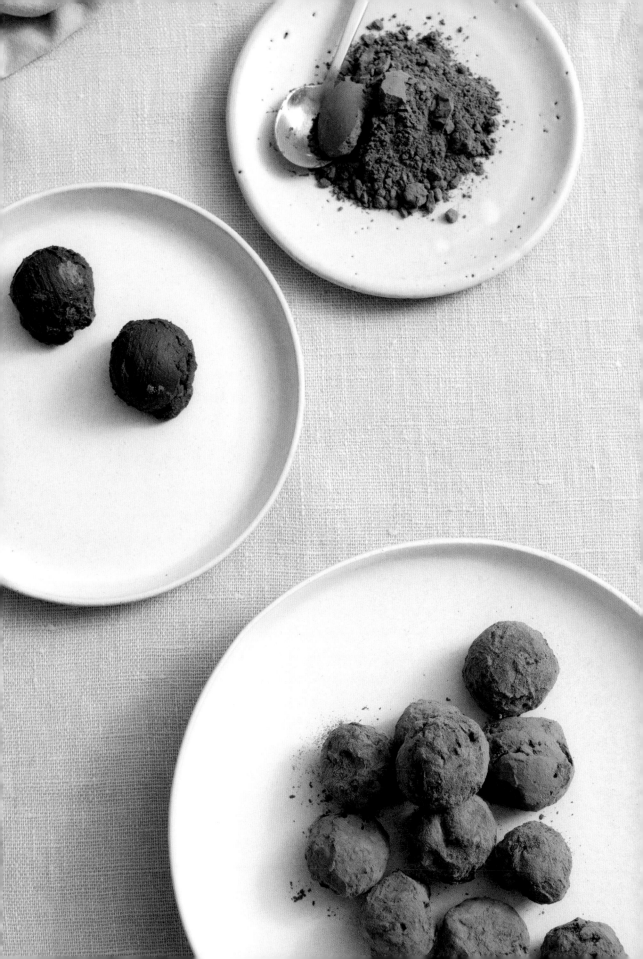

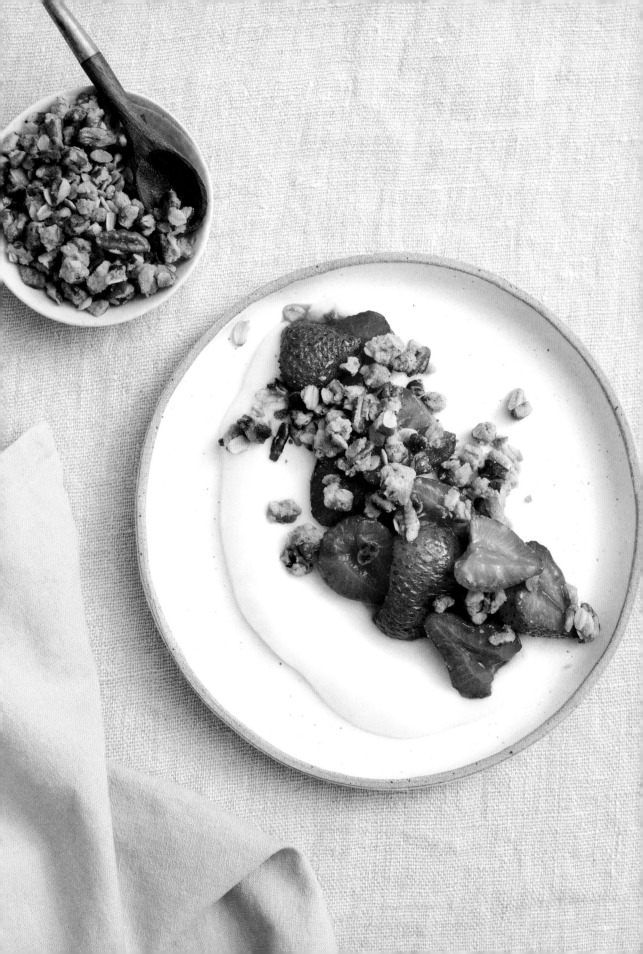

Roasted Strawberries with Yogurt and Pecan Oat Crumble Serves 4

This is an effortless dessert filled with all kinds of goodness. Juicy strawberries, roasted until soft and plump, are paired with a crunchy crumble and perfectly complemented by tart, creamy yogurt. Strawberries are rich in potassium and vitamin C to support healing. It is a sweet, but not an overly sweet, treat. It's also great for breakfast layered as a parfait with hemp hearts for low-FODMAP protein.

DAIRY-FREE • GLUTEN-FREE • LOW-FODMAP • VEGAN

1. Preheat the oven to 350°F (180°C). Line a baking sheet with parchment paper.

2. **Make the roasted strawberries:** In a medium bowl, toss the strawberries with the maple syrup, balsamic vinegar, and salt. Place the strawberries, cut side down, onto the prepared baking sheet. Roast until soft and juicy, 20 to 25 minutes. Be careful not to overcook the strawberries or they will dry out. Watch the strawberries close to the edges of the pan.

3. **Meanwhile, make the pecan oat crumble:** In a small bowl, stir together the pecans, rolled oats, buckwheat flour, maple syrup, avocado oil, and salt.

4. Heat a medium nonstick skillet over medium heat. When the pan is hot, add the crumble mixture. Cook, stirring constantly, until fragrant and the pecans start to brown, 3 to 5 minutes.

5. To serve, add a big dollop of yogurt to shallow bowls or plates. Top with the roasted strawberries and pecan oat crumble.

FODMAP Note If you are not following a low-FODMAP diet, this dish is delicious served with a dollop of homemade Fermented Cashew Yogurt (page 115) on top.

ROASTED STRAWBERRIES

2 pints (1 L) strawberries, trimmed and halved

1 tablespoon (15 mL) pure maple syrup

½ teaspoon (2 mL) balsamic vinegar

Pinch of salt

PECAN OAT CRUMBLE

½ cup (125 mL) raw pecan pieces

¼ cup (60 mL) gluten-free old-fashioned rolled oats

2 tablespoons (30 mL) buckwheat flour

2 tablespoons (30 mL) pure maple syrup

2 tablespoons (30 mL) avocado oil or refined coconut oil

⅛ teaspoon (0.5 mL) salt

Unsweetened plain or vanilla coconut yogurt, for serving

Mediterranean Fig and Walnut Banana Bread Makes 1 loaf

No wonder banana bread is such a family favourite. It's moist, flavourful, not too sweet, and delicious with an afternoon cup of tea or as is for breakfast. I've taken a gut-friendly spin on this classic by using rolled oats, packed with soluble fibre, and protein-rich almond flour to create a tender, melt-in-your-mouth crumb. Figs and walnuts give this loaf a Mediterranean vibe while boosting the fibre, minerals, and omega-3s too.

DAIRY-FREE • GLUTEN-FREE • VEGAN

1 cup (250 mL) gluten-free old-fashioned rolled oats

1 cup (250 mL) almond flour

⅔ cup (150 mL) buckwheat flour

2 tablespoons (30 mL) arrowroot powder

1 teaspoon (5 mL) ground cardamom

¾ teaspoon (3 mL) baking powder

½ teaspoon (2 mL) baking soda

½ teaspoon (2 mL) cinnamon

½ teaspoon (2 mL) salt

1½ cups (375 mL) mashed banana

½ cup (125 mL) pure maple syrup

⅓ cup (75 mL) extra-virgin olive oil

1 teaspoon (5 mL) pure vanilla extract

1 teaspoon (5 mL) freshly squeezed lemon juice

½ cup (125 mL) chopped dried figs

½ cup (125 mL) chopped raw walnuts

1. Preheat the oven to 375°F (190°C). Line a 9 × 5-inch (2 L) loaf pan with parchment paper with extra hanging over the sides.

2. In a food processor or high-speed blender, pulse the rolled oats until a medium-coarse oat flour forms. Set aside.

3. In a large bowl, whisk together the oat flour, almond flour, buckwheat flour, arrowroot powder, cardamom, baking powder, baking soda, cinnamon, and salt until well blended.

4. In a medium bowl, mix together the mashed banana, maple syrup, olive oil, vanilla, and lemon juice until the oil is completely incorporated.

5. Add the banana mixture to the flour mixture and mix until thoroughly combined. Stir in the figs and walnuts. Pour the batter into the prepared loaf pan. Smooth the top of the batter. Bake until the top is golden brown and a toothpick inserted into the centre of the loaf comes out clean, 55 to 60 minutes. Cool the loaf in the pan for 10 minutes, then carefully transfer to a rack using the parchment paper overhang. Let cool completely. As with many gluten-free baked goods, the loaf will firm up as it cools. Slice the loaf with a serrated knife to avoid crumbling. Store loosely covered on the counter for up to 3 days or tightly wrapped in the freezer for up to 1 month.

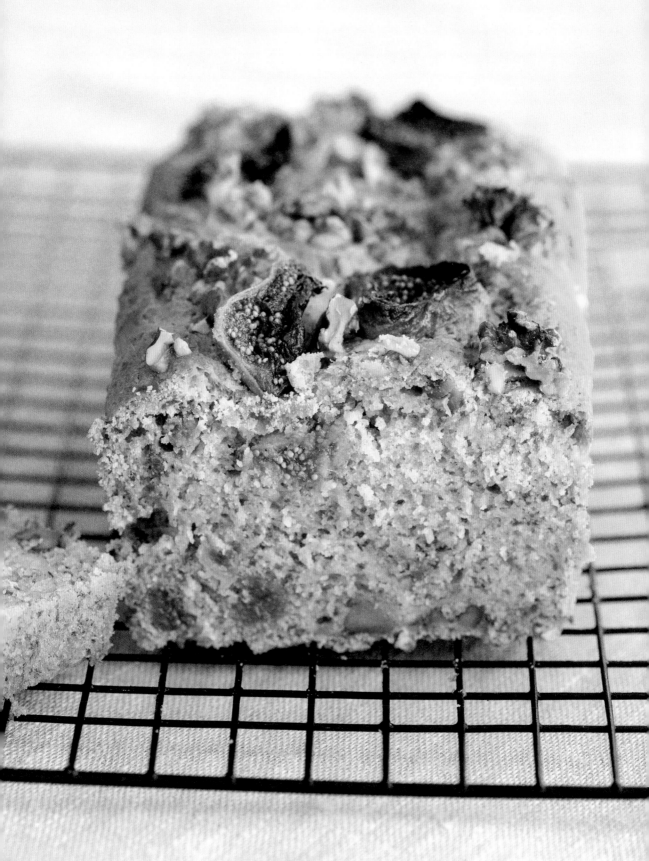

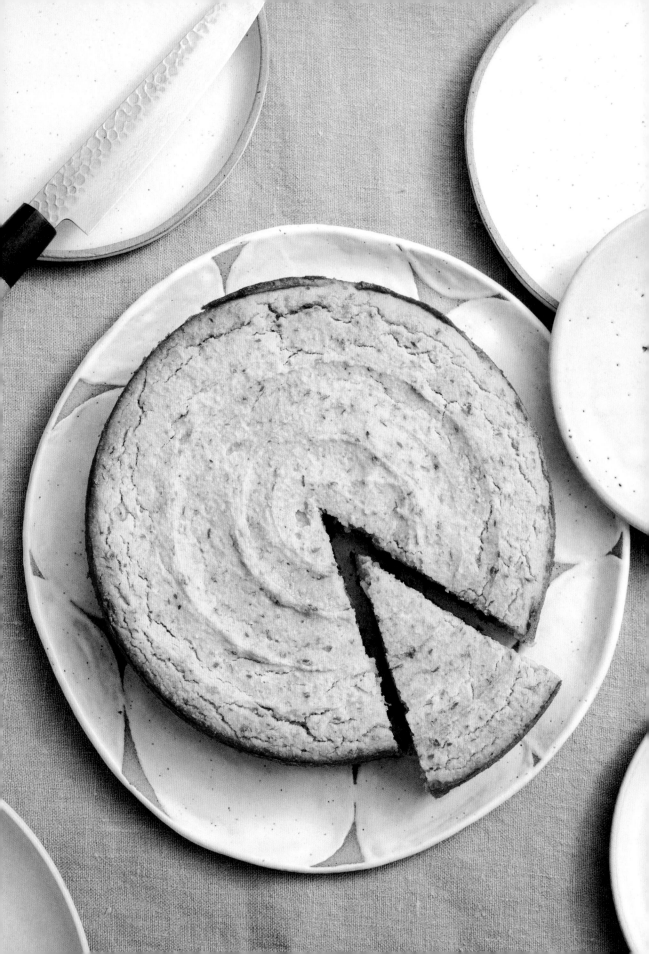

Lemon Olive Oil Cake Serves 8

This is a truly special dessert—the grain-free lemony cake is rich with olive oil and lemon juice and is perfectly sweet. It's deeply satisfying and dense without being heavy. Just twelve ingredients. I could not resist sneaking in a can of gut-friendly beans, which actually lighten up the batter while adding even more prebiotic fibre and replenishing minerals like calcium. Enjoy midday with a cup of tea or maybe even sneak a piece with your morning coffee! It is plant food, after all.

DAIRY-FREE • GLUTEN-FREE • HIGH-FODMAP • VEGAN

1. Preheat the oven to 350°F (180°C). Grease an 8-inch (1.2 L) round cake pan with coconut oil. Line the bottom of the pan with a circle of parchment paper.

2. In a high-speed blender, add the lemon zest, lemon juice, white beans, maple syrup, olive oil, oat milk, vanilla, and almond extract. Purée until smooth, about 1 to 2 minutes.

3. In a large bowl, whisk together the almond flour, all-purpose flour, flaxseed, baking powder, and salt. Add the wet ingredients to the dry ingredients and stir to blend. Pour the batter into the prepared cake pan and smooth the top. Bake for 45 minutes, until the cake is lightly golden on top and a toothpick inserted into the centre of the cake comes out clean. A bit of cracking is normal. Let the cake cool in the pan for 10 minutes. Invert the pan over a plate and tap the bottom to dislodge the cake. Transfer the cake to a rack to cool completely before slicing. Store loosely covered on the counter for up to 4 days.

Coconut or olive oil, for greasing the pan

Zest and juice of 2 lemons

1 can (14 ounces/398 mL) white beans, rinsed and drained

⅔ cup (150 mL) pure maple syrup

½ cup (125 mL) extra-virgin olive oil

2 tablespoons (30 mL) unsweetened oat or soy milk

1 tablespoon (15 mL) pure vanilla extract

¼ teaspoon (1 mL) almond extract

2½ cups (625 mL) almond flour

½ cup (125 mL) gluten-free all-purpose flour

¼ cup (60 mL) ground flaxseed

2 teaspoons (10 mL) baking powder

½ teaspoon (2 mL) salt

Watermelon Mint Chia Ice Pops Makes 6 ice pops

Watermelon and mint is one of my favourite summer flavour combinations. These ice pops offer a few gut-health benefits too. Mint helps to calm intestinal spasms and watermelon contains a bit of FODMAPs at this serving size, which will boost gut bacteria. This refreshing treat is deeply hydrating and low in added sugars. If your watermelon is super sweet, you can omit the maple syrup.

DAIRY-FREE • GLUTEN-FREE • GRAIN-FREE • NUT-FREE • VEGAN

2 cups (500 mL) seedless watermelon chunks

2 tablespoons (30 mL) freshly squeezed lime juice

2 tablespoons (30 mL) pure maple syrup

¼ cup (60 mL) fresh mint leaves, finely chopped

1 teaspoon (5 mL) chia seeds

1. In a high-speed blender, add the watermelon, lime juice, and maple syrup. Purée until it resembles a juice. Stir in the mint and chia seeds and let sit for 5 minutes for the chia to hydrate. Pour the mixture into 6 ice-pop moulds and freeze for at least 6 hours or overnight until firm. The ice pops can be stored in the freezer for up to 1 month.

2. To remove the ice pops from the moulds, gently squeeze the pop as you pull the handle. If it does not release, run the mould under warm water for a few seconds and try again.

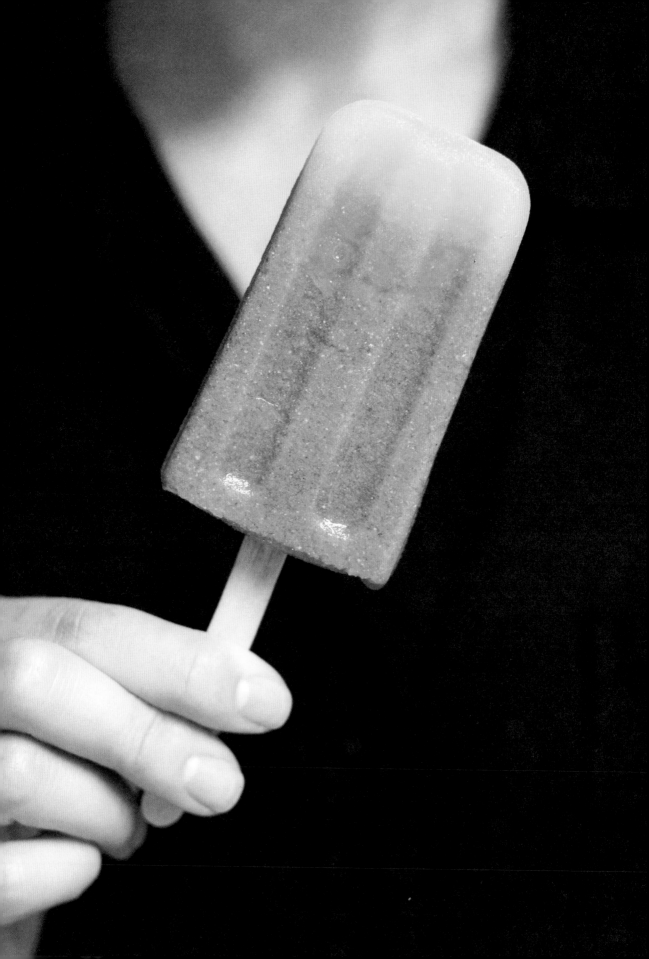

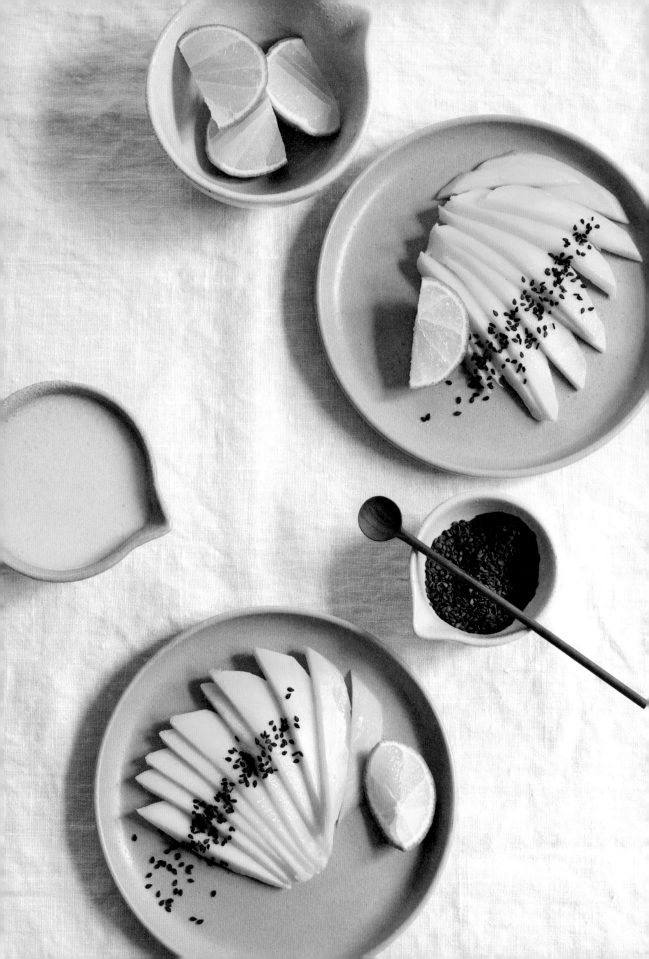

Mango with Salted Coconut Cream Serves 4

Sometimes the simplest desserts can be the most satisfying. Inspired by Thai mango sticky rice, the warm salted mango cream in this dessert pairs with the ripe mangoes for a tropical treat that takes only five minutes to make. Mango is high in gut-boosting FODMAPs and has plenty of vitamin C, as well as energizing copper, folate, and vitamin A.

DAIRY-FREE • GLUTEN-FREE • GRAIN-FREE • HIGH-FODMAP • NUT-FREE • VEGAN

1. In a small saucepan, add the coconut cream, cane sugar, and salt. Bring to a boil over medium heat. When the mixture reaches a boil, remove from the heat. Stir in the lime juice.

2. Divide the mango among small dessert bowls. Pour the coconut cream mixture over the mango. Sprinkle the black sesame seeds (if using) on top. Serve warm or at room temperature.

Tip If you cannot find canned coconut cream, place 2 cans (14 ounces/398 mL each) full-fat coconut milk in the fridge overnight. Gently flip the chilled cans upside down. Scoop out the solid coconut cream into a measuring cup. Add enough of the coconut water from the cans to reach the 1-cup (250 mL) mark.

1 cup (250 mL) canned unsweetened coconut cream (20% fat; see Tip)

2 teaspoons (10 mL) organic cane sugar

⅛ teaspoon (0.5 mL) salt

1 teaspoon (5 mL) freshly squeezed lime juice

2 large ripe mangoes, peeled and sliced

Black sesame seeds, for garnish (optional)

Sophia's Ginger Lime Beer Makes about 1 quart (1 L)

Real-deal ginger beer—not some overly sweet, vaguely gingery soda—is one of my favourite treats. I asked my friend Sophia, who also styled all of the photos in this book, to create this treat for us because she and her partner are major fermenters—they even have kombucha on tap at home. This ginger beer is fresh, spicy, and invigorating, with live beneficial microbes to keep your gut happy. This is perfect for a midday refresher or any time you need to settle your stomach, thanks to ginger's prokinetic power. Ginger bugs are a bit more of a challenging fermentation project but well worth the effort.

DAIRY-FREE • GLUTEN-FREE • GRAIN-FREE • LOW-FODMAP • VEGAN

GINGER BUG

1 cup (250 mL) water

2 tablespoons (30 mL) grated organic unpeeled fresh ginger, plus more as needed for fermentation

2 tablespoons (30 mL) organic cane sugar, plus more as needed for fermentation

1. In a small pot, boil the water for 5 minutes over medium heat. Remove from the heat and let cool for 10 minutes. (Boiling the water helps remove the chlorine that would interfere with the fermentation process.)

2. In a wide-mouth 1-quart (1 L) mason jar, combine the cooled water, ginger, and sugar. Using a wooden or silicone spoon (do not use a metal spoon), stir the mixture. Cover the jar with a layer of cheesecloth or a coffee filter and secure with an elastic band. Wrap the jar in a clean kitchen towel to keep it warm, then place it in a warm spot out of direct sunlight. This mixture is your ginger bug.

3. Each day, feed the ginger bug 1 tablespoon (15 mL) grated organic unpeeled fresh ginger and 1 tablespoon (15 mL) organic cane sugar. Stir the mixture with a wooden or silicone spoon (do not use a metal spoon). Cover again with the same cheesecloth or coffee filter and secure with an elastic band. Repeat this step every day for 5 to 7 days until it is active and bubbly. This means it is ready to use. Use immediately to make your ginger beer or place the lid on tightly and store in the fridge for up to 1 week.

4. To maintain your original ginger bug and keep it ready to make another batch of ginger beer, each week, feed the ginger bug 1 tablespoon (15 mL) grated organic unpeeled fresh ginger and 1 tablespoon (15 mL) organic cane sugar. Leave the ginger bug on the counter for 1 day before using it again.

GINGER LIME BEER

4 cups (1 L) water

¼ to ½ cup (60 to 125 mL) chopped fresh ginger (depending on how spicy you like it)

3 tablespoons (45 mL) pure maple syrup

2 tablespoons (30 mL) organic cane sugar

¼ cup (60 mL) freshly squeezed lime juice (about 2 limes)

2 tablespoons (30 mL) ginger bug (recipe above)

1. In a medium pot, bring the water to a boil for 5 minutes over high heat. Remove from the heat, then add the ginger, maple syrup, and cane sugar. Let cool to room temperature. Add the lime juice and ginger bug. Using a funnel, pour the ginger beer mixture into a 1-quart (1 L) mason jar with a cap or a pop-top bottle. Do not strain out the ginger. Place the lid on tightly. Let sit for 24 hours in a warm spot on the counter, turning the bottle upside down a few times a day to mix.

2. After 24 hours, taste the ginger beer for fizziness. If it is not fizzy, close the lid and let it sit for another 12 to 24 hours, turning the bottle upside down a few times throughout the period. When the ginger beer is fizzy, strain over another 1-quart (1 L) mason jar. Place the lid on tightly. Store the strained ginger beer in the fridge for up to 2 weeks. Serve cold.

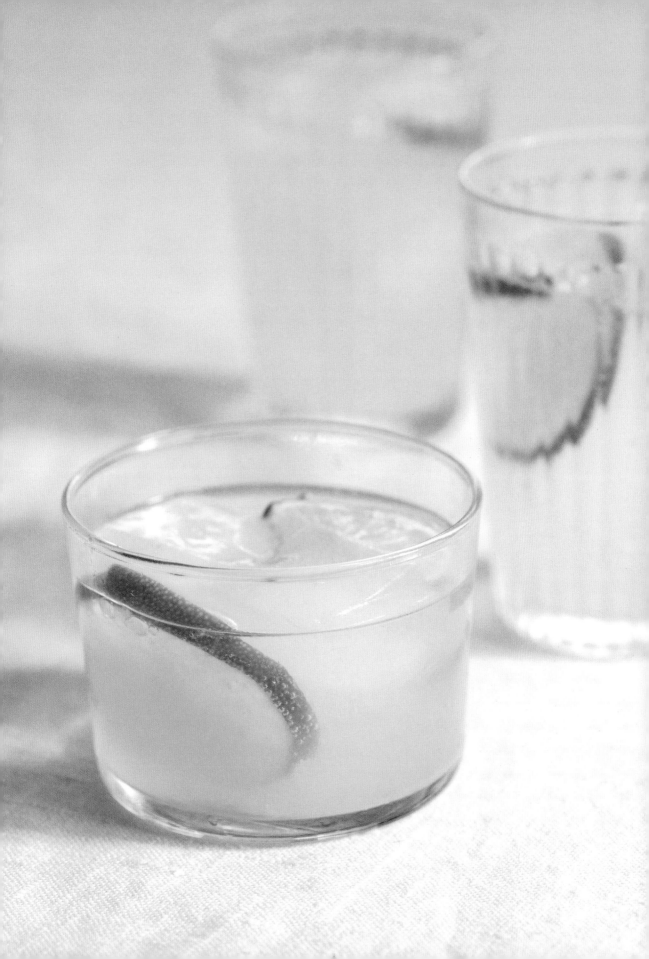

Meal Plans

Seven-Day Protect Meal Plan

MONDAY

   Breakfast Green Smoothie (page 133)

   Lunch Marinated Lentil Salad (page 195) + Easy Asparagus Fritters (page 236)

   Snack Tropical Coconut Trail Mix (page 251)

   Dinner Sheet Pan Harissa Tofu and Veggies (page 169)

TUESDAY

   Breakfast 2 Breakfast Cookies (page 111) + an oat milk latte

   Lunch Marinated Lentil Salad (page 195) + Easy Asparagus Fritters (page 236)

   Dinner Spanish Chickpea and Spinach Stew (page 165)

WEDNESDAY

   Breakfast Calming Rose Smoothie (page 132)

   Lunch Farro, Apricot, and Walnut Salad (page 199)

   Snack Tropical Coconut Trail Mix (page 251)

   Dinner Creamy Tomato and White Bean Soup with Crispy Kale (page 223)
      + 1 slice of Amazing Seeded Grain-Free Bread (page 263)

THURSDAY

   Breakfast 2 Breakfast Cookies (page 111) + an oat milk latte

   Lunch Creamy Tomato and White Bean Soup with Crispy Kale (page 223)
      + 1 slice of Amazing Seeded Grain-Free Bread (page 263)

   Dinner Creamy Mushroom Lentil Toast (page 141)

   Dessert Cherry Pie Nice Cream (page 274)

FRIDAY

   Breakfast Green Smoothie (page 133)

   Lunch Farro, Apricot, and Walnut Salad (page 199)

   Snack Nacho Roasted Black Beans (page 235)

   Dinner Tofu Okonomiyaki (page 145) + Snap Pea Salad with Hazelnuts and Barley
      (page 203)

SATURDAY

Breakfast **Fermented Cashew Yogurt (page 115) + sliced pears**

Lunch **Mediterranean Artichoke Burger (page 161) + Summer Zucchini Salad with Hazelnuts (page 220)**

Snack **1 Breakfast Cookie (page 111)**

Dinner **Baked Eggplant Rolls with Kale and Cauliflower Ricotta (page 190) + Snap Pea Salad with Hazelnuts and Barley (page 203)**

SUNDAY

Breakfast **Pumpkin Oat Pancakes (page 120)**

Lunch **Harissa Spinach Salad with Marinated Tofu (page 207)**

Snack **Tropical Coconut Trail Mix (page 251)**

Dinner **Sunchoke Kale White Bean Gratin (page 166)**

Seven-Day Heal Meal Plan

MONDAY

Breakfast **Cinnamon Orange Bircher (page 127)**

Lunch **Kitchari (page 150)**

Dinner **Silky Broccoli Soup with Sesame Oil (page 212) + Sweet Potato Broccoli Croquettes (page 244)**

TUESDAY

Breakfast **Calming Rose Smoothie (page 132) + 1 Breakfast Cookie (page 111)**

Lunch **Roasted Eggplant and Tempeh Tacos with Cumin Lime Mayonnaise (page 154)**

Snack **Tropical Coconut Trail Mix (page 251)**

Dinner **Sticky Sesame Tofu with Bok Choy (page 185)**

WEDNESDAY

Breakfast **Cinnamon Orange Bircher (page 127)**

Lunch **Kitchari (page 150)**

Snack **Sweet Potato Broccoli Croquettes (page 244)**

Dinner **Gado Gado (page 211)**

THURSDAY

Breakfast Carrot Cake Muffin (page 123) + 1 cup (250 mL) grapes

Lunch Gado Gado (page 211)

Dinner Zucchini Cacio e Pepe Pasta with Pan-Fried Oyster Mushrooms (page 146)

Dessert Magic Turmeric Truffles (page 286)

FRIDAY

Breakfast Calming Rose Smoothie (page 132) + 1 Breakfast Cookie (page 111)

Lunch Roasted Eggplant and Tempeh Tacos with Cumin Lime Mayonnaise (page 154)

Snack Tropical Coconut Trail Mix (page 251)

Dinner Oat Milk Polenta with Burst Tomatoes, Crispy Tofu, and Arugula (page 178)

SATURDAY

Breakfast Carrot Cake Muffin (page 123) + 1 cup (250 mL) grapes

Lunch Lentil Niçoise (page 215)

Dinner Roasted Spaghetti Squash with Chickpeas, Red Peppers, and Kale Pesto
(page 186)

Dessert Roasted Strawberries with Yogurt and Pecan Oat Crumble (page 289)

SUNDAY

Breakfast Pumpkin Oat Pancakes (page 120)

Lunch Miso-Glazed Root Veggie Hash (page 247) + Blistered Dijon Green Beans
with Almonds (page 248) + add pan-fried tofu

Dinner Soba with Napa Cabbage and Peanutty Tempeh (page 153)

Seven-Day Soothe Meal Plan

MONDAY

Breakfast Chocolate Cherry Rebuilder Smoothie (page 132)

Lunch Thai Mushroom and Tofu Laab (page 228)

Snack Blackberry Vanilla Hemp Milk (page 135)

Dinner Zucchini Cacio e Pepe Pasta with Pan-Fried Oyster Mushrooms (page 146)

TUESDAY

Breakfast Cherry Almond Muffin (page 131) + Green Smoothie (page 133)

Lunch 1 Glorious Grain-Free Bun (page 264) + Smoky Red Pepper Hummus (page 256) +
sliced tomato and cucumbers

Dinner Kitchari (page 150)

Dessert Mango with Salted Coconut Cream (page 297)

WEDNESDAY

Breakfast Crunchy Grain-Free Granola (page 128) + Blackberry Vanilla Hemp Milk
(page 135)

Lunch Kitchari (page 150)

Snack Smoky Red Pepper Hummus (page 256) + sliced cucumbers

Dinner Silky Broccoli Soup with Sesame Oil (page 212) + 1 Glorious Grain-Free Bun
(page 264)

THURSDAY

Breakfast Cherry Almond Muffin (page 131) + Green Smoothie (page 133)

Lunch Silky Broccoli Soup with Sesame Oil (page 212) + 1 Glorious Grain-Free Bun
(page 264)

Dinner Tomato Coconut and Lentil Curry with Spinach (page 157)

FRIDAY

Breakfast Cinnamon Orange Bircher (page 127)

Lunch Kitchari (page 150)

Dinner Mediterranean Artichoke Burger (page 161) + roasted sweet potatoes

SATURDAY

Breakfast Crunchy Grain-Free Granola (page 128) + Blackberry Vanilla Hemp Milk
(page 135)

Lunch Spiced Tahini Roasted Squash (page 252) + 1 slice of Amazing Seeded
Grain-Free Bread (page 263) + Curried White Bean Dip (page 255)

Dinner Pasta with Tomato Garlic Confit (page 189)

Dessert Lemon Olive Oil Cake (page 293)

SUNDAY

Breakfast Cinnamon Orange Bircher (page 127)

Lunch Creamy Tomato and White Bean Soup with Crispy Kale (page 223)

Snack Lemon Olive Oil Cake (page 293)

Dinner Soba with Napa Cabbage and Peanutty Tempeh (page 153)

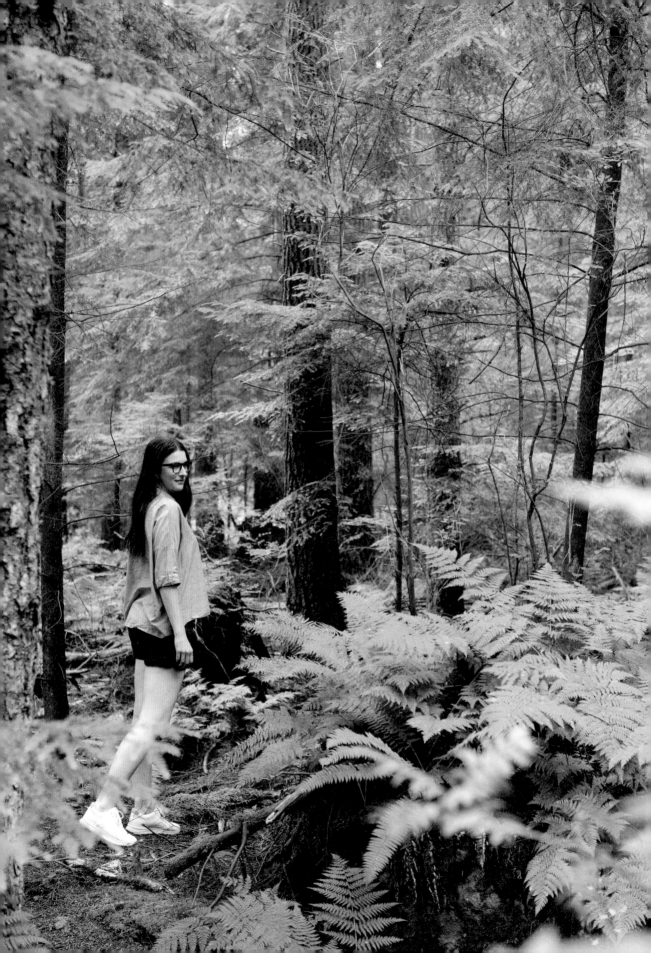

Acknowledgements

Thank you for bringing this book into your home.

I became a dietitian because I believe in the power of food to heal—it is a privilege to watch others find joy, comfort, and healing in food. I am thankful for every day that I have the opportunity to do what I love, but this book you are holding in your hands made me even more aware of this gratitude. More than half of this cookbook was written during the COVID-19 pandemic, and getting up every morning to create these recipes was a safe harbour in a time of uncertainty. On days when I could do little else, I could cook. Cooking carried me away from the doom-scrolling and brought me back into the present moment. Know that these recipes are infused with love and the hope that I can share a bit of nourishment and healing from far away.

To Jim, Elliott, and Iris—our family is magic. Thank you for bearing with me even when I was maniacally trying to create a vortex of focus (AKA ignoring you) with my big headphones as work-from-home life swirled around me. Thank you for eating all the cold food, listening to me blab on ad nauseum about my work, and even cheering me on. I love you more than I can bear sometimes. Thank you for loving me.

Thank you to my mom, Ligia, for isolating with us so we could actually work from home. This book literally could not have been written without you. To our parents, Svein, Wendy, Casey, and Bonnie, for supporting my weirdo dreams and taking the kids every once in a while once it was safe to do so, so we could all get a change of scenery (and work even longer days).

To Willow, thank you for maintaining isolation so you could toil long hours as my kitchen right hand. Chopping and cleaning is way faster and more fun with you around. Thank you for testing so many of the recipes, as if you weren't sick of them already, and always reminding me that a dish could use some pepper. To my friends and colleagues who tested recipes: Megan Leong, Carla Ullrich, and Jess Pirnak—thank you for taking time out of a crazy year to cook.

The shoots for this book were an oasis in a year spent in isolation. Once we were able to gather, Janis Nicolay, photographer extraordinaire, let us take over her beautiful home for no fewer than twelve days spread out over three months. Janis, I cannot thank you enough for your endless support of my work, your utter freaking genius behind the camera, and the endless cups of coffee. I already miss our kitchen parties.

Sophia MacKenzie, you are my kitchen angel. From making every dish look its absolute best at the shoots, to mastering ginger beer when I was tired of struggling with my ferment, to even testing extra recipes. You are a remarkably talented human and I am really glad I finally learned how to ask for help . . . and that you said yes. Thank you a million times over. Also, I cannot look at a papaya without thinking of you now.

Andraya Avison, thank you for signing up for twelve days of kitchen chaos and not batting an eye when the kitchen became two rocks on the beach. Your infectious energy—and your knife skills—made these shoots a lot more enjoyable.

To my agent, Carly Watters, thank you. Thank you for always being willing to go to bat for me, for trusting my weird ideas, and for laughing at my poop jokes. Your work makes dreams come true and I am forever grateful.

To Andrea Magyar, you are the most wonderful editor I could have ever hoped for. Thank you for championing my work and making it better. Thank you for signing on for another nerdy ride with me; I honestly don't know how I got so lucky.

Finally, to the incredible team at Penguin Random House Canada, you are epic and it is an honour to co-create with you and bring a book into the world together a second time around.

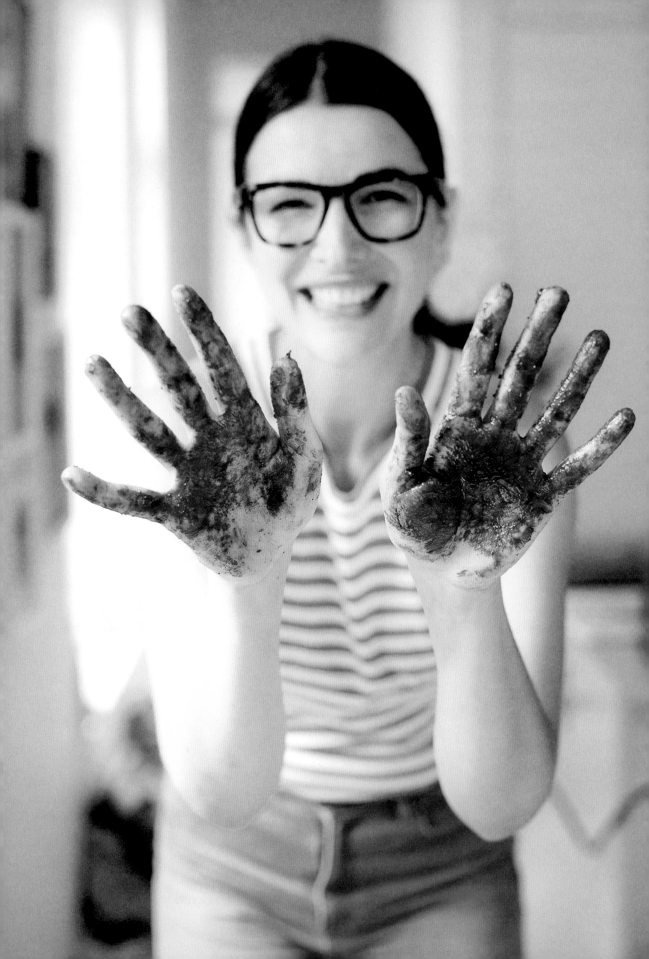

Index